Ouija Medicine

The Dark Side of Energy Medicine

Marci Julin

Ouija Medicine

The Dark Side of Energy Medicine

Printed in the United States of America
ISBN: 979-8-9905751-0-3

Learn more information at:
www.HeartandMindMinistries.com

Dedication

*For all those who will not trade the truth of God for a lie.
To God be the glory!*

Contents

Part 2: What Now? —Moving Forward with Hope

Part 3: Redemptive Testimonies

Appendix

Foreword

O Israel, hope in the Lord! For with the Lord there is steadfast love, and with him is plentiful redemption. Psalm 130:7

At one time, I knew it all. Beyond my notice were limitations of my sight and understanding, and so with great certainty I unintentionally led many astray. It calls to mind the biblical story of Saul persecuting the church. Convinced his zeal was for the work of the LORD, Jesus had to blind the future apostle so that his eyes might be opened. I too required drastic measures for the Lord to open my eyes and change my course.

At the time of this writing, it has been well over 10 years since my repentance from the alternative health practice of muscle testing, which I once considered my lifeline and mission. How could I, a devout Christian who desired with all her heart to serve the Lord by helping others, become a slave to divination? It was simple, really. I had unknowingly traded the truth of God for a lie. My pride provided fertile ground for entrapment by *the snare of the devil.*[i] Now, much humbled, I entreat others to hold these practices up to the lens of Scripture.

What about you? Has something brought you to a place of questioning what you once embraced with great certainty? Questions are good if they lead us to seek answers. Regarding many alternative health

---

[i] 2 Timothy 2:26 All passages will quote from the English Standard Version (ESV) unless otherwise noted.

practices, people should be asking questions, and so I applaud you for doing so.

I have come to treasure the redemptive character of God. Not only has the holy God of the universe shown me undeserved mercy and grace, He has also brought good of my folly. Over the years since I wrote that first series of articles detailing my sinful involvement with muscle testing (AK), I have repeatedly experienced redemption each time God has brought me individuals who wish to discuss how my past might shed light on their present.

As you read this book, therefore, know that the theme is not condemnation or judgment for those seeking to determine if they have wandered astray. On the contrary, it is a story of a patient God who offers redemption for transgressors. Do not be afraid to keep reading, "for although sin is ugly, truth is beautiful."[ii]

[ii] Said by my father-in-law, Stan Julin

Part 1

Removing the Veil
Over
Energy Medicine

CHAPTER 1

My Journey in Deception

The Spirit clearly says that in later times some will abandon the faith and follow deceiving spirits and things taught by demons.
1 Timothy 4:1

Although for me, my departure from the truth can be pinpointed to the specific moment in time when I first encountered muscle testing, the years of illness that preceded that moment, as well as the numerous concessions in thought and deed that followed must also be considered. These first two chapters will share my story, and the chapters that follow will provide a reasoned case for the physical and spiritual concerns regarding many alternative health practices. I write with a humble heart, as one who was deceived, and with great compassion, as one who knows the struggle.

As I now write, over twelve years after the merciful Father first healed me, I find I sometimes forget the consuming illness and pain that characterized my life for decades. Although my past health issues trace back to childhood, the significant downward spiral began during my twenties—from chronic fatigue syndrome and Epstein Barr to parasites and heavy metal poisoning (most likely the souvenirs of mission trips to India and Poland, respectively), from a multitude of female conditions to significant adrenal and thyroid insufficiency, from Fibromyalgia to severe anemia, from allergies to herniated discs, and from pain, explained and unexplained. The list of symptoms and diagnoses seemed endless. As the years progressed, I would at times be unable to eat or drink anything as my body seemed to be simply shutting down, sometimes resulting in hospitalization. For well-over a decade, I lived with literally constant pain. The chronic fatigue, although difficult to manage during the day, at least enabled me to sleep at night. Even then, I frequently woke myself up crying from pain that never ceased. Doctors offered little help and no hope. Despite my Christian faith, despair consumed my private thoughts.

The ability to continually push through pain, fatigue, and weakness came to a screeching halt in 2004. I went to my first ever chiropractic appointment in hope of finding relief from a bulging disc in my neck and instead left with a far worse situation. The doctor's adjustment herniated a disc in my low back. The nerve that disc pinched catapulted me into a new level of misery. I was officially an invalid.

Being unwilling to go the route of prescription pain medications, I sought relief from the pain of the injury by resting on ice or heat in a recliner by my bedroom window for an entire year. With barely strength to walk or stand, that chair became my haven. God had brought me to the end of being able to distract myself with activity. During this period of seclusion and incapacitation, I had plenty of time and motivation to fervently seek the Lord. Staring out the window, hour after hour, day after day, I pleaded with the Lord for answers. He answered through the advice of a counselor who wisely pointed me to the Bible.

You see, my physical brokenness mirrored my spiritual and emotional brokenness. For the decade preceding my complete incapacitation, I carried tremendous burdens of anger and bitterness, sad remnants of a traumatic event. My heart languished continually. Because my 13 diagnosed conditions had medical explanations, I had no awareness that the thoughts and emotions of my heart were powerfully impacting my autonomic nervous system and draining life from every cell of my body. I thank the Lord that by making me an invalid He forced me to deal with the state of my heart, and then He renewed my soul and spirit as I sought Him through the Living Word. As the merciful Savior bound up my broken heart with the balm of His truth, my body also began to heal.[iii]

In the months that followed, God's Word and Spirit radically transformed my heart from one that desperately feared the future, due to my view of a wrathful God, to a heart that swam in the deep waters of God's limitless love. Despite continued problems with pain and illness, a remarkable transformation took place. Joy began to fill my days. Gradually but remarkably I also started seeing physical improvements. How true it is that *a heart at peace gives life to the body*.[iv] By removing the tremendous and previously unending stress response due to the feeling that God was against me, my body began to be rejuvenated.[v] The melodious sound of hymns flowed from my lips as I worked around the house, and changes in my health continued.

A significant detour into deception

As is so often the case when God works mightily, the Enemy doubles his efforts to undermine that work. Such was the case with me in this next phase of my journey. It pains me to admit how I fell prey to Satan's deception, but I choose to share the story anyway because I know the desperation of those who suffer from poor health, and the tremendous temptation alleged solutions present.

Immediately following the time of great healing in my relationship with the Lord, but while I was yet sick, I saw a book on display at the library called, *Say Goodbye to Illness* by Devi Nambudripad. This book detailed a branch of alternative medicine that would open a new chapter in my life that proved costly in its writing. The author redefines allergies in a much broader sense. She explains in the book that *the central nervous*

[iii] For a complete discussion of the biblical and scientific perspective of the heart, and its impact on the body read Chapters 4-5 in my book, *Life to the Body—Biblical Principles for Health and Healing.*
[iv] Proverbs 14:30
[v] My book, *When You Can't Trust His Heart—Discovering the Limitless Love of God*, tells the transforming work of God's Word in bringing me to a place of knowing the personal love of God and trusting in Him.

system reacts to foods or other substances as if they are toxic when they are really neutral or beneficial.[1] The practitioner uses muscle testing as a tool for determining the offending substances so they can then be treated. (Most muscle testing is associated with Applied Kinesiology or AK. If you are unfamiliar with AK, refer to Appendix B.) The quick and painless treatment the doctor created, called NAET (Nambudripad's Allergy Elimination Treatment), purports to eliminate the faulty messages in the brain that rally the body to fight the otherwise harmless substances she calls allergens.[vi] In so doing, Nambudripad claims to *reprogram the brain to perfect health.[2]*

The author provided reasonable sounding explanations to several of my physical conundrums, which traditional medicine had failed to address. Although it sounded too good to be true and a bit "out there," desperation drew me to it like a moth to a flame. After devouring the book, I quickly found a NAET practitioner in my area and scheduled an appointment. Even though the whole thing sounded a bit odd, and the appointment pushed the envelope for what I considered strange, I was desperate.

Initial dramatic results

Shockingly, the initial results were dramatic, even miraculous. Within a couple of hours of my first treatment, I felt like I had the flu. Coming from a history of sensitivity to detoxification protocols, the negative reaction to NAET only served to convince me that there was something to this practice. Returning for my next appointment, I was treated for calcium, and, voila; I suddenly began sleeping better with far fewer aches during the night. At this point, I was convinced NAET and muscle testing worked, but persistent uneasiness troubled me. I prayed and pleaded with the Lord for understanding.

Next came the treatment for iodine, following which my thyroid immediately began functioning normally. I had been on thyroid

---

[vi] For a further explanation of *NAET*® and the clinical studies that have been done on this treatment modality refer to Appendix C.

medication for 2 to 3 years at that point but had to immediately stop taking it because I suddenly became hyperthyroid with my heart racing terribly. According to conventional medical understanding, once an individual is on thyroid medication, that person can never get off it because the natural function of the thyroid largely ceases as the body learns to rely almost solely on the medication. For the first time, even since being on the medication, I had completely healthy thyroid function.

I also discovered in the days, months, and years ahead that all my female related conditions were gone.[vii] I suddenly had balanced and healthy hormones, where once a doctor had declared me "a hormone nightmare." (The doctor's statement was inspired by my lab results, which included a handwritten note in the report indicating that they had retested my results because they could not believe my hormone levels were so low.) You can imagine my shock and joy over what appeared to be such miraculous changes.

Wrestling with a critical question

Not a doubt existed in my mind that muscle testing "worked," but from day one, a nagging uncertainty about how it worked plagued my mind. Like times in my childhood when I had an unexplainable sense of unease before I was even told that a particular activity was wrong, so it was with NAET and muscle testing. From the beginning, I knew that its power was either physical or spiritual. As a Christian who had benefited from the practice, it was important to me to conclude that it was purely physical.

Sadly, the apparent healing of my thyroid trumped all other logic or discernment, and the gentle voice of the Holy Spirit faded as I journeyed further into the labyrinth of energy medicine. I initially concluded that NAET and muscle testing must be a gift from God and proceeded to go to great lengths to convince myself and others that some obscure, unproven physical explanation for it must account for its evident power.

[vii] I will discuss an explanation of this "healing" in a later chapter.

I failed to consider that a merciful and sovereign God might have orchestrated my healing because of changes in my heart towards Himself, IN SPITE OF my ignorant decision to get involved with AK. The grace He extended to me during this time in no way legitimizes the practices with which I became involved, but instead testifies to a loving Father who had mercy on His child as she fumbled in the dark.

I later came to understand that the Holy Spirit tried to warn me through the sense of unease I felt. After all, the Bible calls the LORD, the God of peace,[viii] and says that life and peace characterize the Holy Spirit.[ix] The absence of peace was the unrecognized answer to my prayers for discernment. How I wish that I had realized that at the time.

Witnessing results both great and terrible

Although the first results of the new treatment methodology were dramatic, they gave way to a constant need to retreat previously "cleared" allergies and to treat, for the first time, every conceivable thing I encountered in life. By doing so, I attempted to hold on to a tenuous level of wellness that I believed had been made possible by my strange new healthcare practices. Instead of continuing to pay the provider, I learned to do it all myself, and taught my husband and son as well, so that I could manage the onset of sudden symptoms on the spot. When treating at home, I sometimes attempted to "Christianize" it by praying in place of the standard protocol of speaking to the body. Surely, if there was any cause for concern, praying made it alright. How wrong I was!

By this point, God had healed me of all my traditionally diagnosed conditions, and yet I began constantly reacting in new ways to everything around me. The reactions were often severe and quite bizarre. For example, during spring in Florida, the Live Oak trees drop their leaves and copious amounts of pollen, which piles up along the edges of the streets. A typical allergic reaction to pollen might include symptoms such as sneezing, hives or hay fever. I had none of these because I am not actually

---

[viii] Romans 15:33, 16:20, Philippians 4:9, 1 Thessalonians 5:23
[ix] Romans 8:6

allergic to oak pollen. However, during this period, I did react in a very unusual manner. My legs became so weak that I collapsed from simply stepping on a pile of oak pollen while on a walk. Muscle testing then confirmed that oak pollen was the trigger, and upon treatment, my strength immediately returned. The same thing happened on more than one occasion from walking under streetlights, and so I became convinced that I was extremely sensitive to EMFs (electromagnetic fields). The time spent testing and treating endlessly for everything under the sun seemed a small price to pay for the great relief it brought. Regardless of what peculiar reactions I experienced, a quick treatment could have me doing well in a couple of minutes.

As I became quite proficient in muscle testing, I began using, without charge, the methods I had learned on others in what I deemed to be a ministry to the hurting. During that time, I saw two instances of apparent miraculous results in others. One was with a friend's infant, the other with a coworker.

My friend had refused visitors after the birth of her daughter because her baby screamed almost unceasingly and slept for only minutes at a time. Finally, in desperation, my friend allowed me to drop by when the child was four months old. I was shocked at the state of things. Without delay, I determined through surrogate testing[x] that the child was allergic to the formula they were feeding her. I then treated the baby through her mother, and the poor child finally stopped screaming and fell asleep.

When I came back the next day, I saw a remarkably changed baby. Rather than a red-faced infant, contorted with pain and an exhausted mother who franticly paced and bounced her screaming baby, I witnessed a calm mother and child. My friend reported that, after I left, her baby had an enormous bowel movement and then slept for three straight hours for the first time since she was born. I then tested and treated the infant for the second formula they had been using and left. It was reported to me that the

---

[x] Surrogate testing is used for those who cannot perform the muscle test--small children, the elderly, or those who are too weak. The tester pushes down on the surrogate's arm while he or she makes skin contact with the one being tested.

same thing happened as before, but this time the baby slept through the entire night for the first time. From that next morning forward, the parents reported that she was a different child, with a sweet disposition.

The other seemingly miraculous case was with a man who had muscular dystrophy as a child. Thankfully, the illness went into remission as a teenager. Unfortunately, in his thirties the symptoms seemed to be returning, and he was terrified of the outcome. His pale complexion and sluggish manner at work prompted my inquiry and offer to help. Following my treatment for granola bars, which he had started eating every day, the symptoms disappeared.

Although I failed to recognize it at the time, most of the responses to my muscle testing and NAET treatments produced insignificant results that did not last. However, the dramatic change in my thyroid, the baby's response, and the coworker's recovery fueled my certainty of the amazing power of energy medicine, motivating me to keep on despite several upsetting events.

The worst of these events was the suicide of a close friend following her involvement with AK to treat for bipolar disorder. Upon learning of her depression, I told her about my NAET practitioner, and she decided to schedule an appointment. After initial treatments seemed to bring stability, she decided to quit taking her medication, following which she spiraled out of control. Her original doctor attempted to restore stability through medication, and her husband took time off of work in an attempt to guard her at all times until the medicine took effect. Tragically, she still managed to kill herself. Although I never treated this friend, I did encourage her to try NAET, and therefore felt tremendous guilt at my friend's death and the trauma it brought to her family. Some consequences for sin are greater than others.

It is worth mentioning that to my knowledge, the practitioner who treated my friend never learned of her patient's death. This calls to question how often practitioners of energy medicine are unaware of the tragic results of their attempts to help people. My own continuance with these practices following her death also highlights the blinding nature of deception. If you have been involved with energy medicine, are there things that you too have ignored or excused? I urge you not to make the mistake I made.

One of my attempts to help could have also had a deadly outcome and again highlights a common problem with energy-based treatments—in my experience, the treatments frequently do not last. A relative by marriage with ulcerative colitis allowed me to test and treat her, following which, she seemed to be no longer allergic to dairy. (According to muscle testing she had "cleared" for dairy.) As is so typical of these treatments, the initial apparent improvement reversed, but being unaware of this, she continued eating dairy. After years of being deprived of cheesy pizza and ice cream, she made up for lost time. As a result, she ended up in the hospital for days in grave condition.

I also witnessed a Christian friend with health issues progress into all-consuming environmental illness after I introduced her to muscle testing. Within weeks, she panicked if she had to breathe air outside of her now, heavily controlled home environment. She required everything she wore to be meticulously washed under strict control and ate only the most basic of foods, carefully prepared.

Right before my repentance from muscle testing, I visited her at home because I knew she was terribly ill. Even though at the time, I had yet to fully accept the true nature of energy medicine, upon entering her house, I felt an unholy presence that left me shaken. I felt a conviction that I was not to return there again. As we visited that last time in her home, she told me in all seriousness how she had previously followed the instructions of a remote testing practitioner. The witchy sounding protocol dictated she be treated with the NAET protocol on the night of a full moon while holding a banana in her left hand and with her right foot in a dish of milk.

What I witnessed on that last visit to her home disturbed me greatly. There were piles of laundry everywhere, as her mother could not keep up with having to rewash everything repeatedly to remove every trace of offending substances. Her bed had been pulled out of her room because of some, yet to be determined, sensitivity problem, and she was sleeping on a bare mattress on the floor in the living room. Distraught, she told me how, according to muscle testing, she was reacting to something a neighbor had sprayed on his yard. In response, she had torn apart her house to eliminate any sources of allergens. She looked like a ghostly figure. This beautiful child of God now lived in constant torment. To my knowledge, that torment continues over a decade later as I write this.

Despite my tremendous conviction that these alternative practices were God's gift to the world, the time was coming for the patient Ruler of the heavens to peel back the veil that I *should see with my eyes and hear with my ears and understand with my heart and turn and be healed.*[xi]

[xi] This verse is repeated in Matthew 13:15, Isaiah 6:10, Jeremiah 5:21, Acts 28:27, & Ezekiel 12:2.

CHAPTER 2

The Veil is Lifted

For this people's heart has grown dull, and with their ears they can barely hear, and their eyes they have closed, lest they should see with their eyes and hear with their ears and understand with their heart and turn, and I would heal them.' Matthew 13:15

A year and a half into my involvement with AK, a friend spoke to me of my "bondage" to those practices. She tried to gracefully point out that even though AK allowed me to continue living "normally," it consumed my attention and kept me a slave to it. Although I initially dismissed her comments as absurd, I began earnestly seeking the Lord through His Word. With the loving Savior at work in me, I was unable to rid my mind of the thought that my constant, "allergic" reactions might have a spiritual component.

I began to feverishly read through the Bible chronologically looking for God's thoughts on health. Just as Matthew 13:15 and four other verses in the Bible describe, my eyes, ears, and heart had been closed by sin. However, as I earnestly turned to God's Word, He would open them, and He promised true healing. While reading, I highlighted in blue every verse that spoke of health, illness, or healing. When I came to Jeremiah, several of the Lord's messages to the Israelites through the prophet Jeremiah spoke of God using illness as a means of bringing His people to repentance.

Rather than coming across as diatribes, those passages reveal a deep sorrow on the LORD's part at having to use illness as a tool for restoring His people to Himself. God's heart of grief and longing fill the pages. Furthermore, His warnings often end by expressing a desire to heal them if they would only repent.

While reading the Bible one morning, I came across a detailed, private conversation between Jeremiah and God that spoke directly to me. The passage spoke of the prophet's insistence that he lived righteously and therefore should not be suffering physical pain and illness. The fact that Jeremiah, the seemingly righteous prophet, was sick surprised me. His complaint about his condition dripped with pride for his righteous living, and I related. Surely, I too could make a similar case to God. Look what the prophet said in 15:15-17:

> *Lord, you understand; remember me and care for me...think of how I suffer reproach for your sake. When your words came, I ate them; they were my joy and my heart's delight, for I bear your name, Lord God Almighty. I never sat in the company of revelers, never made merry with them; I sat alone because your hand was on me and you had filled me with indignation.*

Immediately following Jeremiah's self-righteous reminders to God, he asked the question in Verse 18 that I too had wondered in light of my self-assessment: *Why is my pain unending and my wound grievous and incurable? You are to me like a deceptive brook, like a spring that fails.* *Yes!* I resounded. *I have tried to honor you, Lord, in everything. Surely you have wrongly struck me down all of these years.*

But then I read God's response to Jeremiah in Verse 19. Because the prophet's argument so closely depicted my thinking at the time, it was as if I, not Jeremiah, had spoken the protest, and God now answered me directly. *Therefore, this is what the Lord says: "If you repent, I will restore you that you may serve me."* Yikes! Since I had always attempted to do what would please the LORD, I had grown proud and self-righteous, just like the prophet. Just as he wrongly compared himself to the rebellious Israelites and became puffed up, so too had I compared myself to the sinful world around me and become noxious in my self-righteousness, critical spirit, and judgment of others.

Oh, how blind I had been to the significance of my sin and the need for God to use illness to bring me to repentance. There in the privacy of my room that morning, I wept over my pride and sought my Savior's forgiveness.

After I came to understand the biblical connection between sin and illness, I felt overwhelmed and yet determined to discover if those teachings applied to my abundance of allergies. Suddenly, the offense to my pride at such a possibility mattered little. I just wanted to be well and not propped up by frequent treatments.

As a result, I desperately wanted God to reveal any areas of sin in my life that might have made necessary God's discipline. However, I was blind to the deception of my heart, and no sin came readily to mind. I recalled that the Bible speaks of praying for God to search our hearts, so I began to do just that. I encourage you to do the same. I simply began praying daily that God would search my heart and reveal to me any sin that He found therein.

For two weeks I prayed in this way. Faithfully, God answered. He moved in my heart so that I might recognize and confess my sins to the great High Priest, Jesus, as well as to those I might have wronged.

My repentance brought healing.

When God ceased calling to my mind any further areas in need of repentance, I got down on my knees and prayed according to my understanding that repentance leads to healing. I simply prayed in the quiet of my bedroom and asked God for healing from all my "allergic" reactions. At that moment, God miraculously healed me, separate of any treatments.[xii]

I no longer muscle-tested positive for a single "allergy." I now realize that the most likely explanation for my sudden improvement was that God

---

[xii] For a compassionate discussion of the biblical teachings on sin, illness, and healing following repentance, read Chapters 10-12 in my book, *Life to the Body—Biblical Principles for Health and Healing.*

merely required the unclean spirits who had been tormenting me to stop. God responded to my heart's desire for holiness, even though I was still far from attaining the goal. Following that day, I never again needed NAET personally, although still blind to the true nature of muscle testing, I continued to try and help others with those practices, while earnestly praying that God would continue to reveal any other areas of sin in my life.[xiii]

An unwanted presence

Yet, in response to my prayers, the long-suffering Savior began to peel back the veil and reveal to me strong evidence of the demonic forces at work in energy medicine. Some concerning and unexplainable things began to happen. I believe that, because of my prayers, significant spiritual warfare began. Just as in the Bible, when Jesus entered the presence of demons, and they became agitated--doing things that made their presence known, so also the once quiet evil influence became noticeable around me. At least twice that I specifically remember, doors in my house slammed unexplainably while I was home alone. My fourteen-year-old son, who also had a tremendous ability for muscle testing, started having frightening "prophetic" dreams.

One particularly bizarre and unexplainable incident unsettled our whole family. We were on vacation in upstate New York, and I wanted to mail out postcards from a local post office to all my nieces and nephews. While silently addressing the cards with my head down, sitting in the idling car, I listened to my husband and son talk about a symbol painted on the parking lot nearby. I then exited the car and went inside. When I came back out of the building and again sat in the car, my son began telling me of the conversation he and my husband had had.

[xiii] I had, however, developed quite a fear of food because of the pain the previous reactions had created. My negative physical responses to that fear diminished as I used God's Word to transform my mind and make eating pleasurable once again. I share the details on how to overcome a fear of food that God intends to be a blessing in *Life to the Body—Biblical Principles for Health & Healing,* in Chapter 18 on nutrition.

I quickly interrupted and finished telling him, in great detail, about their conversation. Confused, I asked why they were bothering to repeat a conversation that they knew I had already heard in its entirety. They were both perplexed and insisted repeatedly that there was no way that I could have known the details of their conversation.

They both distinctly remembered watching me wait in line through the glass windows of the post office as they had that conversation. I kept insisting that they were wrong and that they most definitely had the conversation while I addressed the postcards in the car. With mutual expressions of concern and confusion, they reiterated that they had waited in silence for me to exit the car before they began talking. How did I hear and know the words voiced in my absence before they were spoken? Perhaps they simply misremembered the order of events, but they were quite insistent. And, because of that unsettling incident, I began praying that God would make it clear if I had opened myself and my family up to demonic influences.

Something else had begun that I was not yet ready to admit to anyone. I suspected that I not only had an uncanny sensitivity for muscle testing but that I had now developed an actual power that could not possibly be explained scientifically. I seemed to know without muscle testing, whether someone would test "allergic" to something. I suspected that this foreknowledge matched up to muscle testing with 100% accuracy but was afraid to test the theory. The ramifications were too frightening.

For the first time, I understood how it is that many practitioners can "muscle test" people on the phone. These clairvoyant abilities defied scientific explanation and pointed to the true source of power. I am ashamed to admit, however, that I liked this capability and resisted the thought of giving it up. Eventually, however, I confessed my suspicion of "special knowledge" to my husband and told him that I feared the practices I was involved in were spiritually based.

I will never forget the night of that confession. My husband, Seth, devised a simple way to test the theory of "special knowledge." First, he named things in the room and asked me if he was allergic to them. As soon as the object was named, an immediate and strong sense of the answer came to me. Perhaps, one could compare it with reading a question on a test and immediately knowing, without a doubt, that you know the correct answer. The sense was so strong that I wanted to laugh at the absurdity of it. Before we did any muscle testing, my husband recorded my predictions regarding how he would test for well over ten things.

When he finished recording my clairvoyant answers, I muscle tested him and found that 100% of the time, my foreknown answers matched the muscle testing results.[xiv] After testing on all of the prerecorded objects with 100% accuracy, Seth calculated the statistical odds of such occurring by chance. It was staggering!

Afterward, we both just sat, rather stunned. The odds were impossible for me to have correctly guessed every time. Our Christian faith has a term for such predictive power: divination. And, the Bible teaches, that *anyone who practices divination...is an abomination to the LORD!*[xv]

Now please understand; even though I can be swayed by emotions, Seth is a logic, fact-based kind of man. Also, we are not charismatic in our theological persuasion. Although as Christians we believe in spiritual forces, we are not of a mentality that sees angels and demons behind every act. Furthermore, we knew that a true believer has the Holy Spirit indwelling them and therefore cannot be possessed by demonic powers.[xvi] It appeared, though, that demonic forces were somehow influencing me outwardly.

Repentance

Following our test, Seth and I called our son in and explained to him what we believed to be the case. As the spiritual head of our home, Seth prayed for God's protection, and then in the name of Jesus, verbally

---

[xiv] Seth is a strong man, and at the time of these events, he was a weightlifter. Short of hanging from his arm, I was not capable of pushing his arm down if he resisted me. Yet, when muscle testing indicated an "allergic" result, I barely had to exert any effort to press his arm down. Therefore, muscle testing him always produced a definitive, binary (allergic vs. non-allergic) outcome.

[xv] Deuteronomy 18:10-12. I will discuss the biblical definition of divination in a later chapter.

[xvi] 1 Corinthians 6:19, Romans 8:9-11, 1 John 4:4

instructed any demonic forces present that they must get out of our home. When he did so, an indescribable and overwhelming presence of fear and evil encompassed me so pervasively that I could hardly breathe. My chest felt like it was being crushed, and I began crying out. Seth again renounced any influence that Satan had on me, and suddenly my fear and physical distress ended.

An urgency to eliminate everything tied to AK prompted us to immediately begin ridding our house of all literature and paraphernalia related to those practices. At first, the trashcan outside seemed sufficient. However, I later experienced a compelling temptation to rescue the stuff from the trash. It was like voices were calling from outside. Recognizing the temptation, I asked Seth to eliminate, once and for all, the possibility of my retrieving the material.

I was afraid to try muscle testing again because I did not want to be guilty before the Lord of returning to my previous sin, but the next day I had to know if perhaps our conclusions about Satan's involvement had been wrong. If my ability was the result of science or even God's, not Satan's, power I should still be able to muscle test as before. So, I tried one final time, and had absolutely no ability, nor did I have any sense of "special knowledge."

Afterward, I went on my routine prayer walk through the neighborhood but felt such overwhelming guilt for my sin that the only thoughts I could think of were the Accuser's. *You have failed too badly this time. God can never use you again. How could someone who truly loves God be so deceived. You have hurt so many others by your sin and deceived so many. Your sin is too great and cannot be forgiven.*

Thankfully, the Holy Spirit cried out in my defense and began to call to mind Scripture for me to cling to as truth. The blood of Jesus is sufficient for all sin![xvii] If God could use Paul—a persecutor of the faith, David—a murderer and adulterer, and Peter—a denier of the Savior, then God could still use me. So, I talked it all out with the Father and took my stand against the Accuser of the brethren in the name that has power over all the powers of darkness—*Jesus.* Just as 1 John 1:9 promises, forgiveness from the

---

[xvii] Isaiah 53:5-6, 11, Romans 3:23-26

Savior comes immediately upon confession: *If we confess our sins, he is faithful and just to forgive us our sins, and to cleanse us from all unrighteousness.*

One problem remained, however; I had also sinned against many people by my actions and led many astray. Besides Jesus' command in Matthew 5:23-24 to go to a brother upon realization of your sin against them, I also ached that those I had led into deception might know the truth and be set free. So, despite the shame I felt, Seth and I decided a letter would be the appropriate way, in most cases, to share why I had repented of the alternative practices I once promoted and to ask for their forgiveness. Only a few required a personal conversation. Thankfully, most received the news well, and I had a burden of sin and shame lifted from my heart. Some did not repent, and, for them, I began considering and praying Paul's words in 2 Timothy 2:24-26:

And the Lord's servant must not be quarrelsome but kind to everyone, able to teach, patiently enduring evil, correcting his opponents with gentleness. God may perhaps grant them repentance leading to a knowledge of the truth, and they may come to their senses and escape from the snare of the devil, after being captured by him to do his will.

Freedom & healing that lasts.

Psalm 107:20 says well what transpired in my life: *He sent out his Word and healed them. He rescued them from the grave.* (NIV) For the first time since childhood, I was truly well! There were no more treatments or planning my life around the constraints of my health. I could run miles on pollen laden streets or take a moonlit stroll with Seth without fear of streetlights. In the days ahead, many a conversation took place between Seth and me as we tried to understand the events of the past two years, as well as to marvel at the healing God had brought about in me. *Praise the LORD, oh my soul, all that is within me praise His holy name! Praise the LORD, oh my soul, and forget not all His benefits. He forgives all my sins and heals all my diseases.* (NIV)[xviii]

[xviii] Psalm 103:1-3 NIV

CHAPTER 3

Muscle Testing Through the Years

Have nothing to do with the fruitless deeds of darkness, but rather expose them. Ephesians 5:11

[xix]"Marci, you need to see this email right away," my husband said with concern as I entered the front door of my house.

Emails from my website came with some regularity, but apparently, this one was more concerning than most.

It read, "May I please call you? I so much need to speak with you about a heart-breaking situation that just occurred. We found your website about two weeks ago, and all hell has broken loose since then."

Pausing to pray for wisdom that I might rightly respond to whatever story this stranger had to tell, I then picked up the phone. An hour and many shared tears later, I closed the call with prayer and, with a heavy heart, said goodbye. The dear sister in the Lord with whom I spoke had shared the tragic story of her family's involvement with a young man that her eldest son had befriended. They had generously shared the love of

---

[xix] The following story is reprinted from *Life to the Body—Biblical Principles for Health & Healing*, ch.17.

Christ in word and in deed with him over the course of a year. He was full of promise, although he had not yet decided to trust Jesus as his Savior.

One evening after eating dinner at their house, the young man described to them a pain in his chest that seemed to come on him whenever he tried to read the Bible. He told them how his mother was proficient in *Body Code*, one of the many alternative health practices that utilize muscle testing, and she used it frequently in his home. So, when this pain would arise, he would ask her to "treat" him, following which the pain would immediately subside. As he described this to the Christian mother of his friend, she felt, with certainty, the Holy Spirit's prompting that this was demonic and told him so. To the surprise of all, he readily agreed, and said he was done with it all. She warned him not to ever have the "treatment" done again.

A short time later the pain again came on him with great intensity, and so he asked his mother to treat him once again. Apparently, it is one thing to be an ignorant participant, but quite another to know of Satan's work and seek it for help. His personality changed suddenly and dramatically following that treatment. He began describing to others that he felt tormented, and thoughts of suicide consumed him. He also started texting disturbing pictures related to his plans for killing himself.

The Christian family fasted, prayed, and pleaded with him to turn to the Lord for salvation. When he went to this family's home, the daughters, who had written and recorded songs that beautifully spoke of the Gospel, would sing to comfort him. Like with King Saul when David played the harp, this young man's torment would cease with the music. Everything indicated that he had become demon possessed as a result of the "treatment" he had received.

A couple of weeks later, he texted his sorrowful, last words to multiple members of their family and then shot and killed himself on a farm tractor.

Satan's power to deceive.

If you are new to my writing and speaking, you may wonder how I ended up in a position of speaking with this woman and why she would desire to share with me the details of such a tragedy. Following my repentance from muscle testing, I hoped to put it all behind me and never talk about it with anyone. After all, who wants to put their failures on display? God, however, had different plans. He began to prompt me to write a series of blog posts explaining why I concluded that the power of muscle testing is demonically based. My husband cringed at the thought of sharing our story.

In the end, we both conceded to the Lord's leading. We desired to follow the biblical instruction, *Have nothing to do with the fruitless deeds of darkness, but rather expose them*,[xx] With Seth's help, I wrote a series of three blog articles and posted them on my ministry website, www.heartandmindministries.com. A few years later, as part of a women's Bible study series, I spoke on the topic in a lesson titled, *11 Reasons Muscle Testing is Divination* and posted the video to YouTube in 2018.

I never anticipated the impact those materials would have! Since their posting, I have received a steady flow of emails and phone calls from people, mostly professing Christians, who have become ensnared by energy medicine. Through hundreds of these stories, my own experiences, and continued research, I have become aware of the pervasive work of Satan to ensnare Christians who are sick. By sharing their stories at the end of this book, some of these individuals have participated with me in this endeavor to expose these deeds of darkness.

Relentless, unending pain has a way of making people desperate, and worse yet is the desperation of the parents of sick children. Traditional medicine often fails to provide solutions to chronic conditions, and so many turn to alternative practices that purport to bring relief. Unfortunately, it is in this realm that Satan has gained a tremendous foothold in the lives of countless Christians who truly love God. The apostle Paul warned that Satan would take this tactic in the end times when he wrote, *The Spirit clearly says that in later times some will abandon the faith and follow deceiving spirits and things taught by demons.*[xxi]

[xx] Ephesians 5:11
[xxi] 1 Timothy 4:1

Jesus also warned that Satan's signs and wonders might deceive even the elect.[xxii]

In the early 2000's, most considered alternative medicine a fringe option that largely appealed to those dealing with chronic conditions. Twenty years later, alternative medicine now claims a broad base, as general discontent and mistrust of conventional medicine surges.

Picture alternative health as one massive tree with numerous large branches. It calls to mind the enormous Live Oak trees of Florida, some of which have one massive trunk that diverges near the ground, forming branches that spread in all directions. Each branch appears a tree in itself.

Similarly, holistic health, natural medicine, functional or integrative medicine, and energy medicine grew out of the enormous trunk of alternative medicine but then diverged to form countless, smaller branches. Within the neutral trunk lies all things natural, giving potential for the growth of good or bad branches. Some of these, in theory, could potentially be safe, both physically and spiritually. (For example, herbs are a part of creation given for our use, but when their use coincides with demonic interference, it becomes witchcraft.) With others, however, spiritual influence cannot be divorced from the practice, although many try. Sadly, even the "safe" branches can easily become entwined with the "unsafe" as undiscerning professionals borrow from other practices and ideologies.

Many alternative practices also fall under the umbrella of New Age medicine, which includes a number of occultic practices that are beyond the scope of this book (i.e., medical mediums, psychic surgery, etc.). Therefore, I will use the name energy medicine to refer specifically to those health practices based on a belief in subtle energies.

One practice, in particular, permeates much of alternative medicine-- muscle testing (Applied Kinesiology or AK), and it, therefore, requires special attention. With an online information search about muscle testing, it becomes apparent that it has numerous names and the way it is defined, explained, and used varies widely among practitioners and individuals. For example, the most commonly used method requires two people and

---

[xxii] Matthew 24:24-25

tests the arm, but sway testing and finger testing look quite different and allow one to self-test. Other methods with different names also exist, some of which do not even require a muscle to be involved in the process. It can be challenging to see past the differences and recognize the common threads present in each one. To that end, it is helpful to start the discussion with the benign, and quite legitimate, original—manual muscle testing.

Manual muscle testing

In the early 20th century, Polio had reached epidemic proportions. In the second stage of this terrible illness, the virus attacked the central nervous system and the motor neurons, resulting in muscle loss and sometimes paralysis. Two individuals, Wilhelmine Wright and Robert W. Lovett, are credited with creating a systematic method to grade the strength of the muscles in polio victims. The goal was not to fix anything but to evaluate. Wright first presented the idea for manual muscle testing (MMT) in 1912 and Lovett expanded the protocol in 1916.

In an article for the physical therapy department for the University of Dayton, the authors describe the continued progression of the development of MMT.

> *Florence Kendall along with her husband Henry Otis Kendall, refined testing positions in the 1940s. The manual muscle testing taught today incorporates the anti-gravity testing methods of Wright and Lovett, with the refinement of Kendall.*[3]

The non-spiritual MMT of Kendall includes a systematic and progressive manner of testing 14 separate muscle groups based on movement and position, while the tester applies force against the muscle being tested. The tester then subjectively grades the muscle response on a scale of 0-10.[4] Some variations among testers are inevitable because the force used by one tester may be slightly different than another and the grading results, although standardized, are subjective. Despite these limitations, MMT proves extremely useful in multiple ways. It helps to isolate (or at least point to) the origin of neurological interference with the muscles, which is helpful in diagnosis. It can also be useful in keeping track of progress during treatment or the progressive weakening in degenerative conditions.

So, how is MMT used today? Suppose you develop tingling in your hands while you sleep at night that interferes with your rest, and you go to your doctor to have it checked out. As a part of the physical exam, he will inevitably ask you to perform some simple physical tests. The physician wishes to observe the strength of the various muscles of your neck, arms, and hands while in different positions. He does so to determine numerous things, one of which is whether there is compression of the median nerve. Based on those simple tests, he may conclude or rule out a diagnosis of carpal tunnel syndrome.

Such physical muscle tests provide valuable information about the neurological function that enervates muscles. (In super simple terms, muscles do not work if something interferes with the signal from the motor neurons.) *Today, manual muscle testing remains the mainstay of muscular assessment in the medical community, including physical therapy and medical schools.*[5]

A variation of MMT is functional muscle testing (FMT), which measures and rates the ability to engage in and perform activities required for daily living, such as walking, bending, squatting, and holding or lifting objects. FMT evaluations take into consideration the ability to balance, bear weight, climb stairs, walk, lunge, and jump or hop from one spot to another. Such tests can be useful after a stroke or head injury.

To reiterate, the purpose of MMT and FMT is simple—to grade literal, physical muscle weakness. These procedures are purely physical in nature, and clinical studies repeatedly show the effectiveness MMT and FMT provide as tools for diagnosis. As you will see, this limited, clinical purpose varies greatly from the muscle testing of Applied Kinesiology.

Applied Kinesiology is born.

Chiropractor, George Goodheart, first established Applied Kinesiology in 1964 by combining his knowledge of multiple medical disciplines (traditional and alternative) and spiritual ideas such as *life force* or *ch'i* with MMT. Then, in 1975, with the help of others who valued his work, he founded the International College of Applied Kinesiology (ICAK), which continues to this day, educating people in AK. Because I am a proponent of using original sources whenever possible, let us consider how ICAK defines its own practice.

Many advocates of AK insist that it is merely based in anatomy and body movement (Kinesiology). This is false. Notice the distinction The International College of Applied Kinesiology makes between Kinesiology and Applied Kinesiology:

> *The term Kinesiology is a word that means the study of movement and motion in the body...They learn bio-mechanics and physical mechanisms of body motion. **The term Applied Kinesiology (AK) is a different thing altogether**... It is a term to describe a technique of using specific muscle testing as a neurologic evaluation of **body function**. A doctor or professional can use this feedback system to **aid in the diagnosis of functional imbalance** as well as assist in the feedback of appropriate treatment of a body **imbalance**.*[6] *xxiii*

Their abbreviated description sounds quite similar to MMT—testing to determine neurologic problems. This quote provides a good example of how a little scientific sounding rhetoric goes a long way in deceiving the unsuspecting. A few of the words I highlighted in the quote hint at bigger goals than anything MMT seeks to achieve—body function and diagnosing *imbalance*. If we persist in searching for understanding, clarity will come regarding these distinctions.

George Goodheart and colleague, Scott Cuthbert, wrote the following (here they borrow the title MMT to refer to AK): *When performed by an examiner's hands MMT **may not be just testing for actual muscle strength**; rather it may also test for the nervous system's ability to adapt the muscle to the changing pressure of the examiner's test.*[7] As you will see shortly, the nervous system Goodheart refers to has a unique scope and meaning.

---

xxiii All use of emphasis within this quote or those to come are mine.

The college's website goes on to explain that over the years, AK has expanded to include over 80 forms, but *the common denominator in all these methods is the simple case of testing a human muscle in order to gain some sort of feedback.*[8] Since muscle testing is the common denominator in the many forms of AK, then what distinguishes AK is muscle testing, and understanding the nature of this practice is critical.

Key differences in AK and MMT

The manual muscle testing of Wright, Lovett, and Kendall has nothing to do with the mystical beliefs of the *innate, ch'i, prana*, or *life force,* by any name. It has nothing to do with acupressure meridians but only with the proven understanding of the neurological systems of the human body as they relate to muscle function. It does not attempt to draw conclusions that connect various organs of the body with the muscle test, as AK does.

In 2003, three chiropractors, Haas, Cooperstein, and Peterson, published an article in *The Journal for Chiropractic and Osteopathy.* The article's intent rings clear through the title: *Disentangling manual muscle testing and Applied Kinesiology: critique and reinterpretation of a literature review.* What was the review to which these doctors responded? George Goodheart and colleague, Scott Cuthbert had published a lengthy review of AK related literature, including clinical studies that had been done. Many in chiropractic and osteopathy found the review problematic. In an attempt to set the record straight, Haas and company meticulously set forth the errors in approach and accuracy in Goodheart's review.

Although I will discuss these two articles at length in the next chapter, for now I want to share one facet of the counter position. Haas and company rightfully distinguish what Goodheart conveniently ignored— that MMT is fundamentally different from AK. The authors state,

> *MMT, as performed by chiropractors, does not necessarily differ in its execution and interpretation from manual muscle testing as performed and interpreted by the standards applied in physical medicine. To either practitioner, a weak muscle might suggest a*

*primary muscular or neurological pathology. **However**, AK technique uses manual muscle testing not just to evaluate the functional integrity of muscle and nerve supply, but also as a means to "diagnose structural [and functional], chemical, and mental dysfunctions."[9]*

The differences lie in purpose and conclusions. In MMT the diagnostic conclusions will be limited to the accepted understanding of the neurological system of the body and what can affect it in particular. For example, when testing the deltoid muscle and finding weakness, a doctor would limit his considerations to things affecting the parts of the Central Nervous System associated with the shoulder. The same test done in AK might lead to conclusions about whether a supplement, music in the waiting room, parasites, a traumatic memory, or spleen function are to blame for the muscle weakness.

At this point I need to make clear the possible difference between a certified, professional applied kinesiologist and many other practitioners who use muscle testing. In order to be a certified applied kinesiologist, a licensed professional, i.e., doctor, chiropractor, osteopath, naturopath, dentist, or veterinarian must complete a minimum, 100-hour curriculum in AK and pass both a written and hands-on proficiency exam. They also must maintain their certification by meeting certain standards. These individuals generally have a tremendous knowledge of anatomy and physiology and incorporate AK into their existing practice. The form of muscle testing they employ might possibly look more like traditional MMT with the testing of many muscles rather than just the arm. However, as previously mentioned, their conclusions will likely be unique to AK.

In contrast to the high, professional standards of AK, one of the earliest off-shoots, *Touch for Health*, took the complex knowledge required with the original and simplified it for the masses. *Touch for Health*, founded by chiropractor John F. Thie, approached Goodheart in 1965 with the idea of making AK accessible to everyone. They later joined forces in establishing ICAK, and by so doing, appealed to both the professional and the general public. Notice the difference in the rhetoric used by Thie in describing his practice:

The Touch for Health System is a practical guide to natural health that utilizes acupressure and massage to improve postural balance and reduce physical and mental pain and tension. It is an approach to restoring natural energies that combines ancient Chinese energy therapies with recent Western developments in kinesiology.

TFH Kinesiology can be easily learned by anyone, with a little practice, without any prior knowledge of muscles, physiology, meridians, etc.... **In TFH we use muscle testing as a method of biofeedback to identify imbalances in the body's energy system.**[10]

It is important to note that when encountering individuals who practice muscle testing, whether a professional Applied Kinesiologist, a general practitioner, or a completely untrained individual, the rhetoric will vary widely, but the practice is the same. As Goodheart said, *the common denominator* is *the simple case of testing a human muscle in order to gain some sort of feedback.*

More variations in muscle testing

Now that I have established the origination and evolution of muscle testing, I will give a general description of how muscle testing is performed, based on the variety with which I became involved (and quite "gifted" at). I will then discuss some of the other, common methods. In a later chapter, I will suggest "red flags" to look for when trying to discern if a particular practice is safe or unsafe.

Practitioners who utilize muscle testing to "diagnose" allergies teach that when the body encounters an allergen, the muscles weaken, indicating an unfavorable response. Strength indicates a favorable response. Performing the muscle test is quite simple. The individual being tested holds a tiny amount of whatever substance is being tested in one hand, while extending their other arm to their side at a right angle. The practitioner then places one hand on the individual's shoulder and uses the other hand to lightly press down on the extended arm. In theory, when used in NAET or *nutrition response testing*, if allergic to the substance or if it is not beneficial to health, the individual's arm muscle weakens, and the arm can easily be pressed down. If it is beneficial, the arm remains strong.

It is also possible to self-test using other techniques, such as sway testing or finger testing, but many cannot muscle test themselves. In sway testing, muscle weakness is evidenced by causing one to fall backwards slightly indicating an unfavorable response. In finger testing, the individual makes an O ring with two fingers and tries to pull them apart using one finger from the other hand. If the O is broken easily, that shows weakness and a negative response.

Many machines have also been invented, which practitioners now use as an electronic form of muscle testing. (I will discuss these at length in chapter 11.) Another variation used by some chiropractors who utilize the Koren Specific Technique is called occipital drop. This is performed on the head/neck of the individual. This form of muscle testing can be done quickly and without the patient even knowing it is being done. The hallmark of muscle testing in all forms is that it gives feedback in the form of a binary response to a question—yes or no, positive or negative, favorable or unfavorable.

Surrogate testing allows for the testing of animals, infants, small children, and those who are too weak to perform the muscle test themselves. A further method of muscle testing that is practiced by especially "gifted" practitioners is done remotely via the telephone. In other words, there is no physical contact with the individual! How do you test muscle strength without exertion by the muscles? I will discuss the tremendous significance of this practice later, but for now it is worth mentioning that testing muscles without exerting strain on those muscles or even touching the individual defies any purely physical explanation.

Can anyone do it?

Although trained kinesiologists may take offense at me making this claim, if muscle testing is scientifically based, the average individual should be able to muscle test. I ask you to consider the matter for yourself. In his book, *Your Body Doesn't Lie*, John Diamond, the founder of behavioral kinesiology, said *The body knows! We have only to know how to ask.*[11] They claim the body reliably gives us this feedback/answer through muscle strength/weakness. In light of these claims, does it not make sense that the muscle will behave consistently, regardless of who is testing? Training and skill may aid in proficiency, but the muscle should still weaken or remain strong consistently from one tester to the next.

Think of playing basketball. I may not be Michael Jordan, but if I try to dribble the ball, it will go up and down because gravity, momentum, and other laws of physics are consistent despite my lack of skill. One thing is certain; the ball will not float when I try to push it down. Lack of proficiency does not alter the laws of science. Similarly, if muscle testing is based purely in science, at least a modicum of consistency must be evident. Pushing an arm down requires considerably less skill than dribbling a basketball!

In light of this, it is worth noting that many cannot test others (the tested person's arm NEVER weakens), which suggests muscle testing is not based on the laws of science but something else. Although some acknowledge their complete inability to test themselves or others, I could muscle test others with great ease. The muscle weakness evidenced quite dramatically with the tested individuals feeling as though I had hijacked their muscle. Although they might will their arm to resist my gentle force, the arm would drop anyway. Oddly, my husband could muscle test me but no one else, and some people could easily perform the test in my presence but not at home. Some have told me that a practitioner required their spouse to leave the room because "their energy interfered" with the testing.

Another suspicious phenomenon associated with muscle testing is the use of substitute substances. In NAET and numerous other practices that utilize AK, the supposed allergen or substances for which testing is done are not typically what is being held by the one being tested. Instead, they hold a vial with a liquid in it that has, supposedly, been electrically charged with the energetic or electrical frequency of that substance. This practice is used in other forms of energy medicine as well and is based on a belief that all things possess a measurable frequency or vibration. (More on this in a later chapter.) It is not based on good science but is easily explained through the ideomotor response (to be discussed later), fraud, or spiritual interference.

Many practitioners also claim to test the appropriate dosages of nutrients or the effectiveness of supplements for an individual. Again, the procedures vary. For example, the practitioner might ask "the body" a yes/no question such as, *would vitamin C be good for you to take?* and then muscle test. If the response indicates "the body" needs additional vitamin C, the practitioner then asks; *How many vitamin C tablets should you take?* He would then count out loud while pressing the patient's arm down. At whatever point the arm weakens, that is the number of pills "the body" knows should be consumed. Because of this practice, I have talked to many who, on the advice of their practitioner, were taking 60 to a hundred supplements a day! Can you imagine the bio-chemical impact this has on the human body!

Muscle testing is also used to determine formulations for essential oil blends or supplement combinations. Both individuals and some supplement companies do this. If muscle testing is demonic, then using that influence to create recipes or formulations is sorcery/witchcraft. Another common practice is to "verify" the effectiveness of an energy-based treatment with muscle testing.

Muscle testing is quick, painless, and immediate in its use, unlike traditional diagnostic methods such as blood work and imaging. Its immediacy affords control and quick answers to the patient, which appeals to many. For these reasons, patients often forgo the traditional testing and place their trust in the practitioner.

The ICAK website explains that muscle testing is one of numerous tools that a trained professional should use to make diagnosis. However, in actual practice, muscle testing often becomes the comprehensive, primary diagnostic and guidance tool. Goodheart himself apparently modeled this behavior from the beginning. Long-term colleague of Goodheart and writer of *Your Body Doesn't Lie*, Dr. John Diamond, stated the following in a tribute lecture about George Goodheart at the ICAK:

Throughout that time, I have never known him to carry out any therapeutic procedure, nor prescribe any nutritional *supplementation, that he did not test for its particular effect on the particular patient at that particular time... However powerful his clinical judgments—and they are as powerful as those of any clinician I have ever known—he **always defers** to the patient's own body as the final arbiter of what should be administered.[12]*

Whether Goodheart's willingness to let muscle testing supersede all else is true of all traditionally trained Applied Kinesiologists, I cannot say. However, my experience, as well as that of many who have contacted me, is that even traditional lab work and imaging are discounted or re-explained if they counter the results of muscle testing. If one is to implicitly trust this practice above all else, then determining the source of its information and power is paramount. If the claim is accurate--it reveals what the body knows is true, then perhaps conventional methods of testing should be discounted. However, if it is no better than random guessing, then one risks bodily harm by following its counsel. Worse yet, if it is often directed by evil forces, then tremendous danger to body and soul awaits! We must ferret out the truth.

CHAPTER 4

Does Science Explain Muscle Testing?

Thus says the LORD: If I have not established my covenant with day and night and the fixed order of heaven and earth.
Jeremiah 33:25

Does science confirm Applied Kinesiology's efficacy? For those who have just been introduced to muscle testing, this simple question generally holds much interest. For those who have been involved for some time, the question seems oddly irrelevant. Why? They have experienced results that have convinced them of its effectiveness, and no amount of evidence to the contrary can convince them otherwise. If you have read my story of involvement with muscle testing, you know that I too could offer evidence that it "works." But, if it works, how does it do so? Does it work purely within the physical realm? If so, great! Science can then measure it and verify its effectiveness. If scientific study does not show it is reliable, consistent, and measurable, then we have learned a very valuable clue in understanding the nature of these practices.

Some professing Christians have criticized me for putting such an emphasis on science. They cite biblical passages that speak of the intersection of the spiritual and the physical as evidence of my mistaken focus. My response is simple: Did not God ordain the laws of science to govern the physical realm? Jeremiah 33:24-26 compares the absolute certainty of the unchanging covenant God established with David to the unchanging covenant God also fixed with the laws that rule the physical universe.

> *"Have you not observed that these people are saying, 'The Lord has rejected the two clans that he chose'? Thus they have despised my people so that they are no longer a nation in their sight. Thus says the Lord: If I have not established <u>my covenant with day and night and the fixed order of heaven and earth</u>, then I will reject the offspring of Jacob and David my servant and will not choose one of his offspring to rule over the offspring of Abraham, Isaac, and Jacob. For I <u>will</u> restore their fortunes and <u>will</u> have mercy on them."*

Although God appeared to have rejected His chosen people by allowing them to suffer in captivity because of their sin, He had not abandoned them, or His covenant promises to them. Neither would he break the covenant established at creation with the physical universe.

God created the laws of the universe and only interferes with these laws on rare occasions to serve a specific purpose. When He does so, it is called a miracle! This is why science is measurable, consistent, and repeatable. However, science is limited. It only measures the *fixed order of heaven and earth* (the physical realm) and not the spirit realm. So, when trying to discern between the spiritual and the physical, science is a good place to begin. By ruling out the one, it points to the other. Doing so does not make science a god or a religion to the Christian but simply a system whereby to evaluate measurable and repeatable physical activities and phenomenon. A useful tool, if you will.

God has allowed Satan, the *ruler of this world,*[xxiv] a time of influence as *the prince of the power of the air.*[xxv] His interference in the physical realm is also spoken of in Ephesians 6. The Bible does not make it clear how the devil and unclean spirits influence the physical but only that they

---

[xxiv] John 12:31
[xxv] Ephesians 2:2

do. In trying to discern if something is physical or spiritual, consider one distinguishing factor. The physical is consistent with God's unchanging laws of nature, whereas the spirit realm in which Satan and his cohorts function is unpredictable because capricious entities move within it. Within that realm one finds personalities with motive. Something may be physical but influenced by the spiritual. When this happens, the tell-tale sign will be that the results are not consistent with the *fixed order of heaven and earth.* Satan can only counterfeit. This, then, is our heads-up.

Aside from considering a spiritual explanation for alternative practices, we should also consider several other possibilities to explain apparent results. Mankind continually makes new discoveries in science and gains new understanding of things that were once mysterious. Could this be the case with energy-based practices? Many would shout, "Yes!" If they are correct and science has yet to explain it, the phenomena will still be consistent and measurable. Some proponents suggest explanations such as quantum physics or energy. If any of these purely physical explanations for muscle testing are correct, then, I reiterate; they will be verifiable scientifically even if the "how" is not yet understood.

Skeptics, who discount everything spiritual, suggest the placebo effect or ideomotor activity (this involves unconscious responses and behaviors), as plausible explanations for the inconsistent results of energy-based practices. How, then, can we know? Again, by looking first through the lens of science for the *fixed order of heaven and earth.* If it is a purely physical practice, then it can be measured repeatedly and consistently.

Yet, another explanation to consider is fraud. We know from history that fraud in the medical realm has been rampant. From the snake oil peddlers of early America to the weight loss scams of today, health deceptions perpetrated on an unsuspecting public are commonplace. Therefore, we must not too quickly dismiss that possibility either.

I will consider these various explanations in greater detail in the chapters that follow. For now, let us begin our quest to discern the truth about energy-based practices by putting muscle testing through the rigors of scientific evaluation.

Blind vs. double blind studies

Many years ago, as a stay-at-home mom, funds were short, and I looked for short-term opportunities to make money. So, when I learned of the chance to be paid to participate in a double-blind, clinical study of a whitening toothpaste, I eagerly enrolled. The participants were given detailed instructions to brush their teeth for two minutes, twice a day using a specific quantity of the toothpaste provided. None of the participants would know whether their toothpaste was the one being tested for expected whitening results or a placebo (non-whitening toothpaste). Each patient and toothpaste were given a number. Only the testing company knew which number correlated with which product. The patients had to return periodically to the dentist office responsible for the study's check-ups to document our results. The dentist, also, did not know which toothpaste the participants were using but only the number. Following this protocol made the study a controlled, double-blind, clinical study.

If the participants had known which toothpaste they were using, questions about the validity of the results could have arisen. How? If one believed they were using the best product, they might brush more vigorously than if they thought it was the placebo and vice versa. If the dentist had known which toothpaste a given patient was using, this knowledge might have skewed his subjective evaluation of the coloring of that patient's teeth. Although these modifications might be unintentional or even unknown to the dentist or participants, subtle changes can be problematic to accurate study. Hence, a double-blind study is the gold standard.

If the patient was unaware of the toothpaste being used but the dentist knew, or vice versa, then it would have been a single-blind study. Understanding the difference between single-blind and double-blind studies is important in discerning the truth in the claims of countless products and practices. Other notable factors in a reliable, clinical study include having a sufficient number of participants, having an unbiased third party implementing the study, and following careful regimentation of scientific protocols. Failure to meet these requirements does not necessarily render a study invalid but does mean that the results may be insignificant without corroboration from other reliable studies that show similar results.

Applied Kinesiology sometimes bears up under single-blind studies but never survives the scrutiny of double-blind studies. In the following pages, I will discuss the studies that have been done and explain why there are different outcomes for single-blind versus double blinds.

A surprising scientific study on muscle testing

A question I always ask when looking at clinical studies is who funded it. Why? I want to know if an agenda might have clouded the accuracy of the study's conclusions. Yes, it is possible and even common for clinical study results to be biased.

In 2013, a group of seven doctors and PhD's published a peculiar, double-blind study on AK. What made this study rather unique was the individuals involved and their conclusions. In researching the potential biases of these individuals, I learned of people who clearly had a favorable mind-set to the AK agenda. Jessica Utts is a parapsychologist and statistics professor at the University of California, Irvine known for her investigation into remote viewing.[xxvi] Stephan A. Schwartz also classifies himself as a parapsychologist. S. James P. Spottiswoode does research on ESP, shape shifting, global consciousness, and other parascience topics. Christopher W. Shade, the chief scientist for Quicksilver Scientific, once said in a lecture that his company "quality tested" all of their products using muscle testing. Also joining the team, Dr. Lisa Tully is the

founder of the Energy Medicine Research Institute (EMRI), whose primary mission is to assess the efficacy of vibrational medicine technologies and therapies. The EMRI specializes in assisting companies in the integrative health and natural product arenas to obtain clinical trials to support marketing claims.[13]

[xxvi] "Remote viewing is defined as the ability to acquire accurate information about a distant or non-local place, person or event without using your physical senses or any other obvious means. It's associated with the idea of clairvoyance and sometimes called *anomalous cognition* or *second sight*."
https://www.gaia.com/article/how-to-remote-view

Last in the study's group of scientists[xxvii] is Ginette Nachman M.D. Ph.D. whose online biography describes her as having a *longstanding interest in helping to educate health care and mental health professionals regarding non-local aspects of consciousness and clinical approaches to exceptional experiences.*[14] She promotes the Parapsychological Association, whose goal is to promote *the study of psi (or 'psychic') experiences, such as telepathy, clairvoyance, psychokinesis, psychic healing, and precognition.*[15]

From this information, you can imagine my shock upon reading the following conclusion from their very thorough clinical study:

> *The research published by the Applied Kinesiology field itself is not to be relied upon, and in the experimental studies that do meet accepted standards of science, Applied Kinesiology has not demonstrated that it is a useful or reliable diagnostic tool upon which health decisions can be based.*[16]

This study met all of the requirements for a sound, clinical study. As one would expect from the scientists' backgrounds, they began with a presumption of AK having diagnostic capabilities and structured the study to answer the following questions:

> *(1) Is there a difference in muscular strength when an individual holds a substance that is inimical to life processes (a poison solution), as compared to a substance that is essential for life (normal saline)?*

> *(2) Is this effect a transaction involving input from both the person being measured and the kinesiologist doing the measurement or is it only the person being measured?*

[xxvii] I was unable to determine the background of one of the 7 persons associated with this study.

(3) As an extension of question 2, is the result the same when different kinesiologists take the measurement or when no kinesiologist is involved?

(4) Does belief, expectation, gender, or time cognition play a role in determining response?[17]

51 participants were each tested by three kinesiologists (one female and two male) and by a hand-held dynamometer that measured grip strength, which provided an unbiased control set. When the kinesiologists tested, the amount of force they used was kept uniform by a tool to measure the pressure exerted. They tested the participants by all kinesiologists and the dynamometer for unmarked vials containing either a saline solution with a salinity level vital to life, as well as a saline solution with a toxic level of ionic hydroxylamine hydrochloride $(NH3OH)(+)$.[18] If the claims of AK are correct, the muscles should measurably and consistently weaken in the presence of the toxic solution.

The results among the different kinesiologists varied, and all were consistent in providing results that were no better than random chance. Upon completion, those responsible for the study also did a review of the literature claims by the Applied Kinesiology field itself and concluded that their claims are *not to be relied upon.* And this came from a group of professionals who were clearly disposed to believe that AK could be relied upon.[xxviii]

Other studies on muscle testing

Some dentists use AK both diagnostically and to test for the materials used in dental procedures. They aim to use only materials that correspond

---

[xxviii] I contacted Dr. Christopher Shade's company, Quick Silver Scientific, by email to ask them about this study and whether they still "quality test" their products using muscle testing. They responded, *We do third party testing on all of our products to ensure they meet our high standards of quality. The change would have been a company wide decision due to growth and **more concrete** practices.*

well with the patient. This noble goal was tested in a double-blind clinical trial. The Department of Conservative Dentistry at a university in Germany conducted a clinical study to test the claim that AK can accurately reveal an individual's (in)tolerance of dental materials. 112 volunteers who were unfamiliar with AK were tested by two dentists trained in AK using the standard method of muscle testing—the deltoid muscle. *In 14 cases, the results of the open and blinded tests matched, whereas in 26 cases they did not (95% confidence interval, 21%-52%; p = 0.98)* indicating that muscle testing was no more reliable in determining appropriate dental materials than random guessing.[19]

Another common use of muscle testing replaces traditional allergy testing. This use of AK has undergone much study. In an article examining the claims of various unconventional methods of allergy testing, including AK, published by University of Zürich in Switzerland, Professor Wüthrich concluded that *these unproven techniques may lead to misleading advice or treatments, and their use is not advised.*[20] He based his conclusion about AK on an Italian test called a DRIA, which involved placing a sublingual, allergenic in the individual's mouth. They then used an ergometer to test muscle strength. *No investigation supported the rational and diagnostic claims of the DRIA test.*[21] Wüthrich reiterated his conclusion by stating, *there is little or no scientific rationale for these methods. Results are not reproducible when subject to rigorous testing and do not correlate with clinical evidence of allergy.*[22]

Many who contact me indicate they use muscle testing for their children's healthcare. Once upon a time, I did the same. Every parent desires to provide the best for their children and yet, like me, few take the time to research whether AK is shown to be effective in diagnosing and treating children. No parent would want to give their child supplements or treatments based on faulty information and yet many do, as the following study indicates.

A unique and insightful study of children in Germany was done over a two-year period. The study sought to evaluate the diagnostic accuracy of AK in determining nutritional intolerances. To do so, it compared traditionally accepted diagnostic tests with AK results. (The tests compared were RAST, lactose breath hydrogen test, and a specific IgG test [Cytolisa].) The study kept track of the care received through AK of 315 children and adolescents, 0-17 years old, with different chronic diseases such as headache, abdominal pain, chronic eczema, hyperactivity, and bronchial asthma. The results of the two-year study clearly demonstrated no inter-tester reliability and no statistically significant agreement with the traditional diagnostic methods of testing.[xxix] The conclusion stated, *AK cannot be recommended for diagnosing nutritional intolerance.*[23]

Although having a large number of participants in a study lends significance to the results, multiple small studies that reveal consistent conclusions also demand attention. A small double-blind study was done to determine if muscle testing could accurately differentiate between wasp venom and a placebo placed in vials. Seven individuals who had clinically confirmed wasp venom allergies (both clinically and allergologically), were muscle tested by multiple, trained examiners. Ten unmarked vials each of venom and a placebo, totaling 20 vials per person were used. Both the participants and the examiners were blind. The results showed unambiguously that AK *as a diagnostic tool is not more useful than random guessing.*[24]

Another small but impressively comprehensive, double-blind study involved 3 trained muscle testers and 11 subjects who were tested with four different nutrients (zinc, vitamin C, thiamin, and vitamin A) and two placebos (pectin and sucrose). The subjects were tested with applied kinesiology, standard nutrient laboratory tests, and with computerized isometric muscle testing. They were tested to determine if nutrient deficiencies existed in the subjects for the four nutrients and then again when supplementation was given to those who were deemed deficient. The thoroughness of the study led to significant results:

[xxix] "We found a moderate test-retest reliability (intraclass-kappa 0.62) but no inter-tester reliability (intraclass-kappa -0.01). Moreover, there was no statistically significant agreement with either RAST and Cytolisa (sensitivity 73.6%, specificity 45.2%) or lactose breath hydrogen test (sensitivity 77.1%, specificity 43.2%)." (https://pubmed.ncbi.nlm.nih.gov/11926427/)

*Statistical analysis yielded no significant interjudge reliability, no significant correlation between the testers and standard biochemical tests for nutrient status, and no significant correlation between mechanical and manual determinations of relative muscle strength... **the results of this study indicated that the use of applied kinesiology to evaluate nutrient status is no more useful than random guessing.**[25]* (emphasis mine)

Single-blind studies

As I searched for any reference online to a study that showed muscle testing proved an accurate, consistent, and valid tool for health, I found only privately done, single-blind studies offering favorable results. For example, a couple of popular skeptics have been given audience through the years with respected applied kinesiologists to test AK. The test scenarios always involved an initial single-blind test scenario followed by a repeat of the first scenario but in double-blind fashion. The results remain consistent—single-blind testing of AK shows some level of reliability while double-blind brings abysmal results. When the one testing knows what is being tested, they tend to alter how they test, thereby producing more accurate results. The same is true when only the one being tested knows what is being tested.

The founder of the Skeptics Toolbox, Ray Hyman, PhD, describes a time when he took part in a test of AK at Dr. Wallace Sampson's medical office in Mountain View, California. A team of chiropractors began the proceedings with a test scenario of their choosing. Based on a shared belief between many natural health proponents that natural sugars are healthy whereas processed sugars are not, the chiropractors chose to test the participants by placing drops of glucose (a "bad" sugar) and fructose (a "good" sugar) on their tongues. In this single-blind test, most of the time the subjects gave the expected muscle weakness with the glucose and strength with the fructose. The chiropractors ended this portion of the test feeling vindicated.

After a break, the tests were repeated, only this time the glucose and fructose drops were administered in a way so that no one knew which sugar was being tested. Sometimes the subjects tested strong and sometimes not, but when the substances were revealed, no correlation between muscle strength/weakness and a particular sugar existed. Hyman related the telling response:

> *When these results were announced, the head chiropractor turned to me and said, "You see, that is why we never do double-blind testing anymore. It never works!" At first I thought he was joking. It turned out he was quite serious. Since he "knew" that applied kinesiology works, and the best scientific method shows that it does not work, then — in his mind — there must be something wrong with the scientific method.[26]*

Righting an inaccurate scientific review

In the last chapter, I wrote of two literature reviews published in *The Journal for Chiropractic and Osteopathy*. The initial review was done by the founder of AK, George Goodheart, and his colleague Scott Cuthbert. The response to that review came soon after from three chiropractors, Haas, Cooperstein, and Peterson who desired to set the record straight. They point out numerous flaws in Goodheart's review, including cherry-picking, but highlight the most significant flaw in their estimation. The authors say,

> *Most importantly, a misunderstanding of the review could easily arise because the authors did not distinguish the general use of muscle strength testing from the specific applications that distinguish the Applied Kinesiology (AK) chiropractic technique. The article makes the fundamental error of implying that the reliability and validity of manual muscle testing lends some degree of credibility to the unique diagnostic procedures of AK.[27]*

Why is this distinction so important? Not a solitary, double-blind, clinical study has been done to date that concludes applied kinesiology is a valid diagnostic tool, a discerner of what the body knows as true about health, or a reliable tool, in any form, for health. However, studies do exist that show the original, manual muscle testing used in numerous traditional medical practices is a valid tool for health. What Goodheart sought to do in his review was to assume ownership of studies that did not test AK but MMT. Do not be deceived by such tactics!

Perhaps some will read this chapter and respond as the previously quoted chief chiropractor did in dismissing the evidence by concluding science itself is the problem. However, I ask you to consider that scientific study has revealed a valuable clue in understanding AK. What we have learned is that muscle testing does not follow *the fixed order of heaven and earth*. As muscle testing forms the basis for treatment by many different alternative medical practices, it is important to know what you are dealing with. If the foundation of muscle testing is problematic, then all practices built upon it are also problematic.

Although it is alarming to think of basing healthcare decisions on something that has been unequivocally proven to be no better than random chance, the anecdotal evidence strongly suggests people do sometimes get results, albeit inconsistently. In fact, many individuals report dramatic changes upon following the recommendations based on muscle testing. Furthermore, it is hard to ignore that the individual's muscle does often, unexplainably, weaken significantly when muscle tested. Why? I shall explore the answer further in the next chapter.

CHAPTER 5

Solving the Mystery of How Muscle Testing Works

They are full of superstitions from the East; they practice divination like the Philistines and embrace pagan customs.
Isaiah 2:6

In the last chapter, I laid out the resounding conclusion from the scientific studies on Applied Kinesiology—It is no better than random guessing. However, if you have participated in this alternative practice, you probably have a story or two to share that suggests anecdotal evidence that AK "works." If you read the stories of individuals in the last section of this book, you will read more subjective evidence. How can this be if science has proved it is not a reliable health tool?

As previously mentioned, multiple explanations for this mystery exist. Some of the reports of the change in symptoms could be attributed to the placebo effect or even the nocebo effect.[xxx] I realize no one wants to think their confidence or lack of confidence in a therapy could positively or negatively affect its impact. Before dismissing the possibility, consider the multitude of clinical studies that have been done that clearly document

---

[xxx] Placebo would be a positive outcome generated by belief, whereas nocebo would be a negative outcome generated by belief.

the powerful impact belief has in making a product, treatment, or surgery produce an effect.[28] The way the brain achieves this is remarkable! One example of how the expectancy-based placebo effect works is by the brain producing its own opioids. One study monitored 27 regions of the brain, which are known to produce pain-reducing chemicals (opioids). It revealed that 14 of those regions showed *significant placebo-induced increases and none showed decreases.*[29]

So, just believing something will produce a positive effect can trigger your brain to produce opioids that reduce your painful symptoms. It stands to reason, then, that a belief in the accuracy of muscle testing in diagnosis and the choosing of supplements could produce short-term, noticeable relief from ailments, hence, the anecdotal evidence indicating AK works.

As for an explanation for why the muscle test itself often "works," some skeptics of AK suggest the ideomotor effect. When one believes something to be true, subconsciously driven, subtle, behaviors exhibit themselves. Body language is the most familiar example of the ideomotor effect. Some suggest that when an AK practitioner suspects a particular outcome, they subconsciously alter the manner they muscle test to produce the corresponding result, i.e., the amount of force used, the direction they push down, their subjective interpretation of the arm's resistance, etc. Although practitioners are reticent to acknowledge this possibility, the fact that only single-blind studies show some consistency strongly suggests that the practitioner's ideomotor effect is influencing the results.

Oxford University performed numerous tests of AK and came to several conclusions, including whether results could be attributed to the ideomotor effect. They chose a unique testing method. They did not test AK as it is used in health but instead tried to determine if muscle testing worked as a lie detector test. They presented truths and untruths while muscle testing and repeated the scenarios in numerous ways. All tests showed a level of accuracy significantly greater than random guessing but did not suggest that a belief-generated ideomotor effect caused those results.[30]

The standard lie-detector test, although certainly fallible, has notable reliability because the body responds physically to the stress of lying. Telling the truth uses four areas of the brain whereas lying uses seven.

Therefore, it is more difficult to do other things while lying as opposed to while telling the truth.[31] As a result, your muscles work less effectively in response to a lie.[32] Make no mistake. The level of accuracy from the Oxford studies did not show that the body reveals hidden truth about itself but that the brain produces a physical response to what an individual believes to be true or false.

Suggestions of spiritual activity

Considering the placebo/nocebo effects and ideomotor effect as explanations for times when AK "works," is it possible, then, that the answer to the mystery resides solely in the physical realm? I do not believe so. Although much can likely be explained by the aforementioned effects, too many other characteristics of muscle testing point to the involvement of spiritual entities. Consider the following:

1. An overwhelming number of Christians describe having a general unease or lack of peace about the practice. (Is this evidence of the Holy Spirit at work warning His people?)

2. The muscle test often cannot be performed by individuals, and the presence of some individuals interferes with the test. (Often this individual is the husband, whom God ordained as the spiritual head and protector of his family.)

3. Distance or remote testing and surrogate testing can be done. (This is not possible in the physical realm so either those who do such testing are frauds, or a spiritual entity is directing them.)

4. Many who practice muscle testing report strange phenomena. (Reports resemble demonic activity, such as frightening or prophetic dreams, onset of suicidal thoughts, poltergeist events, and clairvoyant knowledge.)

5. Many who practice muscle testing become increasingly dependent upon it and progress toward use that clearly takes the place of the Word of God and the Holy Spirit's guidance (Spiritual bondage?).

6. Almost all who practice muscle testing for an extended time have a general trajectory of worsening health with only occasional "good days" or temporary relief. (Satan's goal is to steal, kill, and destroy.)

7. Those who were once proficient in muscle testing report a change upon their repentance and standing against the enemy. They can no longer muscle test and no longer "know" things.

Although those characteristics are not true of everyone and some could be understood by non-spiritual explanations, the list does align with biblical descriptions of spiritual activity.

Surely such things warrant further investigation. Christian practitioners prefer not to discuss the origins and basis for Applied Kinesiology, but someone who wishes to make an informed decision on this practice would be wise to carefully consider those beginnings.

The religious origins of muscle testing

Contrary to what proponents of AK would have you believe, this is not science, but rather pantheism. (The word pantheism itself reveals its meaning. It comes from the Greek roots *pan* (all) and *theos* (God), and so, very simply put, it is a belief that everything in the universe is a manifestation of God. Because of this foundational religious belief, practitioners often talk to the body of the person they are treating as though it is its own separate entity. The pantheistic idea that your body, as a part of god, can communicate mysteriously is rampant in eastern and New Age religions and the health practices that developed from them.

Although the idea that *the body knows* originated with Goodheart, his friend and colleague, John Diamond, wrote the book that firmly established the mantra throughout the alternative medical world.

Repeatedly in his book, *Your Body Doesn't Lie*, Diamond attributes all explanations of how the body knows and reveals hidden knowledge to the thymus gland. In a casual reading of the book, one might wrongly conclude that much science confirms the validity of the thymus gland as the central focus of knowledge about the human body and the reason muscle testing works.

However, in a video Diamond published on YouTube in 2020, he revealed his true thoughts and intentions in writing the book.

*When I wrote my first book, "The Body Doesn't Lie"...**I was really talking about the heart chakra**, but I knew it would never get accepted so I talked about the thymus instead. Because the thymus is the organ that most relates to the heart chakra, which is in front...**The book was really about the heart chakra**.*

*The best part of that book is Appendix 1 where I talk about, what I call, the thymellium, which is like an incense burner, which they put thyme, and this was burned as an offering, an aspirational offering to **the gods. And that is what we have in us**.*

The thymus, as I understand it, is the transducer, the changer of the chi in the atmosphere into electromagnetic energy which is the chi that then flows through the acupuncture system.[33] (emphasis mine)

George Goodheart created Applied Kinesiology by combining elements of psychic philosophy, Chinese Taoism, and ancient Eastern practices such as meridians and chi, with the chiropractic theory of the *innate*. His leanings were not hidden among those who knew him. For example, doctors Kravitz and Pollack remark on the mystery of the origin of Goodheart's comprehensive charts. They said that the charts show:

the effects of specific nutrients and herbs upon specific organs, teeth, acupuncture meridians, and muscles. These are extremely elaborate, and a major question is raised as to how such complex interrelationships could possibly be validated without the efforts of numerous researchers and the production of a great deal of published *research. **When a major proponent of applied kinesiology was queried on this, he stated that Goodheart was psychic (personal communication) and developed his charts by this means.**[34]* (emphasis mine)

Also confirming Goodheart's connection with the occult, his lifelong friend, John Diamond, MD, gave a tribute speech upon his friend's death in 2008. Diamond speaks with admiration of Goodheart's reliance on spirit-led dreams in solving difficult cases.

*Every time we dream, we too are receiving Inspiration from the Beyond, including, of course, **the spirits of the deceased**. As George Goodheart was given. And some of them he recognized and, recognizing or not, he gratefully accepted and used their teaching.[35]*

In another lecture to ICAK by Diamond, he discusses the idea of "life energy" that permeates AK.

As Goodheart has shown, this particular muscle is energized by the chi, the Life Energy, flowing into it through the lung meridian. So any stress factor that reduces this flow of Life Energy will be manifested by the muscle testing weak in certain situations.

Every time we test the muscle, we are challenging the efficacy of the flow of Life Energy through the associated meridian… Only the body knows—and the doctor must humbly ask.[36]

Divination

The mantra, *the body doesn't lie*, forms the basis for a belief that muscle testing reveals true and reliable information about one's health. However, as clinical studies clearly demonstrate, the body does not reveal true and reliable information about health through AK. This fact is also demonstrated repeatedly when proven diagnostic tests counter the results of AK. What the mantra does reveal about muscle testing, though, is that the the father of lies is using the teaching that *the body doesn't lie* to deceive and ensnare people to their destruction.

In direct contrast to this lie from the pit of hell, the Bible says, ***The heart is deceitful above all things and beyond cure. Who can understand it?***[xxxi] The prophet Hosea also spoke of this and the consequence that would follow for allowing the deceitful heart to lead God's people into following idols. ***Their heart is deceitful, and now they must bear their guilt.***[xxxii]

Satan has power and can, with God's permission, use anything for his purposes, which are to *steal, kill, and destroy.*[xxxiii] So, although there is no accuracy or reliability to muscle testing for health in the physical realm, the deceiver gladly couples the temptation for hidden knowledge that muscle testing promises with enough results to lead people astray. I say "hidden knowledge" because it is clear from science that AK fails to provide true information, and yet people who rely on it become obsessed with knowing—What caused this symptom? What supplement should I take? How much of the supplement should I take? What memory from the past is causing this emotion that is making me have this symptom? Does so and so love me? And, the temptation consumes the thoughts with intense desire to know what was previously unattainable or attainable only through expensive tests or waiting on God to direct through the Word and by the Holy Spirit.

Meriam Websters Dictionary defines divination as *the art or practice that seeks to foresee or foretell future events or discover hidden knowledge usually by the interpretation of omens or by the aid of supernatural powers.*[37] If muscle testing is empowered by spiritual entities and not scientific truth, then it is divination.

The desire for secret knowledge goes back to the fall. In the Garden, Satan tempted Eve with a desire to be equal with God in knowledge. The deceiver used the tactic of calling into question God's good plan and suggested that God kept back information from Eve that she had a right to

---

[xxxi] Jeremiah 17:9
[xxxii] Hosea 10:2
[xxxiii] John 10:10

know. *For God knows that when you eat of it your eyes will be opened, and you will be like God, knowing good and evil.* [xxxiv] When Eve considered the matter for herself, she determined the serpent must be right. She fell for the lie, and Adam went along with her bringing death to all mankind.

I have heard from many Christians of how they once used muscle testing as a way to make their every decision. The availability of this method as a replacement for God's Word and the Holy Spirit's guidance clearly reveals it as divination. One might argue that just because a tool can be used wrongly does not make the correct use of the tool wrong. For example, a hammer should be used to drive nails into wood. However, if it is used to kill someone by hitting him over the head, do we conclude the hammer is evil and should not be used as a building tool? No, but we might conclude that evil was involved in the act of using the hammer to kill someone. Satan is not picky about what he uses to steal, kill, and destroy; only that he does. The significant difference in this analogy is that the hammer can be used to accomplish legitimate work in its original design. Muscle testing cannot. It is and always has been a lie based in the occult. Whereas a hammer is neutral; muscle testing is inherently evil. Therefore, muscle testing cannot be redeemed and is off limits to the Christian.

In the Old Testament law God commanded, *Do not practice divination or seek omens.*[xxxv] Through the prophet Isaiah, God speaks of why He allowed the Israelites to suffer at the hands of their enemies. *You, Lord, have abandoned your people, the descendants of Jacob. They are full of superstitions from the East; they practice divination like the Philistines and embrace pagan customs.*[xxxvi]

This forbidden fruit of hidden knowledge could be sought through all manner of practices that provided guidance or information from demons. Throughout history, people have used divination rather than seeking God. As such, God asserts, in Deuteronomy 18:9-14, that not only are such practices an abomination but also those who practice them!

[xxxiv] Genesis 3:5 ESV
[xxxv] Leviticus 19:26 NIV
[xxxvi] Isaiah 2:6 NIV

"When you come into the land that the Lord your God is giving you, you shall not learn to follow the abominable practices of those nations. There shall not be found among you...anyone who practices divination or tells fortunes or interprets omens, or a sorcerer or a charmer or a medium or a necromancer or one who inquires of the dead, for <u>whoever does these things is an abomination to the Lord.</u> And because of these abominations the Lord your God is driving them out before you. You shall be blameless before the Lord your God, for these nations, which you are about to dispossess, listen to fortune-tellers and to diviners. <u>But as for you, the Lord your God has not allowed you to do this.</u>

God-ordained divination

At this point in the argument against muscle testing, some who are familiar with the Bible will stipulate to AK being divination, but they will argue that it is godly divination empowered by the Holy Spirit. They agree that muscle testing is indeed spiritual but equate it with the God-ordained use of lots or the Urim and Thummim from the Bible. In order to address this argument, we again look to Scripture.

God mentions the Urim and Thummim in only a handful of Old Testament passages. They were to be placed on the high priest's outer garment called the ephod. These were occasionally used as a tool for gaining guidance from God as to what the people should do.

Those mysterious objects were by no means the only Old Testament methods God ordained for seeking His direction. By God's initiation, the prophets, lots, and dreams were also commonly used. But, then Jesus, the Word became flesh! Hebrews 1:1-2 lets us know that everything changed with the way God would communicate with His people after His Son's arrival. *Long ago, at many times and in many ways, God spoke to our fathers by the prophets, but in these last days he has spoken to us by his Son.*

In John 14, Jesus told the disciples that He would soon be leaving them but that the Holy Spirit would come in Jesus' place and indwell them.

Jesus explained one of the purposes of the Spirit in Verse 26. ***But the Helper, the Holy Spirit, whom the Father will send in my name, he will teach you all things and bring to your remembrance all that I have said to you.*** God's Word and the empowering of the Holy Spirit to understand that Word became the Father's method of revealing truth.

But, what about the New Testament use of lots, many have asked? Do you know when the last time lots were used in the Bible? It was BEFORE Pentecost when the disciples felt the need to choose a replacement for Judas.[xxxvii] Then, at Pentecost, the Holy Spirit came upon them with fire just as Jesus had promised. Never again were lots to be used as a God-ordained tool for seeking Him. To do so would be divination.

As to the argument that the Holy Spirit uses muscle testing as a means to communicate God's knowledge and direction to His people, we must again consider what the Bible says. As John 14:26 and 15:26 say, the Holy Spirit calls to mind what Jesus already revealed, and the Spirit testifies of Jesus. The Spirit always points us to the Word. In over one hundred references to the Spirit, not one even hints that He uses anything resembling muscle testing to communicate for God.

In contrast, the messages of divination usually come through some object that brings a binary, yes or no answer. Although I will discuss muscle testing as a form of divination in greater length in the next chapter, I wish to end this chapter with some encouragement for the reader whose heart is now broken over the knowledge that they have participated in the sin of divination.

Truth for the repentant

For those who love the Lord with all their heart and desire to please Him, awareness of sin, especially significant sin, can be overwhelming. Satan will seek to accuse you. His condemnation seeks to render you useless, under the weight of guilt, rather than walking in the blessing of complete forgiveness. Stand against such lies in the name of Jesus and cling to the truth of God's Word.

[xxxvii] Acts 1:23-26

Consider what the Bible say about repentance. It says that godly sorrow leads to repentance;[xxxviii] so by the conviction of the Holy Spirit you have rightly begun the process. God also gives us comfort in this godly sorrow, as the Psalms remind us that *a broken and contrite heart, O God, you will not despise*.[xxxix] Praise God that in His unfailing mercy He has, by His Spirit, opened your eyes so that you might repent and walk before Him in holiness. (For a more complete discussion of repenting from muscle testing and energy medicine skip to chapter 15.)

In Psalm 32, David also encourages us with a reminder of the blessing of being forgiven.

Blessed is the one whose transgressions are forgiven, whose sins are covered. Blessed is the one whose sin the Lord does not count against them and in whose spirit is no deceit. When I kept silent, my bones wasted away through my groaning all day long. For day and night your hand was heavy on me; my strength was sapped as in the heat of summer. Then I acknowledged my sin to you and did not cover up my iniquity. I said, "I will confess my transgressions to the Lord." And you forgave the guilt of my sin. Therefore, let all the faithful pray to you while you may be found. (vs 1-6, NIV)

In conclusion, I ask you to remember the story we are told in Luke 7:41-50. A sinful but repentant woman came to Jesus with an outpouring of brokenness and love. The disciples wished to shoo her away, and so Jesus used it as an opportunity for teaching.

He told a parable of two men who owed money. One owed far more than could ever be repaid and the other had a minor debt. In the story, both debts were repaid in full by their master. Jesus asked Peter which of the two would love the master more, and Peter replied correctly: *I suppose the one who had the bigger debt forgiven*. Jesus then turned to the repentant

---

[xxxviii] 2 Corinthians 7:10 *Godly sorrow brings repentance that leads to salvation and leaves no regret, but worldly sorrow brings death.* NIV
[xxxix] Psalm 51:17 NIV

woman and said, *Your sins are forgiven… Your faith has saved you; go in peace.*[xl]

Dear brother or sister, repent so that you too can go in peace.

[xl] Luke 7:43, 48, & 50 NIV

CHAPTER 6

The Body as a Ouija Board

My people consult a wooden idol, and a diviner's rod speaks to them. A spirit of prostitution leads them astray; they are unfaithful to their God. Hosea 4:12

Most people are familiar with the Ouija Board. Whether or not they believe it does anything, they know of its association with the occult. If your doctor pulled out a Ouija Board during your appointment and announced his intention to consult it in order to diagnose your condition or determine your treatment, what would you do? I strongly suspect you would leave immediately.

The reasons for hastily leaving might seem obvious but let us consider the rationale briefly. The clear reason, of course, is that God has forbidden divination and witchcraft.[xli] When divination is used medically, the second sin of witchcraft (synonymous with sorcery) often enters the picture. A witchdoctor harnesses demonic guidance (divination) and power to create a remedy (herbal concoction) to affect someone's health. Aside from the important fact that participation with such offenses separates you from fellowship with a holy and jealous God, another very practical reason exists in avoiding these sins. The intentions of Satan are clear. The lion seeking whom he may devour intends to use deception to

---

[xli] Deuteronomy 18:9-14

steal, kill, and destroy.[xlii] No one wants someone with those intentions involved in his health care.

Knowing this, Satan continually morphs in his approach to deception and destruction. He must be subtle in his tactics, appearing as an angel of light, not as the hideously evil being that he is. Therefore, highlighting a few of his methods of divination throughout time can be helpful in recognizing the incredible similarities they have to muscle testing. As the saying goes: If it looks like a duck, quacks like a duck, and walks like a duck, it probably is a duck.

Just consider a few of the divination practices through the ages, beginning with Egypt. An ancient Egyptian wall mural was found in the Tassili Caves in north Africa depicting a man holding a forked rod, searching for water. The practice of dowsing or water witching has been used in many cultures throughout time to gain hidden knowledge about the location of water or minerals. (The same practice can also be done with a pendulum.) Not limited to just finding water, dowsing has also been used through the millennia to answer yes/no questions.

In ancient Greece, people sought two groups of people for direction from the gods: oracles and seers. The rare oracle was believed to have direct contact with the gods, but accessibility and cost limited those who could attain an oracle's services. Seers, on the other hand, were abundant, but their guidance lay in an ability to read signs from the gods rather than in receiving direct messages. As a result, only yes and no questions could be asked of a seer. For example, following the offering of a sacrifice, the seer might determine the flow of blood from the liver indicated a "yes" response. Another sacrifice would have to be offered to receive a second yes/no response to another specific question.

Taking a giant leap forward in time to the Victorian era, another method of divination, called table tipping, became all the rage in England, and America soon joined the pastime. People placed their fingertips lightly on a three-legged table and asked questions that primarily had yes or no answers. Prearranged behaviors of the table for *yes, no, don't know*, or *uncertain* were defined at the outset. Some also included the letters of the

---

[xlii] 1 Peter 5:8, John 10:10

alphabet in interpreting the way the table tipped and would ask questions that the table could then spell out the answer by tipping this way and that.

The origins of the Ouija Board

Proceeding from the influence of table tipping, an ingenious American, named William Fuld, created a seemingly harmless game that allowed anyone to easily become a seer. In the book, *The Ouija Board: Doorway to the Occult,* Edmond C. Gruss describes the history of the game that would amass Fuld a million dollars but cost him his life. Fuld first patented the board in 1892. By 1967, the board had taken the place of Monopoly as the number one boardgame in America. The clever name Ouija came simply from the combination of the French and German words for *yes* (*oui* and *ja*), but the idea behind the game was hardly clever. There is, after all, ***nothing new under the sun***[xliii] but only Satan's repackaging of old evils.

Fuld's rectangular board lists the numbers zero to nine and the letters of the alphabet, along with the words *good-bye* at the bottom and *yes* and *no* in the opposite, upper corners of the board. The heart-shaped message indicator (called the planchet) is a mini three-legged table on which two operators lightly place their fingers so that it can easily glide across the board pointing to or spelling out answers to the questions people ask. The instructions included with the board state that the operators should do so with concentration and seriousness.

Hardly an eccentric spiritualist, the inventor of the Ouija Board was quite ordinary. As a child, William Fuld admitted that his brother Isaac and he used to tinker with what they called a *spirit board*, so as an inventive adult, it was only natural that he perfected the idea. Although Fuld admitted to consulting the board himself for direction, he also insisted that he was not a spiritualist but a Presbyterian.[38] Satan cared little about the religious label Fuld claimed but only that he was deceived and deceiving others.

[xliii] Ecclesiastes 1:9

Fuld asserted that the board named itself by spelling out its chosen name *Ouija*. He also said that it instructed him to leave his long-time job as a customs inspector and invest heavily in a particular building to produce the game himself. After the Ouija Board had become hugely popular and made Fuld a wealthy man, he ironically died in February of 1927 after a freak accident falling from the roof of the board's factory—the very building the board instructed him to build. Fuld's final words to his children indicated he believed sinister causes created his "accident. He reportedly made his children promise never again to sell the Ouija Board.[39] Clearly, Satan's use for Fuld had come to an end, but despite his attempt to sway his children from continuing to profit from the board, the legacy of deception lives on to the present.

The harmless looking "game" became popular for party fun, as well as for more serious séances. Sales increased significantly during World War 1 with the intriguing and much written about story of Missouri housewife, Mrs. Pearl Lenore Curran. After only casual use of the board, a spirit claiming the name of Patience Worth reportedly began using Mrs. Curran to write copious amounts of history about a woman never verified to exist. Many of the writings were published and sold well, generating much publicity for the Ouija Board at a time when family members longed for contact with husbands and sons who died in the War.

Much later, the board became known as the gateway to the occult in the famous movie, *The Exorcist*, which was based on the well-documented case of the demon possession of fourteen-year-old Douglas Deen.[40] A few of the boy's torments included frequent and unexplainable brandings, violent vomiting, sleep disturbed by unexplained movement of furniture and bedding, and foul language and blasphemies spoken in a voice not his own.[41] When compared with the story of Mrs. Curran, the extreme torment of the boy highlights the vast differences in results and consequences from occult involvement.

Since the time of its creation, the board's sales have waxed and waned, frequently based on times of national stress.[42] After the stock market crash and during World War II, the board's sales sky-rocketed. Fuld, when questioned about its remarkable success, the *Baltimore Sun* reported Fuld saying, *All I know is they (the boards) must work some time, or we wouldn't be selling so many. For the last 18 months the sales have been as large as during the best years of the 20's.*[43]

Although many tried the Ouija Board out of idle curiosity, the desire of people for special knowledge or for contact with the dead has drawn large numbers to it through the decades. Countless newspapers have reported on the strange stories of people's involvement with the board, telling personal testimonies of the progressive nature of involvement leading to obsession, oppression, possession, and a wide variety of other troubles.

I will never forget my own introduction to this "board game" in Mrs. Wortman's fifth grade classroom. As a Christian child raised in the church, the concerns about and the pronunciation of that board (wee-jee) were familiar to me, but the spelling (Ouija) and appearance were not. So, when I encountered the game in the classroom game closet, along with my fellow classmates, I innocently began to explore the simple board with a message pointer. Nothing dramatic happened. In fact, if it were not for the widespread, bizarre, and frightening stories of many who claim otherwise, I could comfortably conclude that the Ouija Board is nothing but a harmless game, rather than a gateway to the occult.

It is worth mentioning, however, that even as a naive ten-year-old, I had a strong sense that something was not right about the "game." In fact, the sense was so strong that I felt compelled to ask my parents about it. They wisely asked my teacher to remove it from the classroom closet. A similar sense pervaded me, when as an adult, I began my journey into the world of Applied Kinesiology. Of the hundreds who have personally contacted me about muscle testing, the vast majority describe feeling the same lack of peace from the moment they first encountered it. This unease causes great concern that leads devout Christians to feel the need to pray for confirmation from the Holy Spirit that the practice is safe. The absence of peace is the answer! By His silence, the God of peace is letting His children know that He does not approve.

The use of divination in medicine

Before describing the similarities between muscle testing and the Ouija Board, I wish to demonstrate the danger of applying any method of divination medically in order to receive a yes/no answer by which to guide healthcare. Dr. Kurt Koch, a noted 20th century German author, theologian, and minister who counseled people worldwide suffering from their involvement with the occult, relates an encounter with a doctor in his book, *Demonology Past and Present*. A medical doctor came to Dr. Koch for consultation. The doctor had progressively developed disturbing problems after repeatedly using, with surprising effectiveness, a variation of the Ouija Board involving a disc and pendulum to diagnose and treat his patients. This doctor "applied" the idea of the Ouija Board to medicine, harnessing Satan's power, as many witchdoctors through the ages have done. After a time, the doctor recognized the seriousness of his error. He confessed to Dr. Koch that since employing the pendulum, he *had developed a violent temper, become addicted to both tobacco and alcohol, started suffering from depressions, and begun to fear that he was going mad.*[44] Never forget, the devil does have power and is willing to apply it with effectiveness when it suits his purposes.

Although most Christians know better than to consider using overtly Satanic practices, those who deal with chronic health issues are often susceptible to questionable practices if they seem to lead to results. Similar to the Ouija Board sales, which increased during times of national stress, so also the undiagnosed and sick are especially vulnerable to the temptation toward special knowledge.

How do they work?

Through the years of the Ouija Board's popularity, the big question has been, "how does it work?". Parker Brothers, who bought the company and all rights to the Ouija Board in 1966 claims, *How or why it works is a mystery.*[45] Sound familiar? Others have formulated explanations. Some suggest that the muscles of the arms and hands are affected subtly by the subconscious, producing accurate information that has been locked away in the body's own version of a black box. Some practitioners make the same claim for muscle testing; however, the scientific evidence strongly points away from this possibility. Also, similar to AK, skeptics claim both the Ouija Board and table tipping work through the ideomotor effect.

However, many believe in an alternate explanation of how the game works, which is that spiritual entities move the pointer across the board by manipulating the operator. Similarly, in AK the muscles of the arm are affected to produce an answer. If spirits are involved, it begs an explanation of how they influence the individual to give a response. I see two possible ways. One possibility is by demons exerting a purely outward force on the individual, causing the hand or arm to move appropriately. Picture an unseen force pushing the hand or arm. The other approach could be by spirits affecting the muscles of the individual through the nervous system. This explanation does not necessarily require demonic possession but manipulation of electrical impulses (neurons).

We know from the Bible that spirits can increase or decrease the muscular strength of an individual, although the biblical examples were in cases of possession. We also know, biblically, that spirits can affect the human body of those who are not possessed. After completing a study on every example in the Scriptures where unclean spirits are specifically stated as the cause of a physical condition, I made an interesting observation: All but one of the conditions are neurological in nature. Take a look for yourself:

- Mental illness: 1 Samuel 11 & 18, Daniel 4:33-34
- Dizziness: Isaiah 19:3-4 & 14
- Seizures: Matthew 17:15-18
- Blind and Mute: Matthew 9:32-33 & 12:22
- Crippled: Luke 13:10-16
- Extreme strength: Mark 5:1-15
- Weakness: Psalm 39:3-10, Matthew 17:15
- Painful sores: Job 2:7

After coming out of energy medicine, my husband and I spent many hours pondering how unclean spirits can affect believers or those who are not demon possessed. Although knowing how they work is not necessary for recognizing demonic activity, it is helpful to the inquisitive mind. Based on the Bible, it appears that they do so in large part neurologically.

Obviously, since I exist in the physical world without line-of-sight to the realm which demons inhabit, the following explanation is just a theory, but it seems to fit the phenomena I personally experienced during my era of muscle testing.

A possible explanation

Characteristic of most forms of divination, the muscle testing "answers" to questions asked of the "body" are revealed in a binary format, meaning that for every question asked, the muscle will give a yes or no (true or false) response. The muscle gives these binary answers by either being strong or weak in response to the question asked of it. When the muscle weakens during testing, there is no odd sensation warning the person that his/her muscle has weakened. Nor is there any sort of sense that someone in addition to the tester is exerting force on the arm. There is only the sense that although the brain is sending signals to apply strength, those signals do not seem to reach the muscle in full force, and therefore the muscle does not respond as it should to the will of the tested subject. It is as if something has suppressed the passage of electrical signals between brain and muscle.

While contemplating these things, I came across a neuroscientist, Greg Gage, who did a fascinating demonstration in a TED talk. Using neuroscience, Gage enabled one individual to hijack control of another's hand. While attaching electrodes and wires to the forearm and hand of a young woman who volunteered for the demonstration, Gage explained what normally occurs in the human body each time a decision is made to move the hand.

> *You have about 80 billion neurons inside your brain right now. They're sending electrical messages back and forth, and chemical messages. But some of your neurons right here in your motor cortex are going to send messages down when you move your arm like this. They're going to go down across your corpus callosum, down onto your spinal cord to your lower motor neuron out to your muscles here*

(inner forearm) *and that electrical discharge is going to be picked up by these electrodes right here* (hand).[46]

For all to see and hear, every time the woman who volunteered clenched her hand, an attached device audibly and pictorially recorded the neurons firing. Gage then requested a second volunteer, and a young man joined the demonstration. This time Gage attached a second set of wires from the woman's hand to electrodes on the young man's forearm. Unlike the woman, nothing was placed on the man's hand. Gage explained that the ulnar nerve runs close enough to the surface of the forearm that it can be stimulated by an outward force. He connected the wires to allow the nerve signals from the woman to be sent to the man's electrode on the ulnar nerve. That, in turn, sent messages to the motor neurons of three of his fingers to contract when the woman contracted hers. As a result, the young man's hand was controlled by the woman, according to the movement of her hand.

Gage explained, *So in a sense, she will take away your free will and you will no longer have any control over this hand. It's going to feel a little bit weird at first; You know, when you lose your free will, and someone else becomes your agent, it does feel a bit strange.*[47] The audience responded with laughter as they witnessed the young man's surprise at the repeated movement of his fingers against his will.

A person, sitting at a Ouija Board with fingertips lightly touching the pointer does not detect the subtle variations in electrical signals traveling to the muscles that maintain the arms' position over the board. That person only knows or senses that without him/her willing it to do so, the marker begins to move, giving responses to questions. Muscle testing works in similar fashion. Perhaps, both are explained through unclean spirits hijacking neural control to the muscles in similar fashion to the facts demonstrated by the TED talk.

Conclusion

Through muscle testing, Satan uses the human body as a living Ouija Board. As the board seems to "work" for some and not for others and as its responses are sometimes disturbingly accurate, so it is with muscle testing. Also, like with the Ouija Board, some have been involved with muscle testing and walked away, seemingly unscathed, while others become embroiled with a host of inescapable problems. By reading the personal testimonies in the third section of this book, one glimpses the huge spectrum of progressive troubles many people experience from involvement with energy medicine. Why is such disparity characteristic of occult involvement? The answer lies in the reality that personalities, whether people or spirits, act with motive. The Bible tells us that Satan's motive is destruction. The devil desires to move individuals like pieces on a chess board to achieve his end goal. Some players are largely ignored, others are quickly disposed of, while others hold much bigger roles in Satan's greater schemes.

The laws of science, however, have no motive. They just are. God-given, natural revelation remains consistent, repeatable, and verifiable because it is based on *the fixed order of heaven and earth* and not capricious entities. Though science is limited, it may be relied upon for many useful things, including distinguishing between the physical and spiritual realms.

The use of divination attempts to gain knowledge otherwise unknowable through science. We know from Scripture that the insight from divination will not be reliable with 100% accuracy because, unlike God, Satan is not omniscient. God told His people in Deuteronomy 18:22 how to recognize a false prophet. As false prophets are also a means for divination, the following principle can be applied to muscle testing. The verse says, *When a prophet speaks in the name of the Lord, if the word does not come to pass or come true, that is a word that the Lord has not spoken; the prophet has spoken it presumptuously. You need not be afraid of him.* God's litmus test for revelatory knowledge is nothing short of complete accuracy! When muscle testing fails to match other scientifically verifiable methods of testing, it fails this test and reveals its true nature.

As established in Chapter 4, science proves that traditional test results do not match up with muscle testing results. It is no more reliable than random guessing. Therefore, when AK claims to reveal accurate knowledge about the body by the body, it is actually promising to reveal secret knowledge or divination. Sometimes the information revealed through divination proves astonishingly accurate. Deuteronomy 13:1-4 addresses this as well:

> *"If a prophet or a dreamer of dreams arises among you and gives you a sign or a wonder, and the sign or wonder that he tells you comes to pass, and if he says, 'Let us go after other gods,' which you have not known, 'and let us serve them,' you shall not listen to the words of that prophet or that dreamer of dreams. <u>For the Lord your God is testing you, to know whether you love the Lord your God with all your heart and with all your soul.</u> You shall walk after the Lord your God and fear him and keep his commandments and obey his voice, and you shall serve him and hold fast to him.*

Whether it be through false prophets, tarot cards, tea leaves, chicken bones, the stars, water witching, palm reading, a pendulum, messages from the dead, a Ouija board, an arm's strength, or you name it, demons gladly adapt to whatever means people contrive to seek hidden knowledge. God has made it clear that such things are detestable to Him and a test to determine if you truly love and fear God.

1 Timothy 4:1 warns believers by saying, *The Spirit clearly says that in later times some will abandon the faith and follow deceiving spirits and things taught by demons.* The angel of light, the deceiver Lucifer, has motive to use the repackaged tool of divination to mislead people, yes, even the elect. If you have participated in this form of divination and, perhaps also, witchcraft, I urge you to repent today and find freedom and forgiveness from God.

CHAPTER 7

A Biblical View of Energy Medicine

For this I toil, struggling with all his energy that he powerfully works within me. Colossians 1:29

Energy medicine continues to grow in popularity as people develop more and more dissatisfaction with conventional medicine. Even more widespread, though, is an increased acceptance of the concept of energy that undergirds energy medicine. Because Christians involved in these practices attempt to sanitize the spiritual sounding jargon inherent in energy, we should familiarize ourselves with what energy medicine claims and its terminology.

It must be noted that outside of Christendom, participants in energy medicine make no attempt to disguise, hide, or diminish the spiritual nature of this field or its clear origins. Consider this description found on the website for Energy Medicine University.

Energy Medicine includes all concepts of energy: light, sound, electro-magnetism, body, mind, and spirit. In addition to concepts central to electro-chemical physiology, older traditions of "life force" or "élan vital" are commonly found in the discourses of energy medicine. From Taoist alchemy and Chinese Medicine comes the principle of Chi, with its Cosmic and Microcosmic cycles and flows through the channels or meridians in the physical body. From Yogic Hinduism comes the breath or Prana, and the principles of multiple energy vortices in the body – the Chakras, and especially the concepts of multiple bodies beyond the flesh and blood physiological body, conceived in various systems as layers such as the etheric body, the astral body, the emotional body, the mental body, and the spirit bodies.[48]

Hopefully, alarm bells tolled loudly when you read this brief summary of the unadulterated origins of energy medicine. As the quote details, many ancient religions spoke of energy by various names. This spiritual concept of energy predated the coining of the word *enérgeia* by the Greek philosopher, Aristotle. Although no English equivalent to *enérgeia* exists, a loose translation means *to be at work.* I will show you later in this chapter that the New Testament writers used the term *enérgeia* to refer to spiritual power at work.

By the 17th century, "energy" began to represent power, although the word itself remained unfamiliar. In 1800, Thomas Young introduced this word into the field of physics, but it was not until 1905 that Einstein's theory of relativity began to popularize the concept of energy. Since then, "energy" has evolved to a much more general meaning referring to zest for life. Interestingly, it would seem that the founders of energy medicine appropriately chose the name based on the earliest, spiritual meaning of the term.

According to an article published in the *International Journal of Yoga*, it was not until the late 1980's that the name, "Energy Medicine," was coined by three researchers who gathered in Boulder, Colorado. The founding definition these men authored was, *any energetic or informational interaction with a biological system to bring back homeostasis in the organism.*[49]

This concise definition has some noteworthy aspects. First, notice what is not mentioned. Although it is a definition for what many consider a medical approach to health, no mention of anatomy or physiology is made other than to point out that this approach applies to living (biological) systems. Instead of anatomy, it speaks of energetic or informational interactions. These *interactions* are not neurons firing and passing information or biochemical reactions but something nebulous. So, if the interactions are not physical, what are they? Good question! That would be one reason why explaining these practices scientifically is difficult at best.

Homeostasis & blocks

Notice the key term in the definition—*homeostasis*. The lay term most commonly used is balance. Herein lies the goal of energy medicine. They teach that when this nebulous thing they call energy is out of balance in a living organism, health suffers. A lack of homeostasis or balance is said to occur from things that block the flow of energy—stress, emotional trauma, toxicity, EMF's, lack of appropriate nutrition or exercise, bad air, people you encounter who have negative energy, your own negative thoughts, certain colors, and just about anything.

This shapeless thing called energy is supposedly in and all around you. Chinese medicine calls this universal energy, *chi*. Although energy medicine addresses physical conditions and often uses physical means, everything is done with the foundational goal in mind of restoring balance to this thing called energy.

Marci Baron and Roxanna Namavar, D.O offer another commonly heard explanation in their article, *What Everyone Should Know About Energy Healing*. They state, *Energy healing is a holistic practice that activates the body's subtle energy systems to remove blocks. By breaking through these energetic blocks, the body's inherent ability to heal itself is stimulated.*[50] (The teaching that the body will heal itself if you just give it what it needs forms a belief that I will address in a later chapter.)

To better explain the practice of removing energy blocks, contemplate a theoretical example that illustrates the difference between the approach used in traditional medicine, whose foundation is mechanical and biochemical interactions, with that of energy medicine whose foundation is energetic and informational interactions. Consider the disease of hypothyroidism. A conventional doctor might recommend thyroid medication to artificially produce a biochemical reaction that meets the physical need for thyroxine. This in turn, should create a biological cascade that hopefully brings a balanced hormonal state in the individual.

An energy medicine practitioner, on the other hand, will assume that the failing thyroid is an indicator that something is blocking the flow of energy. Therefore, energy pathways, known as meridians, will be tested using one or more of a wide variety of energetic practices such as muscle testing or a machine version of muscle testing, intuition, and/or therapeutic touch to ascertain what pathway(s) are blocked. Based on information thus obtained, the focus for treatment will then be determined.

For example, treatment may include emotional therapies using energy practices (NOT psychology or counseling) or perhaps nutritional supplementation, herbs, essential oils, homeopathics, crystals and talismans. Those substances or objects are believed useful in energy medicine for removing blocks because they supposedly have vibrational frequencies. Practitioners may also add supposed frequencies to those substances to make them align better with an individual's particular energy.

Other practices include changing false beliefs, aligning the body, cleansing the individual's environment, detoxification, etc., but every step of the treatment will likely rely on the energetic practice of muscle testing in some form or another. Regardless of the chosen treatment, the purpose behind its use is not for a cellular change but a homeostatic state of energy, which they suppose brings health.

The 6 pillars

A unique couple in the field of energy medicine are thought by many to be definitive experts in that field. The husband, David Feinstein, Ph.D., has a long list of impressive credentials, including teaching at both Johns Hopkins University School of Medicine and Antioch College. As a clinical psychologist and the national director of the Energy Medicine Institute, he has authored seven books and more than fifty professional papers.

His wife, Donna Eden, is a pioneer in the field of holistic healing and among the world's most sought-after spokespersons for energy medicine. According to their website, her abilities as a healer are legendary, and she has taught some fifty thousand people, world-wide, how to understand the body as an energy system. She claims that since childhood she has been able to see the flow of the body's energies. From that clairvoyant ability, she developed a system for teaching those lacking this *gift* to productively work with their body's energies. Her best-selling book, *Energy Medicine*, has been translated into 10 languages, and is a classic in its field.

Feinstein wrote the meticulously documented article, *Six Pillars of Energy Medicine, Clinical Strengths of a Complementary Paradigm*, to explain the beliefs behind this system of thought regarding health. His clinical background is evident in the 6 pillars article as he cites 96 sources, many of which are scientific studies. His intent is clear. He desires to explain what energy medicine is and the evidence for it.

Unlike his wife who focuses much on the spiritual aspects of energy, Feinstein attempts to divert attention from the spiritual foundations and make it sound scientifically plausible by replacing spiritual sounding terms with more neutral ones. By the way, renaming spiritual jargon with neutral or scientific terminology does not change what energy medicine is. As Shakespeare said, *A rose by any other name would smell as sweet*[51]. Unfortunately, renaming is exactly what many practitioners who profess Christianity do and think that doing so eliminates the spiritual danger it brings to the soul.

In order to better understand this system of health, let us consider the three foundational terms Dr. Feinstein identifies: auras (he calls biofields), chakras (local fields), and meridians (energy pathways).[52]

The biofield

The biofield, which most call auras, is said to be an energy field surrounding the body. One must not overlook the fact that a belief in auras is an integral part of the occult, particularly among New Age teachings or witchcraft. Although Donna Eden claims to see auras, her husband attempts to cite scientific measurements of electrical fields around living things to prove their existence. In the 6 Pillars article, a noticeable tension exists as Feinstein goes to great lengths in an attempt to explain energy scientifically but, in the end, repeatedly acknowledges his failure to do so.

His approach is likely familiar to many of my readers—the claim that energy is synonymous with the body's electrical and electromagnetic properties.

No one disputes that living things exhibit electrical properties. What is disputed is whether electricity is synonymous with their concept of energy. Feinstein admits and explains the conundrum in this way,

> *Some of the energies they describe cannot be detected by existing instrumentation. It is also a source of debate whether this is because such energies, assuming they exist, fall along the electromagnetic spectrum but operate in such minute quantities that they do not reach the necessary thresholds for mechanical detection or whether they are of a fundamentally different nature than electromagnetic energy.*[53]

After more attempts in the 6 Pillars article to explain energy electrically, Feinstein offers an honest conclusion:

> *Many of the ancient traditions being revisited via energy medicine were spiritual disciplines as well as healing modalities, and some practitioners speculate that **the energies they invoke are a bridge into the world of spirit.*** (emphasis mine)

Local fields

The second key term in understanding energy medicine is chakras. (Belief in chakras is Hindu in origin.) Again, Feinstein chooses a less spiritual sounding term, *local fields*. Whereas biofields (auras) are said to surround the entire body, chakras, believed to be concentrated, local energy fields found within particular areas of the body. Auras are big (whole body)—chakras are small (part of the body). Hindus believe chakras to be vortexes of biophysical energy, and these are core to the practice of yoga (even if it has been "Christianized") and addressed in a variety of healing systems.

The 6 Pillars article cites studies done at UCLA's Energy Fields Laboratory in the 1970's by Valerie Hunt as possible scientific evidence for chakras. Those studies demonstrated that specific regions of the skin produced very rapid electrical oscillations (up to 1600 cycles per second, as contrasted with 0 to 100 cycles per second in the brain, 225 in the muscles, and 250 in the heart),[54] and that these local energy domains corresponded with Hindu descriptions of the body's chakras.

In spite of Feinstein's desire to defend energy medicine with scientific evidence, he always concludes the discussion with a return to the spiritual. He writes, *Spiritual functions attributed to the chakras are based in the way they are believed to be attuned to metaphysical constructs such as "ancestral memories," "past lives," and "archetypes."*[55] One cannot divorce the spiritual from these constructs.

Meridians

The 3rd foundational term, "meridians," further delves into the spiritual roots smorgasbord of energy medicine. Feinstein writes,

> *A third overarching energy system that seems to regulate the flow of specific energies within the body corresponds with the "energy pathways" referred to as meridians in traditional Chinese medicine and also described in a variety of other healing traditions.*[56]

Dr. Feinstein ends his discussion of meridians by once again drawing conclusions that should not be ignored. First, he admits there is disagreement about the origin of meridians. He suggests that they could be incredibly weak electromagnetic fields, which he states would explain why they **cannot be directly measured**. He does go into detail on the limited studies that he believes show, indirectly, of the presence of meridians but admits that none of those studies directly quantify the existence of meridians.

Secondly, he concludes that meridians *do not correspond with known structures in the circulatory, lymphatic, or nervous systems, nor are the meridians and acupuncture points even stable in their shape, size, or* *location on the skin.*[57] So, not only are meridians supposedly too weak to be clearly measured, but **they constantly shift in location, shape, and size!** Shockingly, he then goes on to admit to something quite telling: *This, however, is exactly what would be expected if the meridian system operates as a field that is somewhat **independent of the physical body it acts upon.**[58] (emphasis mine)

Even though some try to suggest that energy is just another word for the electric nature of things, science well documents the electric nature of living beings. Energy meridians, on the other hand, shift and change, ignoring *the fixed laws of heaven and earth.* This begs an answer to the question, what then is energy?

Like lights in a house

If you research energy medicine online or communicate with people involved in some form of it, you will hear all manner of explanations for what it is and how it works. Let me say upfront that I know from personal experience and also the experiences of others that it is sometimes efficacious and that there may even be some supporting science. Dr. Feinstein meticulously cites the supporting research, and yet he even honestly concludes that energy is far more than explainable, measurable science. So, what are we to think?

My husband, Seth, suggested an analogy worth considering with regard to the mystery of how energy medicine "works." Suppose you are standing outside a house at nighttime, and all of the blinds are closed so that you cannot see any movement inside. Suddenly, you observe a light turn on in a room. Later, that light turns off, but another takes its place elsewhere in the house. You have "evidence" that something is going on in the house, but you have no idea of the motive governing why the lights turn on or off or who is turning the lights on or off. From your outside perspective, you can only determine someone has a reason to manipulate the lights. Imagine that the human body is like the house, and evidence for energy medicine is like the lights turning on and off.

One would be ridiculous to look at the house and say there is no power. The lights coming and going in the house indicate there is real power, but that does not mean that the intelligence behind the power is benevolent. There could be a serial killer in the house! Dr. Feinstein, who is trained in clinical science and medicine, yet has a wife who sees what she believes to be auras, concludes that science and spirituality both impact the health of an individual. He wrongly assumes, however, that the power he recognizes is benevolent.

Energy is spiritual power.

We may say things like, "I have no energy today," and intend to refer only to the degree of zest for life and work that we possess at the time. This modern, colloquial use of the word predisposes people to believe energy medicine is acceptable, harmless, and perfectly scientific. However, it is anything but that!

When looking at the original Greek root *enérgeia*, which was used by the writers of the New Testament, we discover that no true English equivalent exists. As a result, Bible translators often use the word *work* in place of energy because that more accurately conveys the Greek meaning. The noun form of *enérgeia* occurs eight times in the NT – and, except for one time, it always refers to God's energy. It means, *power in action, divine energy, working, action, productive work.*[xliv] It typically refers to God's energy which transitions the believer from point to point in His plan (accomplishing His progressive work).

The verb form of the same word, *energeó,* is used 21 times and means *to be at work, to do again.*[xlv] Biblical writers ALWAYS used both noun and verb forms of the word to refer to spiritual power—good or bad working in us. Neither form of energy is used biblically to refer to human power. Instead, they are used only to speak of supernatural power to accomplish work in or through humans.

See for yourself from a few of the passages where it is used. (The underlined word is *enérgeia or energeó.)*

[xliv] Strongs #1753
[xlv] Strongs #1754

- *God <u>works</u> in us to will and to do for his good pleasure.* Philippians 2:13
- *What is the immeasurable greatness of his power toward us who believe, according to the <u>working</u> of his great might that he <u>worked</u> in Christ when he raised him from the dead and seated him at his right hand in the heavenly places.* Ephesians 1:19-20
- *Of this gospel I was made a minister according to the gift of God's grace, which was given me by the <u>working</u> of his power.* Ephesians 3:7
- Ephesians 4:16 speaks of God's energy showing itself in empowering each individual in the body of Christ to do His work through the church.
- *For this I toil, struggling with all his <u>energy</u> that he powerfully <u>works</u> within me.* Colossians 1:29
- *Having been buried with him in baptism, in which you were also raised with him through faith in the <u>powerful working</u> of God, who raised him from the dead.* Colossians 2:12

Satan's energy in the last days

Biblically speaking, energy is spiritual power; period, and that power energizes a human to effective work for God. One passage, however, speaks both of God's work (energy) AND Satan's work (energy). It is scary and yet very enlightening. The passage is 2 Thessalonians 2:3-11. It foretells of deception in the last days that will be according to *how Satan works*. Verse 3 begins by warning of the coming antichrist. ***Don't let anyone deceive you in any way, for that day will not come until the rebellion occurs and the man of lawlessness is revealed, the man doomed to destruction.***

This passage is a "heads up"—a warning of deception to come. The final day of judgment is coming but not until after the arrival of *the lawless one,* also known as the antichrist. Verses 4 through 7 go on to describe what he will do.

He will oppose and will exalt himself over everything that is called God or is worshiped, so that he sets himself up in God's temple, proclaiming himself to be God. Don't you remember that when I was with you, I used to tell you these things? And now you know what is holding him back, so that he may be revealed at the proper time. For the secret power of lawlessness is already at <u>work</u>; but the one who now holds it back will continue to do so till he is taken out of the way.

For the first time, *enérgeia* —the noun form of energy, is used to refer to Satan's spiritual power to work. Verse 7 says that the secret power of lawlessness is already at work but that the Holy Spirit is holding Satan back so that all will occur at the proper time. Now, as you read Verses 8-10, keep in mind, Verse 7 already said that the power of lawlessness is at work in these last days.

And then the lawless one will be revealed, whom the Lord Jesus will overthrow with the breath of his mouth and destroy by the splendor of his coming. The coming of the lawless one will be in accordance with how Satan <u>works</u>. He will use all sorts of displays of power through signs and wonders that serve the lie and all the ways that wickedness deceives those who are perishing. They perish because they refused to love the truth and so be saved.

The second use of *enérgeia* is in reference to Satan's power (energy) to work for his purposes. What is the way Satan works? *All sorts of displays of power through signs and wonders that serve the lie*. Satan counterfeits signs and wonders.

In the area of health, he cannot bring true healing, but he can provide a convincing counterfeit to deceive. How? Through demonic torment, he can mimic the illnesses and symptoms of true physical conditions. For example, I frequently hear of people involved in energy medicine who have developed symptoms of Lyme disease that are completely debilitating, and yet, no traditional test confirms that they have the condition.[xlvi] What if in these cases demonic torment, rather than a bacterial infection, imitates the symptoms of Lyme? If Satan wishes to "cure" their condition, all he need do is remove the thorn of demonic oppression in coordination with the health practices he controls. This creates a powerful illusion by which many are being led astray. I am convinced this happens constantly in the alternative realm of health.

Take notice of the reference to perishing in the last verse. ***They perish because they refused to love the truth and so be saved.*** One might assume that the use of *perish* here only refers to a man's eternal state, but this is likely a wrong assumption. Often, the Biblical references to life and death are two-fold—including both the here and now, as well as the eternal. This passage's reference to perishing does the same. Why do ***they perish***? Because they ***refuse to love the truth and so be saved***.

If we read on, we see the noun form of *energy* used one last time, but this time it speaks of God's energy. ***For this reason, God sends them a <u>powerful</u> delusion so that they will believe the lie and so that all will be condemned (judged) who have not believed the truth but have delighted in wickedness.***

In God's sovereignty, His energy is ultimately the power behind allowing Satan's energy to work in people in the last days. Why would God do that? God intends to provide a test that will separate the wheat from the tares before the final judgment. Satan's energy provides the means to reveal who, by love of the truth, will not be deceived by a lie.

Concluding thoughts

Energy is far more than the electromagnetic properties of living things. It is and always has been spiritual power at work in humans to accomplish something. In these last days, God has allowed Satan to use his energy to accomplish deceptive work in people that the hearts of mankind might be revealed. This is a test! Will you trade the truth of God

---

[xlvi] I am familiar with the purported failings of traditional Lyme testing and the reasoning behind the methods of testing encouraged by energy practitioners. However, reason exists to question the motive behind the propaganda such individuals propagate questioning traditional testing.

for a lie? You may think that energy medicine is your salvation, but God will judge those who choose a lie over the truth.

God's Word, which is the truth that we must hold to, teaches us the path of life! You may think that God is asking you to give up the lie and will then leave you with no hope of ever getting better. Remember, however, Satan can only produce counterfeit healings to deceive. God's truth brings complete healing!

The question becomes: Do you know the truth? Hosea 4:6 says, *My people perish for lack of knowledge* (NIV). Few in the church teach what the Bible says about health and life, and so parishioners are easily led astray by the counterfeit. I wrote the book, *Life to the Body—Biblical Principles for Health & Healing,* out of a passion to share with others the incredible knowledge in God's Word that healed me of 13 diagnosed conditions. In it, I teach everything the Bible has to say about health—and no, it is not a book about diet and exercise, although it does have one chapter on nutrition. The Bible teaches that the *path of life*[xlvii] is one where the heart is at peace with God, others, and oneself. As Proverbs 14:30 says, *A heart at peace gives life to the body* (NIV)*,* and as Proverbs 4:23 says, *the heart is the wellspring of life* (NIV). The Bible has so much to say about health and life, and yet many choose instead to chase after a lie.

Can it be any coincidence that the Bible warns of Satan's *energy* in the last days, and the rise of *energy* medicine? In conclusion, consider the apostle Paul's words in Ephesians 2:1-2. *And you were dead in the trespasses and sins in which you once walked, following the course of this world, following the prince of the power of the air, the spirit that is now at work in the sons of disobedience.* Surely it is not a coincidence that Scripture calls Satan the prince of the power of the air, and energy is believed to be some nebulous substance in us and all around us? Let us turn from our sin and no longer be counted with the sons of disobedience.

[xlvii] Proverbs 3

CHAPTER 8

Quantum Physics Strikes Again^{xlviii}

For my thoughts are not your thoughts, neither are your ways my ways, declares the Lord. For as the heavens are higher than the earth, so are my ways higher than your ways and my thoughts than your thoughts. Isaiah 55:8-9

As common as bullfrogs bellowing after a summer rain, is the statement I hear from those hoping to justify muscle testing: "But, I was told that quantum physics explains it!" Interestingly, in all such discussions, not once have I encountered anyone who had an inkling of what quantum physics is, let alone how it might provide an intelligible explanation for energy-based practices. A respected blog author who advocates for healthcare consumer protection, Harriet Hall, MD, writes about the propensity for people to misapply quantum science as an explanation for all manner of ideas and practices:

Pseudoscience and new age philosophies frequently invoke quantum theory out of context...If there is a God of Quantum Physics, he ought to smite those who take his name in vain...But quantum theory says strange things can happen, so it provides a convenient excuse for believing ideas that don't make sense to science.[59]

xlviii This entire chapter was edited for accuracy by Dr. Steven Golmer, who holds a PhD in atmospheric physics and is a professor at Cedarville University.

Thankfully, the God who created quantum physics demonstrates much grace towards people who speak with limited knowledge, but *what shall we say then? Shall we continue in sin that grace may abound. God forbid!*[xlix] Ignorance does not excuse one from culpability, so we must uncover the truth and walk in it.

As you will read in this chapter, quantum theory does say *strange things can happen,* but differentiating between the proven science (or even good theory) and conjecture requires careful research. Certainly, popular theories of multiple realities or time travel make for intriguing entertainment, but they are science fiction and should not be confused with good science. When people hear something multiple times, they often mistakenly conclude it must be true. Similarly, most energy proponents, some with intent to deceive but others merely in ignorance, put forth quantum theory as an explanation for their practices. Making little to no attempt to explain or validate their claims, they simply assume that using the now popular word "quantum" will end all arguments.

Consider the following examples. The speaker in one YouTube video I watched emphatically stated, *Energy healing removes quantum charges or energy blockages.*[60] Similarly, one energy-based clinic coined a new name for muscle testing—*quantum reflex analysis*, which sounds simply brilliant and masterfully deflects criticism that otherwise might have been directed towards AK. Consider the following claims made on their website: (The parenthetical comments within the quote are mine and intended to demonstrate appropriate skepticism when reading such claims.):

QRA (Quantum Reflex Analysis), is a simple, safe, yet profound way of allowing the body to tell us what it needs to heal. (Really? How does it do this, I wonder.)

It is the union of science-based kinesiological testing, (What science would that be? Are there sources of these supposed tests listed in the

---

footnotes?) *time-proven ancient therapies,* (Which ancient therapies and proven how? Show me the research.) *systematic analysis of the body's quantum biofield,* (There is no such thing.) *and outstanding nutrition and detoxification breakthroughs of the 21st century... QRA is based on empirical observations in quantum energy* (That certainly sounds impressive, but it is ludicrous! As you will learn in this chapter, a significant problem with quantum mechanics is that the act of observation changes the outcome. So, whatever is going on in QRA, it cannot be from empirically observing quantum energy.) *and the emerging field of quantum physics.[61]* (Merely alluding to science should not be sufficient to satisfy consumers.)

In my research and contemplations for writing this book, I knew that I would have to address the false belief that quantum mechanics explains energy practices but lacking a doctorate in physics meant that I would have to rely heavily on those who do. Another hurdle to overcome in presenting this subject matter includes the realization that the quantum world mystifies brilliant PhDs, to say nothing of your average individual. The summary statement for an article on quantum physics written in the online academic journal, *The Conversation,* reiterates this point by concluding with, *As Richard Feynman, Nobel Laureate and truly brilliant man said: "I think I can safely say that nobody understands quantum mechanics."[62]*

Yet, another difficulty involves the fact that respected physicists do not even acknowledge the claims energy-based practitioners make about quantum mechanics because a basic understanding of the topic reveals the absurdity of such claims. Nonetheless, because quantum physics has become the go-to explanation for muscle testing, remote muscle testing, numerous frequency machines, and energy medicine in general, I will endeavor to accurately provide a fundamental understanding of quantum theory. Hopefully, with these facts in hand, you may settle the matter in your own mind.

Quantum theory's beginnings

An awareness of quantum physics first arose in the late 1800s to early 1900s in response to experimentation with atoms, which appeared to defy the classical understanding of the properties of subatomic particles like photons and electrons. History credits the German physicist, Max Planck, with the birth of quantum theory. In 1890, the German Bureau of Standards asked Planck to make a more efficient lightbulb. To do so, he needed to have a light filament that primarily gave off visible light waves. This required that he isolate the different types of light waves, like ultraviolet, visible, and infrared. However, while basing his predictions on calculations from the accepted understanding of electromagnetic light, Planck repeatedly discovered his experimentation did not match the math. In frustration, he finally chose to disregard the accepted theory of electromagnetics and instead see what the experimental data revealed. In so doing, Planck discovered a new law of physics. Light waves produce energy in packets (quanta), with high frequency light producing large packets of energy and low frequency light producing small packets.

Among the basic discoveries was the realization that matter, and energy can be thought of as discrete packets, or quanta, that have a minimum value associated with them. For example, light of a fixed frequency will deliver energy in quanta called "photons." Each photon at this frequency will have the same amount of energy, and this energy can't be broken down into smaller units. In fact, the word "quantum" has Latin roots and means "how much."[63]

Dr. Don Lincoln, a modern physicist who received his PhD in Experimental Particle Physics from Rice University explains the term, quantum mechanics, in simple terms. Quantum is the smallest unit of something. For example, the quantum of the Sahara Desert, with its seemingly endless sand dunes, is a single grain of sand. He then goes on to explain; *Mechanics is the behavior or motion of something. So, quantum mechanics is the motion and interaction of a collection of individual objects of a bigger collection.[64]*

Einstein later corroborated Planck's theory and expounded on it, furthering the scientific discussion of quantum theory. In 1913 Niels Bohr added to the quantum understanding of the hydrogen atom. Since the early years of quantum physics, much progress has been made in unraveling the bizarre, subatomic world, however, endless mysteries still defy understanding.

Groundwork for understanding

For the sake of clarity, let me eliminate potential confusion about several key terms. Although some technical details differentiate quantum physics, quantum theory, and quantum mechanics, scientists often use these terms interchangeably or simply prefer one over the other because of some personal distinction. Do not be distracted by the various uses of these terms quoted throughout this chapter but consider them synonymous.

Also, keep in mind the scientific meaning of *energy*. Indeed, it was classical physicists who first resurrected the long unused, Greek word *enérgeia* from New Testament times. Physicists adapted the original meaning to refer to an object's potential power or more specifically, the ability to do work or produce heat (thermal energy). Therefore, when you see physics quotes using the word "energy," know this is not referring to the pagan-based belief in subtle energies, life force, chi, prana, etc.

Additionally, know that when physicists refer to frequency, they refer to scientifically proven frequencies measured in hertz (Hz), which are quite different from the unproven claims that everything from universal energy to the organs of your body have specific, measurable frequencies. Energy medicine loves to misapply physics terms. Do not be fooled!

I would be remiss to leave out one final caveat. Classical physics portrays the energy and interactions of matter mathematically. Even more so is the reliance on mathematics in quantum physics due to the reality that the subatomic world can be difficult to visualize, and the mere act of measurement literally alters the outcome. Quantum mechanics is, therefore, a mathematical science of probability—predicting the behavior of the components of atoms. Because it would be tedious and beyond the scope of this book to include these equations, I will not do so. However, understand that without including the math, the explanations provided are not precise but written with illustrations intended to convey basic understanding, which is wholly sufficient for our purposes.

When one begins to study quantum physics, a multitude of imposing terms and concepts threaten to overwhelm. Because the goal of this chapter lies in gaining enough understanding of quantum mechanics to determine if it adequately explains energy-based practices, I will not delve into the specifics of Schrodinger's cat, Planck's constant, quantum tunneling, the uncertainty principle, or many other fascinating aspects of quantum theory. Instead, I will focus on the four fundamental concepts of the quantum world that have bearing on our particular topic, but which are generally bantered about in ignorance: wave particle duality, wave function, superposition, and last but not least, the one that energy medicine gets in a lather about—entanglement. Because it is important to have a basic understanding of the first three to correctly grasp entanglement, please bear with me as I seek to explain these scientific concepts. If you could care less about the scientific explanations and wish to skip to a summary of why energy medicine cannot possibly be explained by quantum physics, you will find what you are looking for in the *conclusions* section of this chapter.

Wave particle duality

Wave particle duality is a physics concept that says that sometimes things can act like both a wave and a particle at the same time. If you throw a ball, it moves forward like a particle, but at the same time, it creates a little wave or "wake" behind it, like a boat does when it moves through water. In the case of the ball's movement, the wake created is so small it is imperceptible.

However, in the subatomic realm, wave particle duality characterizes electrons to a significant degree, making the concept crucial to understanding and predicting their behavior. The early understanding of the atom pictured it containing a nucleus surrounded by orbiting electrons, similar to the way planets orbit the sun. These electrons were thought to demonstrate the single, circular trajectory for which particles are known. Physicists now know that, as electrons orbit around the nucleus of an atom, they behave as both a particle and a wave at the same time. Unlike the ball, the "wake" they create is huge, possibly as big as the atom itself.

Unlike a boat creating a wake as it moves through water, electrons do not move through a physical medium like air or water. Instead, they exist in what is called an "electron cloud," which is a sort of energy field that surrounds the nucleus of an atom. When an electron moves around the nucleus, it does not create waves in a physical medium like a boat does in water. Instead, it creates a wave-like pattern in the electron cloud itself. This pattern is sometimes called an "orbital," and it describes the most likely location where the electron can be found at any given time.

Orbitals are *mathematical descriptions that represent the probability of the electrons' existence in more than one location within a given range at any given time. Electrons can jump from one orbital to another as they gain or lose energy, but they cannot be found between orbitals.*[65]

So, while the electron is not moving through a physical medium like a boat in water, it still has wave-like properties that are related to the electron cloud that surrounds the nucleus. These properties help us understand how electrons behave in atoms and how they interact with other particles. Because of this, scientists cannot really measure electrons as particles moving around the atom, but they can figure out where they are most likely to be based on their energy and how they move.

Wave Function

Within the aforementioned orbitals, subatomic particles often behave peculiarly, motivating physicists' desire to better understand and predict their location. For the sake of illustration, think of orbitals as boxes, within which the electron is guaranteed to be found. There is 0 probability that it will be found outside of these boxes.

After years of brilliant scientists attempting to find a way to mathematically predict wave function, Erwin Schrödinger succeeded in 1926. Based on the nature of electrons, his equation governs the mathematical probability (not the certainty) of where the electron might be found within an atom. Simply put, the equation provides a tool to graphically plot the most probable location of the electron. We know that a wave in the ocean has a physical place and can be measured. But, while an ocean wave is a tangible, physical thing, an electron's wave function is theoretical. When you plot the probability of an electron's location on a graph, it looks like a wave. The regions where the wave peaks or plummets the greatest reveal the locations where one will most likely find the electron.

To borrow an illustration, let us imagine for a moment that a boy you know very well, is locked in his room with a PlayStation, a desk with homework on it, and a bed. Based on your knowledge of this boy, you can come up with probabilities of where you will find him in the room should you unlock the door. He is 80% likely to be at the PlayStation, 19% likely to be in bed, and 1% likely to be at the desk.[66] Similar to how you use your knowledge of the boy to predict his location in the room, the Schrödinger equation allows physicists to use what they know about electrons to determine the probability of its location (wave function). Since the formula has been shown repeatedly to be reliable, physicists generally keep to the math without testing the accuracy and for good reason.

The method used to test the Schrödinger equation is a well-known experiment in quantum physics called the double-slit experiment. In it, an electron is beamed towards a plane with two slits or tiny openings so that after passing through one or both gaps, it then strikes a screen beyond. The classical view of the electron suggested that the electron would only pass through one or the other slit, like a small ball might pass through a hole. However, the double-slit experiment reveals that the electron actually passes through both slits at the same time because in the quantum world, electrons behave as both particles and waves. So, instead of being like a ball passing through one slit, the electron passes through both slits, a bit like how ripples in water can pass through multiple openings in a barrier.

When the electron's wave function goes through both slits, something remarkable happens. It creates an interference pattern on the screen beyond the slits. This pattern shows a series of light and dark bands, which is not something we would expect if the electron behaved only as a particle. The interesting part is that when a detector is placed to observe which slit a particle goes through, the interference pattern disappears. This happens because when we try to observe (measure) the path of a particle, we "collapse" its wave-like behavior into a specific position, and the wave no longer interferes with itself.

Think of measuring as opening the door to the boy in the room. As soon as you open the door, you know precisely where the boy is located. In the case of quantum physics, as soon as that measurement is taken, the wave function collapses, and the particle is limited to one precise location. All quantum mechanical effects of the electron abruptly end, and the particle is only at one location. (This reality is crucial but more on that later! Before discussing the significant implications for energy medicine's claims about quantum mechanics, two more key concepts need explanation.)

Superposition

If we continue to press the boy in the room illustration, we discover a significant breakdown. Whereas the boy can only be in one place in the room at a given time, electrons are in a state of superposition of possible states until the measurement is taken. Electrons, therefore, are like the boy being both at his PlayStation and in bed until the moment you open the door. Superposition is the reality that a particle possesses all possible spin positions at the same time and only takes on a single position upon measurement. Electrons spin on their axis, either clockwise or counterclockwise. Physicists refer to this simply as up or down spin.

One must correctly understand superposition as existing only within the context of the subatomic level. It does NOT apply to large objects.[1] Increasingly popular multiple universes theories attempt to apply the extremely limited reality of the superposition of subatomic particles to the naturally occurring universe as a whole. This may make for interesting movies and lively discussions, but it remains science fiction.

Entanglement

---

[1] Without going into detail, numerous double-slit experiments have only proven the theory of the superposition in subatomic particles like photons & electrons.

Now for the aspect of Quantum mechanics, known as entanglement, that some misinformed individuals specifically point to as the scientific explanation for muscle testing and remote, energetic testing. For those vaguely familiar with the theory of entanglement, their knowledge may be limited to the proven fact that entangled particles respond instantaneously to one another without the lapse of time necessary for information to travel from one to the other at the speed of light. If that explanation was all one knew on the topic, then it is understandable how one might imagine all sorts of ways that entanglement might affect the natural world, including the human body. However, entanglement is not so versatile as some would have you believe.

To begin, you need to understand that scientists must take active steps to entangle two particles. Entanglement has yet to be seen to occur naturally, which is an important fact to remember. Laura Sanders, Ph.D., writer for *Science News,* explains one method of entangling photons, another subatomic particle:

> *One way to create entangled photons is to shine a laser at a particular type of crystal. The crystal will split some of the photons in two — leaving two photons whose combined energy and momentum match that of the original photon. The two are now linked even if they travel far apart.*[67]

Don Lincoln, PhD concisely reveals the limited nature of entanglement by defining it as *two particles with opposite spin and a single wave function.*[68] In other words, with two entangled particles, when one of the two is measured in an up or down position, the other will instantaneously spin in the opposite direction. A simple illustration of this can be seen when flipping a normal coin. If the coin lands on heads, you know that 100% of the time, the other side will be tails. However, unlike a coin that is one object (particle), we are speaking of two separate particles that behave as one. How they do so is a mystery! If scientists measure entangled particle A as up, without fail, B, its entangled counterpart, will be down. Experiments have demonstrated this repeatedly, no matter the distance between the two particles. Additionally, *like a spinning coin that is neither heads nor tails until you catch it* is the spin axis of entangled particles until one is measured.[69]

Einstein referred to quantum entanglement as "spooky action at a distance" because somehow the measurement of A forces B to the opposite position. Some in energy medicine have latched on to Einstein's clever phrase, as though the genius himself gave a stamp of approval for the idea that a union between quantum entanglement and energy medicine exists. In actuality, nothing could be further from the truth. Rather than suggesting his support of some proposed explanations for how quantum entanglement worked, Einstein wrote the phrase as a sarcastic expression of his disbelief in some of the ideas his colleagues bantered about. In a personal letter to fellow scientist, Max Born, in 1947, Einstein wrote the following about prevailing theories of entanglement: *The theory cannot be reconciled with the idea that physics should represent reality in time and space, free from spooky actions at a distance.*

The reason Einstein questioned some explanations of entanglement theory is that his conclusively proven theory of general relativity established that nothing, including information, could travel faster than the speed of light, and yet somehow entangled particle B "knew" the position of A upon measurement.[li] Although Einstein recognized quantum physics, he balked at any conclusions about entanglement that theorized some weird outside interference, rather than time and space, governed matter and energy. It turns out he was both right and wrong. He was right in that information is not being transmitted between the two entangled particles and wrong because somehow the measurement of A does indeed force B to the opposite state faster than the speed of light.

Conclusions

As previously mentioned, the mere act of observation (physicists now prefer the word measurement) collapses the wave function and does so permanently, immediately breaking the state of entanglement. I cannot

---

[li] Entanglement theory suggests that entangled particles respond instantaneously to one another without the lapse of time necessary for information to travel from one to the other at the speed of light.

overemphasize the extreme limitations of superposition and entanglement, so I will repeat myself. ANY outside interference with the entangled particles ends their superposition and their entanglement. *Creating entanglement in multiple shapes and forms isn't that useful if the connection can't be preserved. Entanglement is notoriously finicky, fading away with even slight external disturbance.*[70]

For instance, it is because of this fragility that quantum computers can only function when kept at near absolute zero. The fragile state of entanglement and the end of superposition, upon measurement, necessitate quantum physics being demonstrated mathematically through probabilities that demonstrate which position the particles will take upon measurement rather than with physically measuring the two particles.

The important take-away for us is how this fundamentally disqualifies the claims by energy medicine that quantum mechanics explains their practices. Superposition manifests itself only in the direction of spin. It is a **one time**, **one direction** reality between two entangled subatomic particles, manifested solely in spin direction. Once the entangled particles are interfered with, superposition is lost, and the state of entanglement ends. Don Lincoln, PhD emphasizes the point when he says, *No, this does not mean you can use this (entanglement) to transfer actual information. The collapse of the wave function is still statistical. It cannot transmit a message.*

Let us now apply our understanding of the quantum world, point by point, to the claims of some in muscle testing and energy medicine:

1. *Physiological explanation for muscle testing:*

Claim: Muscle testing provides empirical observations in quantum energy, which reveals energetic information about the health of the body.

Proven truth: The act of measurement abruptly ends all quantum attributes. Therefore, since muscle testing purports to measure health or energy flow in the body, it would negate the very entanglement supposedly needed to transmit that information. Even if entanglement was not abruptly ended upon measurement, it cannot transmit usable health information. And, finally, entanglement does not occur naturally.

Conclusion: The scientifically proven nature of quantum mechanics fundamentally disqualifies it as an explanation for how muscle testing "works."

2. *Remote testing and treatment:*

Claim: Because of entanglement, any minute part (DNA) of the larger system (the body) is connected to the whole; thereby allowing what is done to the part to be automatically transferred to the whole, no matter the distance. i.e., One can test and treat a fingernail, a drop of blood, or saliva because the DNA of the part is entangled with the entire person.

Proven truth: Science has not proven entanglement in large systems, nor has it shown DNA to be entangled. Even if DNA is someday proven to be entangled, the law of relativity guarantees that entanglement cannot transmit usable information, nor can it transmit anything multiple times in both directions. Furthermore, any outside interference abruptly ends all quantum attributes that previously existed, which presents an insurmountable problem for a machine or practitioner with the intention of testing or treating using quantum mechanics.

One cannot observe (measure) quantum energy without altering the outcome, which is why it is a science of mathematical probability. To say that muscle testing, remote testing or treatment, or any other practice of energy medicine can gain information about the health of the body or manipulate one's health through quantum mechanics shows an abysmal lack of knowledge about the basic tenets of quantum physics.

CHAPTER 9

The *Modus Operandi* of Frequency Medicine

in which you once walked, following the course of this world, following the prince of the power of the air, the spirit that is now at work in the sons of disobedience. Ephesians 2:2

In your alternative health pursuits, have you encountered practices based on frequencies or vibrations? Recently, I happened to hear a news report on popular mail-in options for testing food sensitivities. Surprisingly, two of the companies the news anchor discussed claim they base their testing on bioresonance. I have also recently begun seeing adds pop up in social media for a new patch that claims to cure menstrual cramps by rerouting the electrical energy fields of the uterus. Frequency medicine is booming!

To recap, whether you prefer the name energy, *chi*, *prana*, life force, *elan vital*, the *innate*, orgone, vital force, or something else, a belief in subtle energies forms the foundation of all energy medicine. An added belief takes these a step further, creating yet another large branch in the alternative health tree—vibrational or frequency-based medicine. The belief states that *subtle energies vibrate causing a measurable frequency and those vibrations are either healthy or unhealthy.*[71] Although unsubstantiated by science, this claim has produced therapies and gadgets galore, claiming to rebalance one's subtle energies with a specific frequency that matches or resonates with your frequency to promote health. (Chapter 11 will focus specifically on these machines.)

The supposed vibrational aspect of everything accounts for the pursuit of numerous, familiar "healing" practices—From reading auras to wearing certain colors and fabrics, from adding frequencies to supplements or using machines that claim to create various frequencies to eliminate specific illnesses, from eating foods that have been chosen according to their *yin* and *yang* groupings (the macrobiotic diet) to using essential oils according to their supposed vibrational aspect (aromatherapy), from using salt lamps to holding crystals; all these stand on a foundational belief in subtle energies that vibrate.

As energy medicine has surged in popularity so has the interest in defending its cause. Although few participants in these practices can give more than a disjointed, pseudoscientific explanation of the beliefs undergirding them, others, professing themselves wise, have made themselves fools[lii] by authoring books claiming to offer a scientific defense. Indeed, you may be vaguely familiar with the defense. The core argument rests on the undisputed fact that living things have electrical characteristics. You will get no debate from me on this point. That living things regulate many of their functions by means of electrical systems is well-established. These proven aspects are measurable, consistent, and follow *the fixed order of heaven and earth*[liii]. However, the mere existence of electrical function in biology in no way substantiates the subtle energy and vibrational claims of energy medicine proponents.

Therefore, three key questions demand answering. Each one builds on the previous one. First, does science prove the existence of these subtle energies? Second, if subtle energies do exist, does science prove these energies create a measurable electric frequency or vibration? Third, if subtle energies exist and have a measurable electric frequency, can they be successfully manipulated to positively impact one's health? A fourth question should supersede all others, for it warrants serious consideration:

[lii] Romans 1:22
[liii] Jeremiah 33:25

Is this concept of subtle energies in fact a deception from the spirit realm that gives the devil a foothold in the lives of the deceived? These questions demand answers!

The *modus operandi* of energy medicine

As I was sorting through my research on frequency-based health practices in order to write this chapter, I had an epiphany. So, what was this unexpected awareness? I recognized a consistent, deceptive pattern of operation or *modus operandi* that eventually becomes apparent when one extensively investigates the endless therapies and treatments available in energy medicine. I have seen this pattern in all of the alternative practices I have studied but recognizing it yet again brought it to the forefront of my attention.

The pattern of deception goes like this: The explanation and defense for each energy-based practice begins with convincing sounding, pseudoscientific rhetoric based in enough familiar truth to appear believable. This usually involves falsely connecting the practice to proven science with the assumption that few will know the difference. The proponents then offer the research done by founders who appear impressive when one selectively chooses which biographical details to mention and which to dismiss. Because reliable research is always lacking, they heavily pad their case with more scientific sounding verbiage and substantial anecdotal evidence. Sadly, for those desperate for help, this approach is sufficient to convince them to willingly part with large sums of money in hope of achieving the promised healing. Instead, it produces bondage to the deceptive practice.

When scrutiny arises and skeptics bring to light the selectively ignored, biographical details of the founders' lives, as well as the lives of those who later take up the mantel, one discovers strong evidence of occult involvement and/or sheer quackery. And, when the supposed science behind the particular practice is investigated and found profoundly wanting, the truth comes out—an admission by proponents that the practice cannot be measured, for it relies upon spiritual forces.

Researching vibrational medicine, which incorporates radionics, bioresonance therapy, or any frequency-based therapy, one quickly uncovers the aforementioned pattern. Because new energetic-based practices spring up constantly with new names and methodologies, discernment in recognizing them as such can prove challenging. By pointing out what to look for, I hope to not only intelligently warn you about present dangers but to impart wisdom for discernment in the future. To aid in achieving this goal, I will lead you through the *modus operandi* as it is demonstrated in vibrational medicine.

Step 1—Falsely connecting to accepted science.

The practice of comparing apples with oranges while attempting to convince everyone that both are indeed apples undergirds this deceptive pattern. It is an effective strategy in misleading the average Joe who lacks the scientific understanding to recognize such faulty comparisons. After all, only a few have a physics degree. Because countering this deception requires an accurate knowledge of the argument, I must take you through some technical discussion. Please bear with me. Since the core defense of vibrational medicine rests substantially on the irrefutable evidence of bioelectricity, let us begin there.

Most people know or are at least familiar with examples of the electromagnetic detection of body processes: The electrocardiograph (EKG) records an electromagnetic signal from the heart. The electroencephalograph (EEG) registers electromagnetic signals from the brain. Magnetomyograms register electromagnetic pulses when muscles contract. Other examples providing evidence of the electrical nature of life include the fact that sharks detect their prey by sensing the electrical charge living things emit. Some other marine life produces electric charges significant enough to immobilize their prey. Living things are electrical! No one disputes this.

Although the electricity that powers the inventions of the world is produced through the movement of electrons and bioelectricity is produced through the movement of ions (electrically charged atoms or molecules), the net result is the same—energy. The cell membrane alters the electrical charge of a cell by allowing or disallowing the passage of ions. *The elements in our bodies, like sodium, potassium, calcium, and magnesium, have a specific electrical charge. Almost all of our cells can use these charged elements, called ions, to generate electricity.*[72]

These things are established science. The electrical aspect of body processes fundamentally affects health just as the chemical aspects do, and science shows the two are dynamically intertwined.[73] The manner in which these things affect health is quite different from what vibrational medicine suggests, however. For example, hormones such as epinephrine and norepinephrine work as chemical messengers to the heart's SA node, which functions as a pacemaker, activating electrical signals that cause the heart to beat. A multitude of things can cause chemical or electrical deficits in the heart resulting in a heart attack.

The evidence for bioelectricity provides a sufficient measure of familiar truth to which vibrational medicine attempts to attach itself. But wait just a minute! Please take notice. None of the proven examples of the electric nature of life include evidence of the subtle energies said to empower energy medicine nor do they provide a **measurable** electric frequency that impacts health? In fact, as I detailed in the earlier chapter on energy, the evidence for auras, meridians, and chakras (all of which are supposed to be manifestations of such subtle energies) falls profoundly short of scientific standards. And, if the vibrations or frequencies of subtle energies cannot be measured, then how, pray, can one discover a suitable frequency by which to treat the supposed imbalance of energy? Something measurable that exists is not the same as something unmeasurable and unproven to exist. You see, proponents of vibrational medicine assume that you are color blind and will fail to recognize that the apple is actually an orange.

Interlude—frequencies of cells

What if we take subtle energies and the spiritual beliefs that go with them out of the equation and only consider the claim that disease cells and parasites have a unique frequency that can be shattered with an appropriate frequency? You may have heard energy proponents use the analogy of a glass shattering by the voice of an opera singer to illustrate the method of frequencies being used to shatter cancer cells. This is a faulty comparison. According to an article in CA: A Cancer Journal for Clinicians, *although sound waves can produce vibrations that will break glass, radio waves cannot destroy bacteria due to their low energy level.*[74] Again, apples and oranges.

Science does not support the hypothesis that aberrant cells in the human body can be decimated through frequency treatments. In the last 15 years, numerous studies have been undertaken to test various diagnostic and therapeutic uses of radio frequency (RF) and electromagnetic frequency (EMF). An abstract from 2013 said, **While uncertainties regarding efficacy remain**, *there is increasing evidence that some forms of RF EMF exposure* **may be** *beneficial for the diagnosis and treatment of disease.*[75] The only "forms" cited in the abstract as unequivocally successful involved the treatment of insomnia with multiple frequencies[76] and the therapeutic use of frequencies for 8-10 hours a day to increase the healing rates of fractured bones.[77] Obviously, these studies, although interesting, are not the same as shattering disease cells. Again, this is apples and oranges.

Some modern scientists who hold a belief in subtle energies have been researching and testing multiple frequency devices for the treatment of various cancers and tumors. The 2013 abstract mentioned in the last paragraph described some of these studies. These scientists tested various frequency devices using daily treatments in the mouth for one to three hours a day. Two of the men carrying out these small studies have patented the device being tested in the study.[78][79] Although nothing is wrong with this, it does suggest a potential bias, which is why typically a third party would oversee the study rather than the one who might benefit financially from favorable results. The small sample sizes these men employed, and their potential motive for bias necessitates larger sample sizes, double-blind controls, and independent studies before one can come to reliable conclusions on the effectiveness of their particular frequency devices. The efficacy of frequency-based treatments over chemotherapy has not been proven.

However, other advances in research using frequencies continue. For example, ultrasound for treating cancer shows great promise.[80][81] Unlike the studies mentioned in the last paragraph, the research on ultrasound is not based in a belief in subtle energies that resonate but rather an awareness of the proven medical applications of frequencies. In the case of ultrasound, two drawbacks have stymied significant progress until recently: The sound levels required for therapeutic ultrasound frequencies produce significant heat in the body, and they kill both cancer cells and normal cells in the area being treated. New methods that address these problems reveal significant potential in overcoming the obstacles.[82] However, you must understand something—although ultrasound uses frequencies, scientists are not attempting to match some hypothesized frequency of a cancer cell with the frequency of the ultrasound. No, ultrasound simply destroys the cells like fire does wood.

Although I will continue this discourse in the next chapter, my analysis of the current research leads me to two conclusions: First, whether or not aberrant cells have unique frequencies is probably irrelevant, as it is doubtful such frequencies could ever be exploited in a therapeutic manner. Second, whether or not time and further research will eventually reveal new treatment options involving specific frequencies for specific disease cells, all attempts to date have proven inconclusive at best.

Each time you learn of "scientific" studies or evidence that every disease, parasite, or toxin emits a distinguishable frequency, look closely and ask questions. For example, is the proponent making a giant leap from accepted science to unproven hypotheses? Have the studies that proponents claim proves vibrational medicine been repeated successfully by others? (If a study is a ground-breaking, monumental study with remarkable results, then you can be certain other scientists will attempt to repeat the study. Repeatability is a hallmark of the scientific process.) Do the explanations bear up under scientific scrutiny, or do they rely on pseudoscience and anecdotal evidence?

Step 2—The Use of pseudo-scientific rhetoric

In addition to energy proponents falsely connecting to proven science, they also use pseudoscientific rhetoric in an attempt to make their theories sound amazing yet credible. Because of this, one must be familiar with the characteristics of pseudoscience. Wikipedia offers the following detailed definition:

> *Pseudoscience consists of statements, beliefs, or practices that claim to be both scientific and factual but are **incompatible with the scientific method**. Pseudoscience is often characterized by contradictory, exaggerated or unfalsifiable claims; reliance on confirmation bias rather than rigorous attempts at refutation; lack of openness to evaluation by other experts; absence of systematic practices when developing hypotheses; and continued adherence long after the pseudoscientific hypotheses have been experimentally discredited.[83]*

My research has taken me to countless websites for various energy-based practices. These sites utilize scientific buzz words, while making grand claims that have little to no proof. They generally provide no sources by which their claims can be verified. These are all hallmarks of pseudoscience. For example, consider the following quote promoting vibrational medicine.

> *We are all vibrational beings sharing a magnetic resonance at a quantum level. Even planet Earth emits a measurable frequency termed the Schumann Resonance. Our environment and lifestyle effects the vibrational frequency emitted.[84]*

In this quote, the author drops the buzz word, "quantum," which sounds deep and scientific and, as discussed in chapter 7, has become the favorite explanation for energy-based practices. The "quantum level" referred to, however, is code for subtle energies and is an "exaggerated" and "unfalsifiable claim." The opening lines to the article, *Alternative Medicine & the Laws of Physics*, by Robert L. Park, PhD provides a noteworthy summation. He says, *The mechanisms proposed to account for the alleged efficacy of such methods as touch therapy, psychic healing, and homeopathy involve serious misrepresentations of modern physics.* Considering Dr. Park earned his doctorate in physics and served as Chair of the Department of Physics and Astronomy at the University of Maryland for 4 years, we can confidently assume he has a grasp on the topic.

Continuing on in our analysis of the previous vibrational medicine quote, we notice the attempt to tie into proven science—Schuman Resonance—as though it is an equal comparison to or proof of "magnetic resonance at a quantum level." According to NASA's website, *Schuman Resonance* is the name of the vibrational waves that encircle the earth due to lightning (electrical storms). The frequency they emit are *some one hundred thousand times lower than the lowest frequency radio waves used to send signals to your AM/FM radio.*[85] The existence of the Earth's electromagnetic vibrations in no way supports the claims that people share a "magnetic resonance at a quantum level," or that "our environment and lifestyle affects the vibrational frequency emitted." Apples and oranges. This is purely pseudoscientific rhetoric.

Let us consider another quote:

This discovery of {resonant frequencies} *reveals why the ideal resonant frequency of each cell can only be sustained or regained by consuming nutrients that are also at their ideal resonant frequencies. This dynamic interaction between the cell and the nutrient creates a highly beneficial, harmonic resonant effect in which the cell is able to ingest not only the nutritional factors but can also absorb the higher resonant frequencies embedded in the nutrient.*[86]

Boy, oh, boy, where to start with this one! In order to understand why this quote's incorrect use of resonant frequency is pseudoscientific rhetoric, one must understand resonant frequency. *Toppr*, a leading edtech platform, explains the physics concept this way: *Resonance is the phenomenon at which natural frequency coincides with the driving force and gives the maximum response. The resonant frequency is the frequency at which resonance happens.*[87] The site goes on to illustrate the definition with the example of you pushing a friend on a swing. *If you push the swing randomly, the swing will not move very well, but if you push the swing at a specific time, the swing will get higher and higher.*

In essence, the quote advocating bioresonance wants you to suppose that your cells are like the friend on the swing, and the foods you eat, and your environment are like the force pushing the swing. If you eat things that mesh well with the vibrations of the cells of your body, then they will resonate optimally and work better and better.

How do we determine if this is apples and apples or pseudoscience? To do so, let us consider whether or not proven instances of resonant frequency support the theory that the frequencies of nutrients affect cellular resonant frequency. To begin, it is necessary to prove that cells vibrate and have a resonant frequency. They do not. In the words of Harriet Hall, MD, a respected Air Force physician who retired with the rank of Colonel and then wrote for "Science Based Medicine," *cells don't vibrate, don't resonate, and don't have frequencies. A tuning fork can vibrate, and a radio station can have a frequency, but a pancreas can't.*[88]

Second, one must prove that nutrients all have unique frequencies, and the knowledge of those frequencies is accurate. Without proof that an accurate knowledge of all these supposed frequencies exists, how can one know if this or that supplement will produce the desired resonant frequency in your body? So, has science proven these things? To answer, let us separate fact from fiction.

The human body as a whole has a frequency of 9 -16 Hz and many industrial illnesses are thought to be caused by vibrations that do not resonate well with that frequency.[89] (There is nothing subtle about the vibrations caused by industrial machinery.) It is like pushing a friend on a swing with random, choppy pushes. The vibrational impact jars the body and understandably interferes with health. If you have ever worked for a length of time with a power tool that vibrates, you probably noticed that it made your arm ache in some way or another. The vibrational frequency of the tool (the *driving force*) works in opposition to your body's natural frequency and therefore resonant frequency does not result. As you can see, true examples of resonant frequency have nothing to do with subtle energies.

What about at the cellular level, does proof exist that cells resonate if provided with optimal frequencies? Although proponents point to the research of Abrams, Morrell, and Rife as individuals who studied and proved various cellular frequencies, each of these individuals' work did not stand up to the scientific method, which requires independent verification and repeatability and was, therefore, discredited by science. (I will go into much greater detail on these men's work in the next chapter.)

Author and retired professor, Robert T. Carroll, PhD, writes the following about vibrational medicine.

> *We all know, or should know, that sunlight provides energy (real energy, not subtle energy) and that a chemical reaction in the body converts some of that energy into vitamin D. Vibrational medicine thinks this process has to do with vibrations; it doesn't. There may be vibrations in the skin and in photons, but the vibrations themselves are neither healing nor harmful.*[90]

Since I do not possess a degree in physics, I look for insight from those who do. In a physics forum I came across, members discussed resonant frequency and the human body. Part way into the discussion someone, who clearly wished to sort out the claims of bioresonance, posed the following questions,

> *Is there anything that can measure the overall frequency of the human body? Or certain organs or body parts? I'm wondering if there is a frequency difference between healthy and unwell human tissue. Also- Is there a frequency difference between humans in different emotional states, and how could you scientifically measure these things?*[91]

A physics mentor on the forum responded tersely by writing, *This sounds like nonsense. We do not discuss nonsense here.* Another individual, marked as a gold member, also responded.

That does sound kind {of like} something woo-woo describing what you have heard or read as a misrepresentation by someone {who says that} everything has a natural frequency, and a healthy body has a rhythm in tune with the yada yada. Be discriminatory with some information out there.

Although the teachings of bioresonance *claim to be both scientific and factual,* they *are **incompatible with the scientific method.*** The claims are *characterized by contradictory, exaggerated or unfalsifiable claims; reliance on confirmation bias rather than rigorous attempts at refutation,* and there is continued adherence *long after the pseudoscientific hypotheses have been experimentally discredited.*[92]

Step 3—Presentation of questionable founders

In addition to false connections with proven and familiar science, as well as an abundant use of pseudoscientific rhetoric, proponents also deceptively present their founding scientists or doctors. Judge for yourself as we consider the founder of radionics, Dr. Albert Abrams. Radionics has nothing to do with radio waves, unlike the implication of the name. Since it is the precursor to other frequency-based practices such as vibrational medicine and bioresonance, it is of particular importance.

The Bioregulatory Medicine Institute defines radionics:

As applied to medicine, radionics is an art by which diagnostic data is obtained through use of equipment which enables a trained operator to detect and measure differential radiations by the different organs and tissues of the body. Other uses of radionics equipment include detecting and determining the location of disease in the body, measuring the amplitude of various types of pathology and health conditions of tissue, and locating and measuring any foreign micro-organisms, and other irritant factors that contribute to disease.[93]

The man credited with founding radionics, Albert Abrams, was born around 1863 in San Francisco.[liv] Proponents of his work herald him a genius and, indeed, his career did begin with much promise. His impressive credentials included multiple medical degrees from the United States and Germany, the first of which he earned at only 19 years of age. He also earned several respectable positions and affiliations. Certainly, one cannot question Abrams' devotion to meticulously studying the workings of the human body for, truly, he worked tirelessly. Borrowing ideas from multiple disciplines like chiropractic, osteopathy, Chinese medicine, and radiesthesia,[lv] his own particular theory on the workings of the human body evolved as his studies progressed from 1900 until the time of his death by bronchial pneumonia in 1924.

Initially, Dr. Abrams focused on the interaction between the spine and the autonomic nervous system with the certainty that living things are electromagnetic. He believed that each part of a living thing has a unique electrical frequency. He taught, as most energy-based practices today do, that when these subtle energies go askew, disease results. He named his work the Electrical Reactions of Abrams (ERA). His book, *Human Energy*, published in 1914 leaves no doubt that he equated vibrations with energy and promoted an energetic view of the body.

At this point, however, it is difficult to speak of Abrams' work without making him sound silly for his unconventional approach. After all, he made his patients bare their chest and reveal their midriff while facing west and holding both arms out from their sides, all the while standing barefoot on a metal plate as the good doctor thumped on their bodies hour after hour. To what end you might wonder? He listened for subtle changes in the sound of the thump as he percussed the patient's abdomen. Such differences in sound proved too subtle for most he sought

---

[liv] Sources disagree on his exact birth date.

[lv] Radiesthesia *is a sensitiveness held to enable a person with the aid of divining rod or pendulum to detect things (such as the presence of underground water, the nature of an illness, or the guilt of a suspected person)* (Merriam-Webster.com)

to train in his methods, so he began inventing electrical machines to aid in the process.

Although some deemed his method scientific due to his meticulous testing (thumping), he was actually melding science with a new brand of dowsing. Think water-witching. His research into radiesthesia (dowsing) influenced his percussive approach because foundational to radiesthesia is a belief that *there is interaction or resonance between the mind of the dowser and the object or information being sought.*[94]

It quickly became apparent to Abrams that sick patients grew tired of his methods, and so he employed surrogates (called *reagents*) to stand half-naked for hours while holding a metal cup (called a *dynamizer*). In this cup, attached to wires and switches, was placed something representing the actual patient. *A drop of blood, a piece of preserved tissue, or even a photograph or sample of handwriting was all that was needed for a diagnosis to be made, because they all possessed the vibratory rate of the diseased person.*[95]

This approach conveniently allowed Abrams to "test" people from all over the world who mailed him one of the aforementioned items. His all-too-frequent diagnoses were syphilis, tuberculosis, and cancer with many patients being told they won the bad-health lottery and had all three. Not to worry, though; they were also informed that for a certain fee, they were completely curable through the good doctor's most popular machine (called an oscillocast).[96] He claimed the machine could target the disease cells with high frequency charges to destroy them.

As Abrams' work progressed so did his fortune and his eccentricities. He claimed he could determine the paternity of a child, one's religion, race, and even location in the world, as well as diagnose disease—all from a sample of handwriting placed in the *dynamizer* and held by a reagent as his abdomen was thumped.[97] The American Medical Association (AMA) reported the case in their journal of a fictitious man who was diagnosed by an osteopath using Abrams' methods. His serious diagnoses included metastatic cancer of the liver and right colon, syphilis, tuberculosis, and streptococci infection of the gall bladder. It turns out the unfortunate patient was a healthy, female guineapig.[98]

The Food & Drug Administration also claimed to have secretively tested Abrams' accuracy by submitting for testing wrongly identified specimens. Reports included the following:

A blood sample from a man who had lost his right leg elicited a diagnosis of arthritis in the right foot and ankle. The blood of a dead man brought back a diagnosis of colitis, and that of a rooster resulted in a report of sinus infection and bad teeth![99]

One highly suspicious practice also surrounded the use of Abrams' inventions that came to be known as "black boxes." His most famous machine, the oscillocast, could only be rented after signing a contract promising not to open the machine for inspection.[100] When the AMA later inspected an oscillocast, they found no components that could accomplish what Abrams claimed the machine could do. During an investigation by *Scientific American*, an oscillocast was examined and said to contain two electromagnets, a device similar to a metronome that makes a ticking noise, a light to indicate it is working, and some other components that fail to generate any appreciable electric current.[101]

Celebrities of the time, including American novelist Upton Sinclair and Sir Arthur Conan Doyle, the British author of *Sherlock Holmes*, became staunch supporters of Abrams' work. As a result of the doctor's fans writing to *Scientific American* about his work, the magazine began an almost ten month and $30,000 investigation.[102] Their first article in a series of ten began with the following:

At this point the <u>Scientific American</u>, urged by the large volume of correspondence regarding the E. R. A.[lvi] which has been received during the past few months, has entered the controversy not to take sides but to act as an independent investigator. It is our intention to listen to the arguments of the believers and the skeptics, review alleged cases of cure as well as alleged cases of failure to cure, conduct a series of tests with the Abrams method of diagnosis and

---

[lvi] Electronic Reactions of Abrams

treatment, and undertake a critical examination of the apparatus employed.[103]

The magazine soon discovered numerous challenges in what they originally presumed would be a simple investigation. First, Abrams made himself unavailable, although he did supply a list of personally approved practitioners. These individuals, although happy to have their methods put to the test, often tweaked those methods to improve perceived weaknesses. The magazine quickly discovered that countless individuals had joined the cause with an eye for possible fortune. Each touted Abrams' belief in radionics but then promoted their own machines as superior to his in some regard. As a result, coming to a meaningful conclusion became far more difficult than anticipated.[104] *Scientific American* was limited to working with numerous ERA doctors, as Dr. Abrams never allowed himself to be directly tested. He did, however, spend much time corresponding with the magazine. The magazine's committee tried numerous tests with several doctors approved by Abrams. All tests failed miserably.

Abrams died of bronchial pneumonia before the conclusion of the magazine investigation. Sadly, he failed to heal himself with his ERA methods just as he failed to heal his two wives who both died of cancer. So much for knowing the frequencies of bacteria and cancer and then being able to shatter the aberrant cells with his machine. At the end of their investigation, the committee emphatically stated their final verdict:

This committee finds that the claims advanced on behalf of the electronic reactions of Abrams and of electronic practice in general are not substantiated; and it is our belief that they have no basis in fact. In our opinion the so-called electronic reactions do not occur, and the so-called electronic treatments are without value. Signed William h. Park, Walter c, Alvarez, Robert c. Post, j. Malcolm bird, Austin c, Lescarboura."[105]

Step 4—Focus on anecdotal evidence.

After inaccurately connecting energy practices to proven science, using pseudoscientific jargon, and misrepresenting the founding fathers to sound like misunderstood geniuses, the next tactic in the proponents' *modus operandi* is to overload their claim with anecdotal evidence. For any who are suffering and desperate for help, this is often the only step that matters and persuades them to act. No matter how much one might hold scientific understanding in high esteem, personal testimony produces optimism bias—a willingness to disregard anything negative and hope for the best. Is it reported that this or that treatment, machine, supplement, or therapy helped people? If so, many gladly toss reason overboard and plunge into the murky waters.

Abrams had no shortage of patients who touted the amazing accuracy and results ERA produced for them, hence, the doctors, celebrities, and average people encouraging *Scientific American* to write about Abrams' work. Similarly, the majority of those who have contacted me first encountered energy medicine and muscle testing because of a friend or family member's testimonial. Such stories provide compelling hope.

As I discussed in an earlier chapter, nonspiritual explanations for these testimonials do exist—the placebo or ideomotor effects, the body's own healing independent of treatment, and numerous other possibilities. Belief, desire, and hope are powerful in creating temporary anatomical conditions that produce positive results. If improvement comes from such things alone, then who cares whether science proves it truly works? If a sugar pill cures me, then I would take that over a drug with side-effects any day. However, if energy-based practices invoke demonic power, buyer beware! Now, you are dealing with forces whose goal is to destroy you and those you love and to separate you from your Lord and Savior.

Step 5—Admission of the spiritual component.

The ultimate end of the *modus operandi* of energy medicine often comes after scientific scrutiny exposes a lack of sound evidence. Take, for example, Abrams' story. In the final article in the *Scientific American* series on Abrams, the magazine described their work with a particular ERA doctor and discussed at length the problems encountered with the ERA method not bearing up under scientific scrutiny. The magazine suggested scenario after scenario whereby the scientific test might validate ERA. The doctor repeatedly admitted that he himself had already tried each one of the suggested tests and all failed.

He then said, *This ERA technique works miracles at times and then fails completely at others. At present I cannot do the experiments which you propose with any certainty of success.*

The magazine continued to press the doctor for some avenue of testing to which he responded,

I am afraid there is nothing I can do. I know the reactions are there, but there is no way I know of to show them to you.[106]

That doctor's description reveals a notable characteristic seen in all branches of energy medicine—that the techniques fail under the rigors of the scientific method yet produce inconsistent but often remarkable results, suggesting spiritual involvement. The fact that they produce "miracles at times" points to more than just the placebo effect. By this, I refer to outright cures or dramatic changes rather than minor improvements. Power resides in these practices that has no measurable or predictable source. Professing Christian practitioners reach out to me, whether in agreement with my conclusions or in criticism, and they confess a recognition of spiritual power behind energy medicine. Those professing to be Christians blindly suggest God is the spiritual force.

The author of the best-selling book, *Vibrational Medicine*, Richard Gerber, MD, openly asserts his belief in the spiritual component of subtle energies. He says,

Vibrational medicine is the first scientific approach I've seen that is able to integrate science and spirituality, something which has unfortunately been left out of the medical model. It's only by viewing the body as a multi-dimensional energy system that we begin to approach how the soul manifests through molecular biology, if you will. Ultimately, that comes down to the whole issue of reincarnation and karma.[107]

Many accuse me of labeling energy medicine as demonic simply because I do not understand it. This is incorrect. Belief in the frequencies of subtle energies is not just a belief in something that science has yet to measure and understand, but a belief in the realm of *the prince of the power of the air*. Ephesians 2:2 says, *In which you once walked, following the course of this world, following the prince of the power of the air, the spirit that is now at work in the sons of disobedience.*

Our bodies do not function upon subtle energies. However, there most certainly is an unseen realm of spiritual forces under Satan's rule. By participating in these practices, you open yourself up to forces intent on your destruction. Have you been disobedient to the Lord and participated with the spirits of the air through frequency-based medicine? I urge you to repent and turn to the Lord. He will not cast you out.

CHAPTER 10

A Closer Look at Ruth Drown & Royal Rife

Thus says the Lord:
"What wrong did your fathers find in me that they went far from me,
and went after worthlessness, and became worthless? Jeremiah 2:5

In the end, the scientific method proved Abrams' devices were quackery, causing him to be dubbed the "dean of twentieth century charlatans"[108] and the "dean of gadget quacks."[109] However, such labels did little to dissuade loyal followers from creating their own variations of Abrams' black box. When considering alternative health practices, the discerning will not ignore the illuminating histories of each modality. As such, in order to gain further insight, I will continue the progression through the timeline of frequency medicine. Ruth Drown and Royal Raymond Rife became the next rising stars in this saga.

Ruth Drown, an American chiropractor born in 1891, established a thriving practice in Los Angeles. She created numerous machines, which she claimed could diagnose and cure illness. Unlike Abrams, who attempted to promote his work as science, Drown reveled in the spiritual teachings of the Kabballah, energy-based ideology, and psychic revelation.[110][lvii] After decades of practicing frequency-based health, she died of cancer in jail while awaiting trial in 1965.[111]

Fraud revealed

In spite of her methods and machines being proven fraudulent numerous times during her career, Ruth Drown continued to bring harm to individuals through her fake treatments.[112] In 1949 she gave a demonstration of her methods at the University of Chicago, during which she grossly misdiagnosed a patient. In 1951, she was convicted and fined for selling a misbranded device across state lines.[113] Finally, in 1965 Ruth Drown and her daughter, Cynthia Chatfield, also a chiropractor, were arrested for grand theft as a result of the work of an undercover agent with the California State Department of Public Health.[114] The agent, a 22-year-old Mrs. Jackie Metcalf, paid Drown and Chatfield $150 for three diagnoses ($50 each) garnered from three blood spots Metcalf told the chiropractors came from her sick children. The two doctors diagnosed chicken pox and mumps for the unfortunate "children." They proceeded to instruct the agent on how to use a $588 machine they sold her to eliminate the illnesses. In reality, the three blood spots came from a turkey, sheep, and pig.

Drown's frequency machine had a unique distinction among radionics devices of the time. She describes her unusual machine in *Drown Radio Therapy*.

> *Machines using electricity are not like our Drown instrument...The Drown instrument uses only the subject's own energy, and the Radionics machine uses electricity as its carrier wave...The patient is both the 'sending set' and the 'receiving set' with the Drown instrument, as all energy returns to its source.[115]*

[lvii] *Ruth was later to tell Riley Crabb, of Borderland Sciences, that her pioneering radionic work was psychically inspired* (see source #98).

Although today many energy treatments do not involve electricity because of the belief that the practitioner and the patient provide the energy needed, in Ruth Drown's day this was highly unusual. Her radionics machine had nine dials with ten settings possible for each dial. She based the frequency rates used in tuning the dials of her machines on numerology from the Kabballah, an esoteric school of thought in Jewish mysticism. John Nauss, a Toronto radionics practitioner and colleague of Ruth Drown, attests to her reliance on the Kabbalah and cites another close colleague of theirs, David Tansley, who further explained her reasoning:

> *Drown would reduce her rates to one number that corresponded to each station of the Kabbalah and the angelic force behind it. David Tansley said there was no logical reason, except in her own mind, for using sacred numerology and making the vibrational link. It is the practitioner who helps to set the pathways to healing and, depending on their connection, in harmony with the client, spontaneous healing occurs. She was a light bearer.[116]*

Tragically, the spiritual nonsense of Ruth Drown impacted many thousands before she could be stopped. Just imagine the damage done based on the figures Ralph Lee Smith states in his article, "The Incredible Drown Case (1968)": *At the time of their arrest, Doctors Drown and Chatfield had treated 35,000 persons from all over the country and had sold their devices to other fringe practitioners who had treated an unknown number of other patients.[117]*

During the grand theft trial, a witness dismantled Drown's machine and showed how the nine dials with ten settings each were all connected in such a way that it made no difference whatsoever the setting used.[118] Numerous individuals testified at the trial who had been harmed by the false diagnoses and treatments by the mother/daughter team. As deputy district attorney John Miner said in his trial summary, *Quackery can kill and the use of fraudulent instruments such as these devices in the courtroom is dangerous to human life.[119]*

Royal Raymond Rife

A contemporary of Drown and another Abrams imitator and famous name in the retinue of "black box" creators was Royal Raymond Rife (1888-1971).[lviii] Because his work in supposedly discovering the frequencies of pathogens has become the gold standard for frequency medicines and the basis for many of its expensive gadgets, I have spent countless hours researching Rife. He claimed that cancer is caused by a virus, or is it bacteria? Welcome to the confusing world of researching Rife! While reading article after article about him, I began to notice significant inconsistencies, like whether it was bacteria or a virus that he claimed caused cancer[lix] or if Rife had a PhD or even something as simple as when he died or if he cured 16 people of cancer in 1934 or if the president of the AMA tried to buy Rife's research and when refused conspired to destroy Rife's work or if anyone besides Rife himself ever confirmed his elaborate microscopes worked, and the list goes on and on.

Little seems to be known about his education, although he is often referred to as a doctor. It is reported that Rife claimed a PhD for himself from Georgia Tech, but the university says otherwise.[120] Some of his followers report he gained an honorary PhD from the University of Heidelberg for his work developing photomicrographs for their *Atlas of Parasites*.[121] This claim is peculiar in that,

> *neither here nor in the United States was there known to be a single extant microscopical preparation worked on by Rife, Gonin or anyone else. With the possible exception of one picture of a phage*

[lviii] A <u>Daily Californian</u> article by Del Hood, *Scientific Genius Dies; Saw Work Discredited,* indicates Rife died in 1971 as it was published the day of Rife's funeral and dated August 1971. However, according to Rife's partner, John Crane's, article, *The Crane report*, Rife died in 1972 and according to other articles by various followers he died in '73 o4 '74. Based on the sources, I find the obituary article the most likely to be correct and so used that date.
[lix] It turns out that he claimed a particular bacteria changes form into a virus that then causes cancer. He used the analogy of a chicken laying an egg to describe the change. He called it *bacillus x* or *bx* (cancer carcinoma) or *bacillus y* or *by* (cancer sarcoma).

there is no proof that any photomicrographs were ever taken with any of the Rife microscopes.[122]

I noticed that articles written by proponents who hail him a hero for finding a cure for cancer, which was then conspiratorially suppressed, consistently used specific statements in their claims as though they were all quoting from the same source. However, none listed sources to back up their claims. Unverifiable details and significant inconsistencies met me at every turn. Why? On what were all of these claims based? In order to separate fact from hearsay, I always strive to reach the original source. So, I kept looking for a way to validate all information. Lest my reader think I fell prey to the misinformation of those who desire to squelch knowledge of anything outside of mainstream medicine or big pharma, I was eventually able to read court transcripts, Rife's deposition, personal letters, and listen to recordings of Rife speaking. I used these and other original sources to gain a more solid understanding of Rife's history.

It turns out that one primary source has created the many inconsistencies repeated endlessly by followers. In 1986, Barry Lynes, an investigative journalist with a passion for astrology,[123], wrote the book, *The Cancer Cure That Worked, Fifty Years of Suppression*. To gain the necessary information for the book, Lynes joined forces with one of Rife's former partners, John Crane, who, incidentally, went to prison for three years because of his work with Rife.

Others close to Rife judged Crane to be manipulative and determined to push Rife's work forward in an undesirable manner. For example, John Marsh, another partner who also went to prison, wrote the following about Crane in a personal letter: *He had kept Rife in alcohol with the front of friendship, thus taking everything he could from Rife when Rife wasn't alert to John's intentions...Crane was and is so money-mad that he couldn't see these finer things in Rife."[124]*

Despite Royal Rife's inventive genius and dogged scientific work, he met an inglorious end. His work was discredited. Because of selling Rife's unproven machines, the producer of his therapeutic machines, the Beam Ray company, endured a lengthy trial in 1939. Two of his partners (John Crane and John Marsh) were arrested and charged with grand theft, while

Rife hid out in Mexico.[125] Rife slowly declined into alcoholism.[126] Lynes, however, resurrected Rife's work over two decades later and promoted an intricate story of conspiracy to account for Rife's fall from favor.

Although I consider it plausible that various government agencies and mainstream healthcare organizations might seek to manipulate information that could interfere with more lucrative cancer treatments, the evidence of conspiracy against Rife stands solely on the word of those who stood to benefit financially from Rife's unproven work. An article detailing unproven cancer treatments describes what I found to be true regarding Lynes' book:

> *The book, written in a style typical of conspiratorial theorists, cites names, dates, events, and places, giving the appearance of authenticity to a mixture of historical documents and speculations selectively spun into a web far too complex to permit verification by anything short of an army of investigators with unlimited resources.*[127]

What can be verified of his life includes the following: Rife was born and raised in Elkhorn, Nebraska. After marrying, he moved to San Diego to work as a chauffeur and mechanic for the Bridges family. The widow Bridges was the daughter of the wealthy founder of the Timkin Roller Bearing Company in Ohio. Having greatly impressed both the widow Bridges and her affluent father through his engineering skills, Rife gained long-term benefactors in them both. They generously funded his laboratory and research for many years. This substantial funding allowed Rife to carry out his research in a laboratory that rivaled any other of the time. Although the details are fuzzy, some sources also report that Rife worked in Germany before the World War for an optics company (maybe Zeiss or Leitz?) making lenses or microscopes.[128]

Unusual microscopes

Royal Rife invented five or possibly six unique microscopes by which he claimed he could see bacteria and viruses moving and changing forms (pleomorphism). Much mystery surrounds Rife's phenomenally complex microscopes, and as these were the tools used to ostensibly prove that bacteria, viruses, and fungi have specific frequencies, we must carefully weigh the evidence. The Universal Microscope, his masterpiece and third out of five, had 5,682 parts, fourteen lenses and prisms made of block quartz that polarized light, allegedly allowing Rife to see the color signature (auras) of microorganisms. Rife claimed his microscopes could magnify objects up to 17,000 times (all other light microscopes, past and present, magnify 40-2,000 times).[129] His incredibly complex microscopes were also said to be capable of taking pictures (photomicrographs), although only one of these pictures exists today, and what it shows *was identified as a well-known artifact of optical systems known as "coma"* rather than a virus. [130]

All of the claims about his microscopes are beyond remarkable due to the magnification limitations innate to light microscopes. For instance, the greater you magnify something, the more light is eliminated. Many distortions also occur at high magnifications due to the nature of light waves. The book, *Molecular Biology of the Cell,* describes some of these problematic distortions:

> *The interaction of light with an object changes the phase relationships of the light waves in a way that produces complex interference effects. At high magnification, for example, the shadow of a straight edge that is evenly illuminated with light of uniform wavelength appears as a set of parallel lines, whereas that of a circular spot appears as a set of concentric rings. For the same reason, a single point seen through a microscope appears as a blurred disc, and two-point objects close together give overlapping images and may merge into one. No amount of refinement of the lenses can overcome this limitation imposed by the wavelike nature of light.[131]*

Another oddity of Rife's claims counters the accepted understanding of the transparency and colorless nature of microorganisms. This transparency affords marvelous views of the innerworkings of bacteria and viruses but does require careful staining and preparation to see microbes distinctly. Yet, Rife claimed that due to his novel microscope design, with multiple quartz prisms, a special light source that he patented, and a unique filtering process of the bacteria itself, he could distinctly see natural, brilliant color.[132]

Still another difficulty arises when focusing at high magnification on a moving organism. We get just a hint of the significance of this problem in photography when zooming in on a faraway subject. Focus cannot be held if the subject moves about unless the camera has features to automatically track the subject. The greater the magnification, the more focusing problems such movement will cause. Only light microscopes can see living organisms, and their magnification limit for doing so is currently 2,000 times. Microscopes that magnify to significantly higher degrees, such as the electron microscope, can only view dead organisms that have been carefully stained.

However, Rife claimed to see the following, even at significantly higher magnifications than all other light microscopes (8,000-17,000 times):

We see them swimming through the field. They're highly motile...So, we see these beautifully turquoise-blue bodies swimming through the field...We place a Coren bacillus under this monochromatic light and there we have a reddish-brown organism...We place the filterable form of the bacillus of tuberculosis, and we have a jade green.[133]

He believed that the distinctive colors of the various microbes he saw revealed the unique frequency they possessed. It was then a laborious task for Rife to determine the matching, killing frequency by endlessly tuning another of his machines, called the Rife Ray machine, to different frequencies until he found one that worked. He said, *I check on that thing* [a bacteria/virus] *and look through that microscope hour after hour day after day...to find something that will kill that bug.* Upon determining the right frequency, he claimed his machine could throw *an electronic frequency through the tissues of the body that simply devitalized the bacteria with no harm to normal tissue.*[134] This is how he claimed to "devitalize" cancer cells, cataracts, tuberculosis, and all manner of pathogenic illnesses.

Rife did not himself claim to cure cancer. Others made that claim for him. *He told his cohorts never to say "cure" when talking about the research. "Devitalize" was vague enough to suggest something positive.*[135] Because he made no claims for curing cancer, nor did he ever personally treat anyone, Rife successfully avoided prosecution when those around him were not so fortunate.

What did others see through Rife's microscope?

Because Rife's "frequencies" solely rest on what he claims he saw through his microscopes, it is reasonable to ask whether anyone else ever verified that Rife's microscopes worked as he stated. His supporters insist that many doctors and scientists did so. One of the purported witnesses, Dr. Arthur Isaac Kendall, was a microbiologist who worked with Rife with the intention of using his microscope to prove that Louis Pasteur's germ theory was incorrect. Dr. Kendall had created a unique medium for culturing bacteria, and with this "K-medium," he and Rife claimed advances in showing illness can come from within the body and not just from outside germs. They would examine the cultured bacteria, in its filterable state, with Rife's microscopes.[ix] An article in *Science News*, published in 1928, stated Dr. Kendall saw the turquoise-blue bodies of the typhoid bacteria in their filterable state with Rife's microscope.[136]

Lynes and Crane also claim in *The Cancer Cure that Worked* that Dr. Edward C. Rosenow of the Mayo Clinic's Division of Experimental Bacteriology saw a demonstration of the Universal microscope and personally saw it worked as alleged. In Rife's deposition for Crane and Marsh's 1959 trial, a July 1932 report by Dr. Rosenow in the Mayo Clinic Bulletin is mentioned but without indication as to what it said.[137] Today, all that remains of the article (that mysteriously disappeared) is a

---

[ix] A filterable state simply denotes the size of the particle as being small enough to pass through a particular filter.

transcription copy by an unknown source.[lxi] Proponents claim Dr. Rosenow described that he saw colorful moving bodies through Rife's microscope. As with numerous other assertions in Lynes' book, most records supporting his claims have vanished or, as he alleges, were destroyed by those wishing to suppress the cure for cancer. Often, only hearsay remains.

In contrast, numerous documented reports exist of others who tried and failed to confirm that the microscopes worked. Rife made five or possibly six microscopes, but aside from Dr. B W Gonin in England, no one but Rife owned these microscopes during his lifetime. In 1976, the daughter of Dr. Gonin donated her late father's Rife microscope to the London School of Hygiene and Tropical Medicine. For fourteen years the microscope was housed at the Wellcome Museum of Medical Science in London, along with a number of papers and notes about its history compiled by various individuals living at the time.

Dr. Gonin's daughter reported that her father claimed to have spent a "king's ransom" to purchase Rife's number four scope but insisted that it was missing key elements and never worked properly.[138] In response to the doctor's complaints, Rife then sent a colleague to England with the number five scope in exchange for the ineffective number four model. According to the daughter, her father *was unable to obtain useful results with either No 4 or No 5.*[139]

In 1978 a Professor of Physics from the Imperial College in London visited the Wellcome Museum to thoroughly test the donated microscope and stated that while *using all the original optics it was quite impossible to obtain an image.*[140] This confirmed Dr. Gonin's earlier complaint that it never worked.

A pathology professor named Hubbard, from the State University of New York in Buffalo, also took a keen interest in Rife's microscopes

---

[lxi] The link at https://rife.org/journal-magazine-articles says the following about the report from the *Proceedings of the Staff Meetings of the Mayo Clinic,* -- *"Observations on filter-passing forms of Eberthella typhi (Bacillus typhosus) and of the streptococcus from poliomyelitis",* by Edward C. Rosenow, July 1932. **Because a copy of the original journal version has not yet been located, this document is a transcription of the original article, the transcriber unknown.**

beginning in 1948. Hubbard visited the Wellcome Museum to inspect and disassemble the microscope in 1978 and went to significant lengths to confirm how and if the microscopes worked. The curator of the museum at the time interviewed Hubbard and wrote the following with regard to their discussion, as well as with regard to the copious research notes Hubbard shared with him on Rife's microscopes. (Hubbard donated his notes to the museum.)

> *Bausch and Lomb said that they had tried to see the Rife microscope but there was so much secrecy that few people, and most of them non-microscopists, had been able to get to it. The few microscopists who had been able to see it were not well-versed in microscope theory and could, therefore, give no worthwhile opinion of its virtue. The company had never been able to get evidence to substantiate announcements that the instrument exceeded the limits of resolution which theory indicated. The Spencer Lens Company, later taken over by the American Optical company, had tested a Rife microscope, in 1936 according to Hubbard, its performance had been no better than an ordinary instrument of similar numerical aperture...* [141]

It could be theorized that, as the inventor of an incredibly complex microscope, perhaps only Rife (and possibly a couple others under his direct instruction), had the patience and skill to make these instruments work. We do know from Rife that he would spend countless hours trying to focus his microscope. In the early 1930s, an eye doctor insisted Rife limit his viewing to two hours a day due to eyestrain, and by 1936 he reportedly could not use his microscope due to the condition of his eyes. [142]

Most importantly, though, one should not minimize Rife's claim of seeing the color signatures of microbes, which caused him to conclude that each possessed an individualized frequency. Past and present, many who openly flaunt their occult powers claim to see auras indicating unique frequencies. What they see is not a unique frequency, but an optical manifestation provided by demons. Although Rife claimed no spiritual source, based on the weight of evidence concerning the true capabilities (or rather, incapabilities) of his microscopes, I suspect that what he actually saw was similar in nature to what others claim to see through spiritual power—auras, indicating demonic involvement. This is conjecture on my part but seems consistent with what I observe throughout the world of alternative medicine. My theory also suggests a reasonable explanation for what Rife claimed to see with his devices in spite of defying proven science regarding the properties of light and magnification.

Curing cancer

As a result of what Royal Rife claimed to see through his Universal microscope, he set out to create a machine that could destroy pathogens through frequencies. At first, he used and modified numerous pieces of machinery already available. Later, he partnered with electronics engineer Philip Hoyland to invent therapeutic machines, which rivaled the technical complexity of his microscopes. The machines produced multiple audio frequencies at the same time to supposedly "devitalize" offending organisms.[143] In the early years of his work (1930s), the Rife Ray machines contained many boxes and highly technical parts. His partners John Crane and John Marsh later tried to manufacture, sell, and patent much simpler versions of the Rife Ray machine from the 1950s-1980s, and for which they went to prison for grand theft.

After years of tedious experimentation with white rats and guinea pigs, Rife joined forces with his powerful friend, Milbank Johnson M.D., to begin human trials. According to the accepted story, Milbank had both medical and political connections in Los Angeles and was able to rent the Scripps House in La Jolla, California as a treatment and research clinic with sixteen cancer and tuberculosis patients. Barry Lynes says the following regarding these early human trials in *The Cancer Cure That Worked*:

In the summer of 1934 in California, under the auspices of the University of Southern California, a group of leading American bacteriologists and doctors conducted one of the first successful cancer clinics. The results showed that: a) cancer was caused by a micro-organism; b) the micro-organism could be painlessly destroyed in terminally ill cancer patients; and c) the effects of the disease could be reversed.[144]

According to Lynes and Crane, many respectable doctors participated in the clinic and announced their confirmation of 16 patients who were cured in 90 days. Per Lynes, records were poorly kept, and the doctors involved were later intimidated and threatened into silence because of a lawsuit against the Beam Ray Company, who began manufacturing Rife's machines in the late 1930s. Lynes and Crane also claim these records were destroyed in raids on Rife's laboratory and offices. As with every other aspect of researching Royal Rife, proposed scenarios abound to explain the loss of clinical records supporting the ostensible results of the 1934 clinic. I find it telling that before Rife died, he made no claim to having cured cancer but, instead, stated to a friend: *The most important thing I ever did was build a microscope.[145]*

During Rife's lifetime and in the years since, many have continued to manufacture and sell machines they claim are based on Rife's frequencies and discoveries. During the Beam Ray trial, the engineer for the early machines, Philip Hoyland, gave testimony that the frequencies programmed for subsequent machines by the Beam Ray Company were alterations from the original.[146] To date, much controversy exists over which set of Rife frequencies are the ones used in the 1934 Scripps clinic. It appears that even Rife did not know the answer to this mystery,[147] so imitator companies feel free to make a case for whichever frequency list they prefer.

I find it illuminating, that, from 1935 until Rife's death in the 70's, he and his many partners attempted to make so many significant changes to the machines. Why significantly alter the frequencies and method of delivery if they worked successfully in 1934? In the 1950's, Robert P. Stafford, M.D. began using the Rife Ray machines and wrote a letter to colleague Edward Jeppson, M.D. of the disappointing results they both encountered.

I am writing you at this time partially because John Marsh informs me in a recent letter that you may be somewhat disheartened or at least worried about your role in the experimentations with the Rife Machine. Believe me, Dr. Edward, I know how you feel, for I too have been through this same feeling with this matter. I have observed clinical results after treatments with this gadget which I can scarcely believe myself. Yet, despite these good results, I have been confused by some rather simple failures...I sent the results to John Marsh and asked for clarification and to be very frank I am not satisfied with John's excuse of the failure as described by Dr. Rife. I am afraid I'm not a very good apostle... I really wonder if this ultrasonic kills bacteria and virus at all or does it work like other forms of ultrasonic and merely stimulate the tissue in some unusual manner thereby improving the circulation and secondarily enhancing the body's defenses against infection.[148]

I find Stafford's commentary on the inconsistent results noteworthy. As discussed in the last chapter, practitioners who used Albert Abrams' machines also found some results remarkable and, yet, at other times, confusingly abysmal. Such is true of many energy-based therapies, and therein lies the mystery. Stafford suggested that the results might be explained by the generic stimulation of bodily tissues. Later, he also postulated that the placebo effect produced the inconsistent results seen. Dr. Stafford stated this in a report sent to Rife, Marsh, and Crane regarding his experiences with the AZ-58 Rife Machine.

As yet, we have failed to "cure" any case of advanced, terminal malignancy. It appears in several instances that we may have impressed the disease favorable, temporarily. It is difficult to rule out the psychological, morale booster effect to the terminal patient when some definitive effort is made again in his behalf.[149]

Having now spent beyond forty hours poring over endless documents, writings, and recordings on or by Rife, I ask myself what conclusions can be drawn regarding this man's work? One thing is certain, most, if not all, subsequent machines claiming to be based on Rife's frequencies are not, for even his own machines used an ever-changing method and frequencies.

By Crane's own admission, he never succeeded in gaining a patent for any machines based on Rife's work because he repeatedly failed to prove the machines did what he claimed.[150] Numerous others in the last five decades, who have manufactured and sold machines claiming to be "Rife machines," have also been successfully prosecuted for fraud because they too failed to demonstrate the machines performed as claimed.

Most importantly, the fact that the basis for Rife's frequencies was the color signatures of microorganisms, when all other science indicates the impossibility of this, leads me to conclude Rife fell prey to the deception of the evil one. As Romans 1:22 describes, ***professing themselves to be wise they become fools*** (KJV).

God's children must be very careful not to trade the truth of God for a lie. May God's words through the prophet Jeremiah not be said of us: *Thus says the Lord: "What wrong did your fathers find in me that they went far from me, and went after worthlessness, and became worthless?* Jeremiah 2:5

CHAPTER 11

Evaluating the
Devices of Energy Medicine

*So I tell you this, and insist on it in the Lord, that you must no longer
live as the Gentiles do, in the futility of their thinking. They are darkened
in their understanding and separated from the life of God because of the
ignorance that is in them due to the hardening of their hearts.*
Ephesians 4:17-18

Although Albert Abrams receives credit for being the founder of
radionics, his gadgetry was not the first of its kind. Over one hundred years
earlier a Connecticut MD, Elisha Perkins, received a patent for a
therapeutic device he called "metallic tractors." His device stemmed from
a discovery by Luigi Galvani, an Italian doctor, physicist, biologist, and
philosopher. Galvani's research with dead frogs serendipitously led to a
discovery in 1780 that electric current animates the muscles. He coined
the name, *animal electricity*, to describe the electrical animation of life.[lxii]
During his lifetime another physicist, Volta, became fascinated by animal
electricity and repeated many of Galvani's experiments. The two scientists
achieved similar results but arrived at very different conclusions: Galvani

---

[lxii] Over a hundred and forty years later, Abrams named his metal cup used in
Electrical Reactions of Abrams (ERA) a *galvanizer*.

believed the frog legs' movement stemmed from electrical current coming from its pelvis, whereas Volta believed it came from the two different kinds of metals used for the rods employed during the experiment, creating a current to pass through the frogs' leg muscles lying in between the rods.

Based on these men's research, Dr. Perkins created and began selling a simple device in 1796 consisting of two, teardrop shaped metal rods—one brass and one iron, which he claimed could cure all manner of medical conditions. All one had to do was place the rods on opposite sides of the problem area, and voila, the symptoms would cease. In spite of the $25 price tag ($500 in today's money), they became all the rage! Even President George Washington owned a set.[151]

Many doctors and scientists questioned the tractors' success and undertook to put them to the test. One of them, Dr. John Haygarth designed a controlled study with five individuals suffering from rheumatic pain. Following Perkins' protocol for the use of the tractors, he treated the patients with a set of look-alike tractors made of wood. The patients believed Haygarth used authentic, Perkins' metallic tractors and afterward reported very specific improvements to their pain lasting from two to nine hours. The following day the same five patients returned for another treatment, only this time Haygarth used the real tractors. Although the patients knew nothing of the change in tractors used, they reported almost identical results as the previous day.[152]

In Haygarth's publication of his results, he stated,

This method of discovering the truth distinctly proves to what a surprising degree mere fancy deceives the patient himself; and if the experiment had been tried with metallic tractors only, they might and most probably would have deceived even medical observers.[153]

Following the publication of the study, the tractors became objects of public ridicule and soon fell out of fashion. The story highlights, however, the power of the placebo effect, resulting from a device one believes to be effective. It also demonstrates how easily one can garner anecdotal evidence from the placebo effect. Lastly, it explains how the temporary benefits of a placebo can create a powerful bondage to a false treatment, at the expense of lasting help.

FDA regulation

Within the alternative health realm, a certainty of belief exists that conventional medicine and big Pharma seek to prevent alternative health options from being available because of money and control. Although evidence for abuses of power does exist, that does not mean that unregulated healthcare is preferrable. Unlike the times of Perkins' tractors, the FDA now regulates any device that claims to *diagnose, treat, cure, or prevent any disease.*[154] Although imperfect, the FDA's role in requiring a company or individual to substantiate their health claims provides a safeguard to the consumer. After all, no one wants to spend thousands of dollars to be defrauded and have their health put at risk.

Dr. Stephen Barrett, founder of Quackwatch.com, has spent much time researching and testing the devices of energy medicine and has corresponded much with the FDA regarding their regulatory role of this industry. Because many alternative medicine machines are, in fact, used for diagnosing and treating illnesses, it is helpful to understand the FDA's classification in order to be a more discerning consumer. Barrett explains,

> *The FDA classifies "devices that use resistance measurements to diagnose and treat various diseases" as Class III devices, which require FDA approval prior to marketing...***No such device can be legally marketed in the United States for diagnostic or treatment purposes.** *A few companies have obtained 510(k) clearance (not approval) by telling the FDA that their devices will be used for biofeedback or to measure skin resistance, but this does not entitle them to market the devices for other purposes.*[155] (emphasis mine)

Because of this, the official literature for most alternative diagnostic and therapeutic devices strategically avoids making any direct claim that places their machines under the jurisdiction of the FDA. They do not want to have to prove their device works! Instead, the increasingly savvy makers of such gadgets dodge legal scrutiny by making generalized claims involving energy balance, enhancing the immune system, or promoting health to the whole person. These types of claims currently remain outside FDA regulation. Please understand, this tactic means they do not have to prove their device does what it says. Practitioners who offer scans and treatments from these devices, on the other hand, often tout the credibility and unsubstantiated claims without concern for legal repercussions. Both the manufacturers and the practitioners tend to focus on personal testimony.

Remember, it is financially advantageous to them to convince you to use the device. This market exudes deception and fraud. Only God knows the intentions of the heart, but the lure of significant wealth from inventing and selling unproven health gadgets might easily cloud the best of intentions. How ironic it is that the majority of individuals purchasing these unsubstantiated machines are people who fear traditional medicine and write off Big Pharma as being only concerned with their profit margin. These individuals prefer to place their trust in unregulated companies selling a wide assortment of outrageously expensive machines believed to measure health and disease states in the body and/or treat for parasites, toxins, and diseases. If you are such an individual, please continue reading before continuing to place your trust in these gadgets.

An overview of energy medicine devices/machines

Many thousands of different energy medicine devices have been and are being sold throughout the world. I cannot possibly write about each of them. Instead, I will discuss the types of devices and the pseudoscience behind them in the hope that my readers can then apply that knowledge to the vast array available. Despite ducking FDA scrutiny, some are primarily used for diagnostic purposes and some for therapeutic ones. When used for diagnostic purposes, they often replace muscle testing, but are no less concerning.

In the previous two chapters, frequency-based treatment machines were discussed. These included Abrams' Oscillocast, the Drown instrument, and the Rife Ray machine, all of which were proved useless during court trials. Because those particular "black box" devices were covered previously in detail, I will limit my discussion to currently marketed types. However, keep in mind, the research and "technology" of Abrams and Rife formed the faulty foundation upon which most subsequent devices are built.

For classification purposes, there are three main types of energy devices that I will cover: frequency machines for treatment, therapeutic electrodermal patches, and electrodiagnostic devices (EAV). To aid you in better understanding each category of gadgets and the marketing tactics employed to promote them, I will provide two detailed examples of each. There are many others that could be discussed but two should be sufficient to aid you in recognizing concerning devices.

The Rife-type frequency machines that claim to have therapeutic benefit include the *Biocharger* (produced by Advanced Biotechnologies, LLC) and *Somavedic* (produced by Somavedic Technologies Inc.). The second category of devices are electrodermal patches that claim to treat pain and assert other therapeutic benefits through frequencies. The third category of energy devices are classified as electrodermal testing devices (EAV). These include the popular ZYTO machines (ZYTO Technologies Inc. sells numerous machines and a patented hand cradle, all of which I will henceforth simply refer to as ZYTO), and the iTOVi scanner and app produced by iTOVi, LLC. These EAV devices are used to determine what is "out of range" or balance and what would best restore balance. (The use of vague terminology skirts the FDA's prohibitions against unproven claims to diagnose or make recommendations for treatment). Because most of these devices are linked in one way or another to pseudoscientific beliefs about frequencies, I will briefly revisit that topic.[lxiii]

Frequency—fact or fiction?

Like the words "quantum" and "energy," the term "frequency" gets bantered about in energy medicine like a beach ball at the seaside. Toss in "biofield" and one has a truly meaningless mix. In *Frequencies and Their*

[lxiii] See chapter 10 for a lengthier discussion of frequencies.

Kindred Delusions, Dr. Hariet Hall explains the true, scientific meaning of frequency:

> *The definition of frequency is "the number of repetitions of a periodic process in a unit of time." A frequency can't exist in isolation. There has to be a periodic process, like a sound wave, a radio wave, a clock pendulum, or a train passing by at the rate of x boxcars per minute. The phrase "33⅓ per minute" is meaningless: you can't have an rpm without an r. A periodic process can have a frequency, but an armadillo and a tomato can't. Neither a periodic process nor a person can "be" a frequency.[156]*

Energy medicine promotes the false belief that EVERYTHING has its own unique frequency. From that premise, they extrapolate that the frequency signature of something can be replicated and used in place of the original object, person, or substance as if the two are the same. Additionally, they wrongly teach that there is an optimum frequency for cells, and that our cells can be "recharged," like a cellphone battery, to better fuel the health of the individual. All of this is pseudoscientific nonsense.

As discussed in the previous chapter, Rife used questionable microscopes to supposedly see the color signatures of microscopic substances and by that to determine their frequencies. This dubious research forms the basis of many frequency lists in energy medicine today. Science, on the other hand, does not substantiate this. Nonetheless, versions of the Rife machine can still be purchased for hefty sums today.

Therapeutic device example #1—*BioCharger NG*?

Other forms of frequency machines, whose primary purpose is for therapeutic treatment, are also on the market. Another name for them is "subtle energy" device. They may, like a Rife machine, claim to use "frequencies" to kill aberrant cells, bacteria, viruses, or toxins, or they may claim to rejuvenate the cells of the human body. The method employed for creating frequencies varies but may include crystals, light, sound, or magnets. Having already covered at length the faulty foundation of frequencies on which energy medicine's gadgets are based, we can now consider the marketing approach of two examples. You decide if they are deceptive.

The *BioCharger NG* by Advanced Biotechnologies, LLC is a modern example of this device class. On the company's website, the inventor, Jim Girard, claims the machine uses frequencies, harmonics, pulsed electromagnetic field energy, voltage, and light to accomplish all manner of nebulous health benefits. In 2024, the website explains that the device cycles through one of over 1200 energy-frequency combinations intended to provide a broad spectrum of frequencies to stimulate cells with weak vibrations to return to their original, healthy frequency and resonate. Dr. Hariett Hall remarks on this by saying; *Never mind that cells don't vibrate, don't resonate, and don't have frequencies. A tuning fork can vibrate, and a radio station can have a frequency, but a pancreas can't.*[157] According to the website, up to six individuals at a time can sit in a circle around the device for twelve to fifteen minutes at a time. With a price tag of just under $17,000, the company insists it is a great deal compared with other such machines.

The *BioCharger* website also offers a number of articles on the "scientists" who provided ground-breaking research upon which the device is based.[158] These include Nikola Tesla, Georges Lakhovsky, Royal Raymond Rife, and Alexander Gurwitsch. Tesla and Lakhovsky supposedly collaborated to create a frequency device that used a Tesla coil that demonstrated beneficial results in treating cancer. Not mentioned on the website, however, is the important detail that this research and device failed to produce any verifiable results, and, as a result, fell out of fashion like so many other blackbox devices. As to the fourth name mentioned, Gurwitsch, the website touts a specific area of his research as credible without mentioning the fact that other scientists made over 500 unsuccessful attempts to replicate Gurwitsch's published observations.[159] The *BioCharger* website makes no claims of any clinical studies that have been done to substantiate their instrument, which is not surprising considering the research on which it is based.

Therapeutic device example #2--*Somavedic*

Another frequency-based device called *Somavedic* claims wide ranging therapeutic benefits like improved quality of sleep and mood, positive effects on the number of negative ions, restructuring water, and significantly blocking EMFs.[160] Their devices contain various minerals and crystals housed in a colored glass globe with an LED light. Supposedly the unit creates an energy field that produces the various aforementioned benefits.

Rather than a marketing plan that focuses on the foundational scientists or past research, their website provides summaries with links to an enormous amount of current, supposed scientific studies. It strategically states the number of pages for each study next to links to the pdf files, ranging in length from three to sixty-eight pages. The average consumer will be duly impressed with the scientific pictures and graphs, lengthy research articles, and "certifications" presented. "Go big" is definitely this company's approach to convincing individuals to fork over roughly $500 to $5,500 for one of their devices.

When researching scientific evidence for practices, devices, or supplements, one must always consider the biases possibly motivating those involved in clinical research. Possible biases are supposed to be stated at the end of a clinical study's abstract. Therefore, when you consider the weight of conclusions from a particular study, the first thing to notice is whether it was conducted in-house by the very people who stand to benefit financially from positive results and conclusions. Now, bias does not mean a study's results should be discounted, but only that it should be scrutinized carefully and demands replication by those who are unbiased. In the case of *BioCharger NG*, I mentioned that the scientist, Gurwitsch reported favorable results, garnering much excitement in the scientific community, but that his results were unable to be replicated. This is how the scientific process works. Science, by nature, is repeatable and measurable.

I am occasionally surprised and particularly interested when someone with a significant bias concludes what is not in their favor. Such is the case with a detailed and lengthy review of *Somavedic* by August

Brice, founder of *Tech Wellness*. According to her website, she is a *former Emmy, Gabriel, and Gold Mic Award-winning investigative journalist who has been studying this issue seriously and collaborating with the most informed scientists in the world in this space* (EMF research) *for most of my adult life.*[161] Her worldview does not appear to be Christian, and she actively participates in numerous energy-based practices. She also states that she suffers from electromagnetic sensitivity and purchased two different devices from *Somavedic* in hopes of experiencing the promised benefits.

Because of the extensive clinical "evidence" from *Somavedic*'s website with claims for positive results, Brice's extensive review led her to consult with professor of neuroscience, Olle Johansson, PhD, *who has authored over 600 papers in the EMF space and has been published in the world's top scientific Journal, "Nature," to give us a detailed analysis of the research and claims.*[162] After an in-depth analysis of the clinical studies listed on the company website, Johansson stated his expert opinion as follows:

> *They are all uncontrolled and dependent. Furthermore, data is lacking in regards to how the standardization was done, how the samples were collected, how the fields of vision were selected, what kind of biomedical statistics that was used, no internal controls are presented, no calibrations met, no blind-coding regiment described, etc...*[163]

Scientific study must adhere to certain standards that are well-documented so that others can follow those same protocols to determine if the observations are repeatable. Failure to maintain those standards and documentation in a clinical study seriously calls into question the reliability of their conclusions. Small sample size and failure to include a control group also lends itself to results based on the placebo effect. Upon taking the time to read the largest clinical study posted by *Somavedic* (68 pages) as of 2024, one discovers it is only an outline of a proposed study, rather than one that has been completed. Numerous other problems found in the website's science section are also discussed in Brice's review. The company seems to count on the consumer being sufficiently impressed by the appearance of quantity and not knowing what to look for in the lengthy pdf files.

Brice's review also included her purchase of an ion meter to replicate the exact conditions of a picture posted on the website supposedly proving their claim that the device increases negative ions. Her test revealed no increase in negative ions but a significant **increase** in EMFs radiating from the *Somavedic* device itself. Brice also did some digging into the company, IGEF that provided the "seal of approval" certification for the reviews on these devices. Although such a certification sounds impressive, Brice states that the International Association of Electrosmog Research (IGEF) appears to mainly be *a vehicle for "certifying" frequency devices that claim to harmonize, neutralize or protect from 5G or EMF.* Their certification can be found in abundance on countless pendants, stickers, quantum pouches, and magnetic cards.

However, for the Christian, the most concerning information I found on *Somavedic* comes from statements made by the inventor, Ivan Rybjansky, during a YouTube interview. When asked how he came up with the idea for the device, he responded by saying; *About ten or fifteen years ago, I discovered that I could diagnose and heal using a pendulum…Over time I've learned the perspective of Chinese medicine, that there are chakras, meridians, and energy blockages in the organism that can be overcome.*[164] He then goes on to describe how he learned from others that semi-precious stones have energy and that by placing them in a pyramid, they create more energy than they could individually. He also states that his device restructures water to try and erase "water memory," which is a scientifically disproven claim that has its roots in the spiritual. (This will be discussed in greater length in the next chapter.)

Finally, he begins explaining a surprising goal of his machine, which is not listed on the website. He discusses his belief in "psychosomatic zones" which he says are spirits that arise when someone is dying.

In summary, I'm trying to neutralize such zones. There are many people who claim they hear someone in their attic but there is no one. Or, their doors or windows open or close suddenly…Some time ago,

I visited a lot of such places to learn to recognize the correct frequencies and feed them into the Somavedic. I dare to say that after switching the device on, 99% of clients have gotten rid of these zones and manifestations of this type have no longer occurred.[165]

Clearly, this device is more than meets the eye.

Therapeutic electrodermal patches

Sellers of the next class of devices employed by energy medicine make claims similar to frequency machines. Therapeutic electrodermal patches are small, wearable, and easily transported patches or discs that ostensibly have frequencies embedded in them to reduce pain and inflammation and energetically bring general health benefits.[lxiv] Some companies manufacturing these products target chiropractors and physical therapists as the purveyors of these devices, which are to be used in combination with other therapies. However, many other energy patches, discs, bracelets, and rings are sold directly to the individual to use as they determine. One company coined a scientific sounding name for the therapy using their expensive discs—*amino neuro frequency treatment.*[166] In case you have not already noticed, the use of the word "frequency" should immediately sound off alarm bells in your mind. Dr. Hariett Hall has this to say about all such devices:

You can't embed a frequency. You might be able to embed something that would produce vibrations or electromagnetic waves with a frequency, but it would require a power source. If a product contained a frequency generator, so what? It requires a phenomenal leap to imagine that exposing the body to that frequency would have a specific beneficial effect on an individual organ or that it would somehow improve human health.[167]

[lxiv] These should be distinguished from TENS devices, which use an actual, electric current to stimulate the nerves to block pain or change the perception of pain. The clinical study conclusions on TENS are mixed in its effectiveness for various conditions. https://www.ncbi.nlm.nih.gov/pmc/articles/PMC9611192/

Patch example #1--*Luminas*

Hopefully, by now, you have become savvier at picking up on the pseudoscientific babble found in the claims and explanations found in energy medicine. See how you do with the description found on the website for a pain patch called *LUMINAS,* created by LUMINAS Energy LLC .

> *Our proprietary technology allows us to capture these unique electric field signatures from 100s of natural remedies used to relieve pain and inflammation. These unique signatures are then modulated onto a resonant carrier wave allowing us to transfer these unique signatures onto the patch. Once applied to the skin, the patches are activated and energy from the 200+ remedies are released to support the body's own innate, natural healing process.*[168]

Really? What red flags does this description raise for you? It should arouse in you an abundance of questions such as how did they determine the "electric field signatures" from natural substances? How did they manage to "modulate" those "signatures" onto a "resonant carrier wave" (and what on God's green earth is that anyway?) and then contain it on a patch? Then, how, exactly, is that information released, without a power source, and received by the body?

Should you simply ignore all such questions because no explanations are needed in light of the results from the posted "clinical study" where patients were asked to rate their pain before and after using the patch.[169] Definitely not! If you have been tracking with me, more questions should immediately come to mind when looking at such a study. Who carried it out? How many patients participated? Was there a control group following the same protocol but using a fake, look-alike patch? Unfortunately, you would find no answers to these questions in 2024 on the *LUMINAS* website.

Instead, the website provides an abundance of pictures from the "study" testing the effectiveness of their patch. They used thermographic cameras to provide "objective results" of the difference their patches produced in reducing inflammation (heat). These images only show body shapes with colors indicating varying degrees of temperatures on the skin. But do such images mean anything? Dr. David Gorsky, a surgeon with a PhD in cellular physiology comments on *LUMINAS'* use of thermography in an article lambasting another instance of what he terms, "quantum magic": *I also know from my previous studies that thermography is very dependent on maintaining standardized conditions and a rigorously controlled room temperature, as well as on using rigorously standardized protocols.*[170]

I found no indication that those conducting the "study" did anything to maintain controlled standards, and manipulation of the pictures can be a simple matter. For example, were the participants fully clothed in all pictures and was the room temperature always the same? Let us suppose the initial thermographic picture was taken with no patch present but while wearing a shirt. The skin temperature would quickly cool following the participants removing their shirts for the patch to be applied. If the shirt was not replaced, the heat sensitive photography would show an increasingly cooler skin, regardless of the patch. Without recorded details of their study's protocols, the results cannot be replicated or verified. Conveniently, *LUMINAS* does not feel the need to share the specific details or procedures of their "clinical study," nor can I find any evidence of its existence in peer-reviewed literature or that it was registered on ClinicalTrials.gov. Without further information, the results are inconclusive at best.

Not surprisingly, the woman credited with product development, Sonia Broglin, has deep roots in energy medicine and is a certified *EnergyTouch* practitioner who graduated from the *EnergyTouch* School of Advanced Healing. Consider this explanation of her training found on the *EnergyTouch* website:[lxv]

[lxv] The first two quotes were originally found on their website and quoted in Dr. Gorsky's article on *LUMINAS* patches. The website has since changed their description, and in May of 2024 includes the third paragraph I quote.

EnergyTouch is distinctive in the field of energy healing in that the work takes place in a more expanded energy field allowing the practitioner to work on a cellular level. Our work includes accessing an energetic hologram of the physical body, which is a unique and vital aspect of EnergyTouch Healing. This energetic hologram acts as a matrix connecting the energies of the outer levels of the field precisely with the physical body on a cellular level.

EnergyTouch practitioners are skillfully capable of moving fluently throughout the levels of the human energy field, to access and utilize outer level energies to clear blocks and restore function at the most basic cellular level.[171]

The Human Energy Field is a dynamic system of powerful influences, in unique relationship to physical, emotional, and spiritual wellbeing. This system consists of, in part, the Aura (made up of multiple levels of the Field), multiple chakras (energy centers that correspond to these levels), the energy of the organs and systems of the body, and the Pranic Tube (our connection to Universal and Earth Energies and Guidance).[172]

Once again, we are reminded that energy medicine stems from a world view that is contrary to a biblical one. These companies may attempt to put on a scientific facade, but when you begin to pry it back just a bit, you always find a New Age belief system that cannot coexist with the Bible.

Patch example #2-- *Taopatch*

The next example for your consideration gets a gold star on making The next example for your consideration gets a gold star on making nebulous claims, guaranteed to prevent FDA regulation. *Taopatch,* created by UPGRADE BIOTECH LLC, headlines their website with the following: *Realign your body, boost your performance, and upgrade your life with the world's 1st nanotechnology light therapy device. The human upgrade device.[173]* It claims to be a patented nanotechnology device the size of a nickel that is worn on the skin and lasts up to two years. They claim it is backed up by fifty years of research, although what this research includes is unclear. Yes, the name comes from the ancient "wisdom" of Chinese philosophy—Tao. The inventor of the patches, Fabio Fontana, claims the devices contain "quantum dots" and nano technology that work by emitting "biophotons" that:

> *help the nervous system to communicate more efficiently, achieve the correct posture, and improve mental focus and immunity, and proprioception, defined as the sense of self-movement and body position. This device "up-converts" the natural infrared radiation from the body into beneficial light waves.*

> *These quantum dots "pick up" infrared radiation from the body and emit radiation in the range of visible light, like that used by low-level and ultra-low-level laser therapy.*[174]

The videos posted on their website show promoters of the products testing people for strength and balance before and after placing the discs on their bodies. The shock on the people's faces at the improvement following the disc's placement appears real and reminds me of the responses people had when I used to muscle test them. Could it be the placebo effect? Possibly. But, having personally witnessed the immediate and shocking change that can come from demonic power, these videos certainly raised concerns in my mind. Remember though, when we wish to discern between the spiritual and the physical, scrutinizing the science can be helpful.

Dr. Samuel Pinches, a materials scientist with a PhD from the University of Melbourne, writes a blog sharing his reviews on products that claim to bring pain relief because he recognizes that the average individual lacks the knowledge to evaluate the scientific, marketing claims made by manufacturers. In his review of *Taopatch* he explains that *while biophotons are a known phenomenon, there is no evidence that these play a role in intracellular communication, or that by simply adding more similar photons that any healing effect can be achieved.*[175] Dr. Pinches expounds further on the scientific claims by saying:

> *Yes, Quantum Dots are a real thing too, but they do not create free energy out of anywhere… they certainly can't create more energy than they receive! Yes, low-level laser therapy is also a real thing too, but there's a big difference between low-levels they use (typically ~5W/cm2) and, well, zero! As you can see, Taopatch® mixes current scientific research, scientific buzzwords, and complete fabrications, to present as a technology that seems 'miraculous' but yet almost plausibly believable.*[176]

Similar to the marketing approach of *LUMINAS*, *Taopatch* attempts to wow the consumer with an abundance of supposed, clinical research. Dr. Pinches also evaluated, at length, each of the studies the company cites. What he discovered should not surprise you at this point. He found low-quality studies with few participants, the names of supposed doctors who do not appear to exist, plagiarism, a "master's thesis" by more non-existent doctors, weak results in a study that does not even mention *Taopatch*, duplicate studies, *a bogus article studying patches on plants*, and a poster instead of a study.[177] These are the kinds of tactics commonly found in the realm of energy medicine machines.

EVA devices

The next class of frequency devices has many names and acronyms, including the following: electrodiagnostic device (EDA), electrodermal testing device, electrodermal screening (EDS), Electroacupuncture according to Voll (EAV), bioelectric functions diagnosis (BFD), bioresonance therapy (BRT), bio-energy regulatory technique (BER), biocybernetic medicine (BM), computerized electrodermal screening (CEDS), computerized electrodermal stress analysis (CDCSA), electrodermal testing (EDT), limbic stress assessment (LSA), meridian energy analysis (MEA), or point testing. I will refer to them as EAV devices, as that is the most commonly used name.

The name Electroacupuncture According to Voll (EAV) comes from Reinhold Voll, a West German physician who combined his practice of acupuncture with galvanic skin differentials to produce devices in the 1950s. Using one of his early "electroacupuncture instruments," he believed to have found connections between internal organs and "acupoints." *EAV is a method of measuring the electrical impedance of acupoints. It utilizes an electronic ohmmeter designed to measure the skin's electrical resistance.* [178] So, once again, we have devices that are based on the false beliefs in Chinese meridians and energy blockages causing disease.

Although significant variations exist in what these devices look like or how they function, in general, the device emits an electric current to a brass cylinder covered by moist gauze, which the patient holds (This may also be a metal plate or cradle on which the patient rests his or her hand.). The tester touches "acupoints" on the patient with a probe attached by a second wire to the device, thereby completing a low-voltage circuit. The information is registered by the device to a gauge or computer that provides a report. In reality though, they are just *fancy galvanometers that measure electrical resistance of the patient's skin when touched by a probe.* [179] Because these modern machines are galvanometers connected to computer software programmed to link certain readings with health conditions and then make health recommendations, it is important to understand the galvanic skin response (GSR or more frequently called, electrodermal activity, EDA). Although the history of EDA may seem unimportant, it is actually crucial in understanding why EAV devices do not do what they claim to do.

Galvanic skin response

At the start of the chapter, I described how Galvani discovered "animal electricity" in 1740 when a dead frog's legs jumped when he placed metal rods on either side of them. A hundred years later, a German scientist, by the name of Dubois-Reymond discovered that human skin was also electrically active. Another thirty years passed before Swiss scientists, Hermann and Luchsinger, made the connection between EDA and sweat glands. *Hermann later demonstrated that the electrical effect was strongest in the palms of the hands, suggesting that sweat was an important factor.*[180] Then, in 1879, French psychologist Vigouroux was working with "emotionally distressed patients" and made a fascinating connection: EDA is tied to psychological activity. Building on that knowledge, eight years later, the French neurologist Féré demonstrated that skin resistance activity could be altered by emotional stimulation and that skin resistance activity could also be inhibited by drugs.[181] For example, science revealed that certain things, such as pain or emotions, elicit

a sympathetic response by the sweat glands, increasing secretion. Although this increase is generally very small, sweat contains water and electrolytes, which increase electrical conductivity, thus lowering the electrical resistance of the skin. These changes in turn affect GSR.[182]

And so the cumulative research continued to build as more scientists studied EDA further. In the early 1900s, the connection between the galvanic skin response and the subconscious was also established. The famous psychoanalyst, Carl Jung, used a *meter to evaluate the emotional sensitivities of patients to lists of words during word association. Jung was so impressed with EDA monitoring, he allegedly cried, "Aha, a looking glass into the unconscious!"*[183] According to Wolfram Boucsein, *by 1972, more than 1500 articles on electrodermal activity had been published in professional publications, and today EDA is regarded as **the most popular method for investigating human psychophysiological phenomena**.*[184] (emphasis mine)

All of that history has firmly established that the galvanic skin response is one measure of autonomic nervous system activity (ANS). (The ANS is responsible for maintaining bodily functions that do not require conscious thought, i.e., heart rate, digestion, sweating, etc.) The fingers, palms, and soles of one's feet have a great concentration of sweat glands. Have you ever noticed that when you get nervous, your palms sweat? Sweat is your ANS responding to an emotion—fear. Psychologists have found that using a galvanometer can effectively reveal to a patient an **emotional** trigger of which they may be unaware. As Jung declared, EDA is *a looking glass into the unconscious!* Because the body responds to the stress of lying, a galvanometer is one component of a lie detector polygraph test.

Other factors besides emotions can also affect the readings of a galvanometer such as temperature, humidity, medications, and hydration, providing inconsistent results. Furthermore, the skill of the operator comes greatly into play, as the amount of pressure and consistency of pressure can change the results.[185] This important detail makes sense since *pressure reduces electrical resistance and makes the current flow better from the probe to the skin.*[186] Unlike the unproven claims of Voll who wished to connect the health condition of human organs to theoretical acupressure points, a great deal has been firmly established scientifically regarding galvanic skin response.

In light of the abundance of proven research on EDA, consider the applications to the electrodermal testing devices prevalent in energy medicine. Suppose that you go to a practitioner to have a scan done by one of these devices, and you had an upsetting encounter on your drive to the test. Yes, you have a bit of road rage! We know scientifically that the results will be vastly different than if you were at ease. Or suppose the first time you have a scan done, you are apprehensive about how it will work. The next time, however, everything seems familiar, and your apprehension is gone. Again, the results will be vastly different. Or suppose one time you have the scan done on a cold day and another scan when the summer humidity could be cut with a knife. You get the idea; the results will again vary greatly. The differing results have absolutely nothing to do with the health of your organs and everything to do with your autonomic nervous system responding to your surroundings and your emotions. Oh, and do not forget, the one performing the test or you can also alter your results by pressing too firmly. Voila! Quantum magic strikes again!

EVA devices—*iTOVi* & *ZYTO*

Since Voll's invention of his EVA device, the *Dermatron*, countless others have followed. The two currently most popular devices are the ZYTO machine, created by ZYTO Technologies Inc., which uses a hand cradle rather than a probe, and the iTOVi, created by iTOVI LLC, which uses a hand-held scanner that connects to a smartphone containing a corresponding app. iTOVi focuses their marketing on using the results of a DNA test in combination with the galvanic skin response received from the scanner to create a "wellness plan." They claim it uses *subtle electrical frequencies and GSR technology...*[that] *tests and records your body's real-time responses to natural wellness products!*[187] Not surprisingly, no published clinical studies demonstrate iTOVi results are of any clinical value or that they are reproducible, but instead that they vary from minute to minute.[188] Since I have already covered the pseudoscience of everything having a measurable and unique frequency and the diagnostic challenges of galvanic skin response, I do not need to spend more time on the *iTOVi*. Obviously, the results from this device are unreliable.

The founder of ZYTO, Vaughn R. Cook, is a doctor of oriental medicine and an acupuncturist from Utah. While working in the 80's in marketing and sales for the Esion Corporation, the maker of an earlier EDA device called the *Interro*, Cook gained experience that prepared him to break away and create ZYTO.

Unlike the iTOVi, which is fairly inexpensive and targets personal use, at the time of this writing, ZYTO's cheapest option runs $400. However, the primary device required for a scan is only accessible through providers who have purchased them at roughly $10,000 or $15,000, depending on the chosen software package, plus a monthly subscription fee. For a device in that price range, targeting healthcare professionals, one would expect a serious attempt by the company to offer scientific proof of some sort. Not so.

Instead, they offer a compelling business plan that allows these providers to use computer software connected to the ZYTO device to make recommendations for products and services that particular businesses wish to sell their clients. The patient pays the provider for the scan and walks out the door with a very expensive goodie bag of all the recommended products. Who needs proof that the product works when patients can be separated from their money so easily!

To illustrate the significant fluctuations in results when using an electrodermal testing device, let us consider what Dr. Stephen Barrett of *Quackwatch* discovered after personally testing a popular ZYTO machine using their Elite 5.0 high-end software. He described the purpose for the three series of tests he ran—*a basic scan that supposedly evaluated my organs and advised what products would bring them back "in range." The other two were nutritional "biosurveys" to determine what foods I should or should not eat.*[189]

Before revealing Barrett's results, let us consider what ZYTO has to say for itself on the website. *By getting a ZYTO biosurvey, you can find which Virtual Items associated with products your body is most coherent with, thus reducing the guesswork and subjectivity that comes with choosing supplements and other personal wellness products.* These "Virtual Items" are simply software programming that has been chosen to represent over 40,000 actual items such as homeopathic remedies, supplements, essential oils, and therapies, *internal body systems as well as external Virtual Items which are called stressor Virtual Items.*[190]

A *biosurvey* typically tests for the "coherence" of both positive items (i.e., supplements & services) and negative items, called stressors. These "stressors" can include organs, vertebrae, teeth, meridians, parasites, toxins, allergens, EMFs, chemicals, foods, and even "lifestyle choices."[191]

How do you suppose they get the information on 40,000 products in order to make these "Virtual" "associations"? Although they would have you believe that "digital signatures" represent actual items, in truth, the means for ZYTO's programming decisions became a matter of public record following an FDA inspection.

ZYTO Technologies Inc. has a long history of warnings and inspections by the FDA beginning in May of 2015, again in 2019, and most recently in June of 2023. In the 2023 warning letter from the FDA to ZYTO's founder Dr. Cook, it states some interesting details about how the company makes its associations between "Virtual Items" and actual items, as well as there being no documentation indicating any true association between the two. The warning letter references information gained during a follow-up inspection in 2019.

> *Our investigator documented that the virtual items are added to the library in house using a machine referred to as the "Tower". Your representative explained that to create a library item, your firm places the item in front of the Tower and the Tower then scans and identifies the item with a generated code from the system **which it associates with the energy of that item**. This becomes a virtual library item. In addition, your firm's promotional materials indicate that the hand cradle can now perform this function as well, so that users can add their own virtual items...*

> *During our inspection, **your firm's attorney stated you have no documented validation of use of the Tower to identify and add virtual items to the library. He further stated there would be no way to test the process used to input these virtual items**...*

> *You have been marketing this product since at least 2019 with no evidence that this design review requirement has been met. We reviewed your response and determined your response is inadequate...[192]* (emphasis mine)

It remains unclear as to ZYTO's response to the FDA's warning, but I did find the following disclaimer on a sample scan posted by the company.

> *ZYTO software has not undergone FDA review for effectiveness. ZYTO technologies are not intended to be used in the diagnosis, cure, treatment, mitigation, or prevention of any disease or medical condition. The diagnosis and treatment of medical conditions should only be undertaken by qualified medical professionals. ZYTO professional software provides general wellness information and should not be used without the involvement of a licensed healthcare professional. **ZYTO products have not been the subject of controlled clinical trials to establish their effectiveness** and their use is not a*

generally accepted medical practice by the traditional medical establishment.[193] (emphasis mine)

Nonetheless, the ZYTO *biosurvey* claims to test for stressors and balancers to determine which "Virtual Items" are most likely to bring stressors back into range, or balance. The following is how the company describes the way their product works:

During the scan, ZYTO software takes baseline measurements of the galvanic resistance to low-voltage electricity through the palm and fingers of the test subject and sends product codes to the hand cradle so the body can supposedly respond to product "signatures" as though the test subject had ingested the products. The system re-measures the galvanic resistance of the test subject and then calculates the difference between the "baseline" and second measurements. This process is repeated over and over again through the product line(s) selected by the practitioner.[194]

Knowing what you have learned in this chapter about galvanic skin response (EDA), it will be no surprise to learn that Dr. Barrett's 43 tests over a ten-day period garnered vastly different results. He performed a general scan to determine which organs were "out of range." Although his gallbladder had been removed, the scan identified it as being "out of range" four times and within range eight times. The rest of his results were as follows:

The organ with the highest "out-of-range" score, positive or negative, also differed from test to test. Four reports highlighted my adrenal glands, three chose my small intestine, two chose my heart, two chose my thymus, and the other six tests each identified a different, supposedly problematic, organ. Only four of the sixteen scans had any organs "within range."[195]

The meaningless results continued as Barrett completed two nutritional surveys, which included twelve food-category tests and fifteen individual food assessments. The results showed numbers indicating the foods that tested "positive," which should be included in the diet, and the "top negative foods" that should be avoided.

> *The food-category scores disagree so much from test to test that Cohen's kappa is zero (complete randomness)... As with the basic scans, the individual-food scores were wildly inconsistent, with many foods scoring "positive" (recommended) on one test and "negative" (not recommended) on another administered a few minutes later....*

> *My basic scan results were so inconsistent that they could not possibly be clinically meaningful. In addition to being inconsistent, my food-category biosurveys recommended excluding so many foods that the resultant diets could be extremely unhealthful.[196]*

As stated previously, the company makes no claims that the coding is based on clinical studies. In fact, their website does not even have a "science" section. According to Dr. Stephen Barrett, his personal study is the only published, clinical study done.[197] It is disturbing to realize that thousands upon thousands of people around the world base their health decisions on the apparently random results achieved during a ZYTO scan.

Spiritual evaluation of energy medicine machines

Clearly, the machines employed within energy medicine do not measure up to scientific scrutiny, which is reason enough not to waste one's money on them or to use them as the basis for health decisions. Additionally, like energy medicine as a whole, participation with these machines may have spiritual concerns. We are told that Satan desires to steal, kill, and destroy and that he is the father of lies.[lxvi] Is it not apparent how the enemy of our souls can accomplish those goals through these machines? By believing a lie, individuals waste God given funds on worthless machines, products, and godless therapies. By believing a lie,

---

[lxvi] John 10:10 and John 8:44

individuals injure their health by consuming products that they do not need, grow convinced that they have health conditions that they do not have, avoid foods that God intends for them to enjoy, and avoid legitimate healthcare that they need. By believing a lie, individuals become slaves to a machine and do not truly seek the Creator for His infinite wisdom regarding their health issues.

One further spiritual concern arises in using these devices. Can the results be directly manipulated by demons? This is a question that I cannot answer with certainty, but a biblical case can be made to suggest the answer is yes. In a previous chapter, I discussed the observation that almost every human illness or condition that is specifically attributed to demons in the Bible could be caused through the person's nervous system. I also proposed the method by which demons work through muscle testing is by manipulating the nervous system. Most of the devices of energy medicine have direct ties to pagan or New Age belief systems, which open wide the door to demonic involvement. Many of these devices rely on the galvanic skin response, which is a proven measure of the autonomic nervous system responding to an electrical current. If demons can manipulate the nervous system, could they not create responses through the machine to achieve Satan's goals?

If you have been using any of the devices of energy medicine, I urge you to repent. If you own them, do not sell them to others who may then also be led astray, but rid your home of them in spite of the cost. Let the early believers who were saved out of sorcery be your example. (Acts 19:19)

2 Peter 3:15b-18 offers applicable wisdom and encouragement in these matters.

Paul also wrote to you according to the wisdom given him, as he does in all his letters when he speaks in them of these matters. There are some things in them that are hard to understand, which the ignorant and unstable twist to their own destruction, as they do the other Scriptures. You therefore, beloved, knowing this beforehand, take care that you are not carried away with the error of lawless people and lose your own stability. But grow in the grace and knowledge of our Lord and Savior Jesus Christ. To him be the glory both now and to the day of eternity. Amen.

CHAPTER 12

Hahnemann's Homeopathy

Abstain from every form of evil. 1 Thessalonians 5:22

It was every parent's nightmare. Overwhelming OCD, violent outbursts, passing out, temporary paralysis, and many other all-consuming symptoms began following a young boy's treatment through muscle testing. This avalanche of devastating symptoms prompted the boy's mother to reach out to me from across the globe. For many years after, the family searched traditional and alternative modalities in hopes of finding a diagnosis and a cure. Although conventional medicine offered no helpful insights, alternative practitioners agreed on a diagnosis of Lymes and PANS. Numerous treatments ensued.

After years of exhausting turmoil and suffering, they began consulting with a respected homeopath. The beleaguered mother described the experience to me. "When my son takes even the smallest amount of a homeopathic remedy, he reacts dramatically. It brings back big, bad symptoms! I have to take two little pellets and dissolve them in eight ounces of water, then take one teaspoon from that glass to put in another eight ounces of water, and then only give him one teaspoon. He is so sensitive, which makes it difficult! We've had remedies that have brought him back to us with no symptoms for three days and then just like that, it's back to PANS hell."

Recently, a friend also described to me her first and only experience with homeopathy. While attending an outdoor event, a bee stung her on the foot. The pain was great until a friend gave her one tiny homeopathic pill, and the pain disappeared! The immediate and sudden end to the pain surprised her, and so she questioned a doctor in the family. With certainty, he explained to her the power of the placebo effect as responsible for the noticeable improvement. She was skeptical of the doctor's explanation.

During my years of utilizing energy-based practices, my family and I also tried our first homeopathic remedy— *Oscillococcinum* for the flu. Just as it claims on the box, our miserable, flu-like symptoms lessened in severity and ended after two to three days.

Similar to most alternative modalities, the anecdotal evidence for homeopathy is abundant, but is there cause for concern? Is it energy-based, and if so, can one simply sidestep those aspects and still benefit from its use? As I have previously stated, just because something works, we cannot assume it is safe, so let us dig deeply into the history, scientific research, and information available on this popular, alternative branch of medicine.

The origins of homeopathy

At a time in medicine when bloodletting, purging, and the use of leaches were commonplace, a German physician, Samuel Hahnemann, founded a far more desirable approach to the treatment of illness. After receiving his M.D. degree at Erlangen in 1779, he practiced medicine for about five years. Frustrated by the medical practices of the day, he largely abandoned his field for research and earned income by translating into German the lectures of a respected doctor, William Cullen.

One day, while translating, Hahnemann encountered a passage in which Cullen discussed the use of a Peruvian bark, called Cinchona, used to treat malaria. Cullen concluded that the bark's bitter and astringent properties were responsible for its effectiveness. Considering that many herbs were bitter and astringent and yet ineffective for treating malaria, Hahnemann became intrigued regarding the real reason for Cinchona's effectiveness. (Unknown to them at the time, Cinchona contains large amounts of quinine, which is effective against malaria.) Desiring to test his own hypothesis, Hahnemann began repeatedly ingesting Cinchona in large doses and observed the development of symptoms that he claimed were similar to malaria, such as chills and fever. Although there is good reason to believe an allergy to quinine was the actual cause of these symptoms, the young doctor wrongly concluded that large doses of the bark caused the same symptoms of the illness it effectively treated at smaller doses.[198]

For the next six years, Hahnemann experimented on himself and his friends. They called these tests "provings," whereby they ingested countless substances and then catalogued every symptom, no matter how small, that followed in the minutes, days, and weeks to come. Hahnemann desired to prove his hypothesis that "like cures like"—*similia similibus curantur.* He believed that the same substances, which in large doses and in healthy people, produced the symptoms of a particular illness, can be used effectively in miniscule doses to treat illnesses with those same symptoms. (For example, coffee creates awakeness in large amounts, and so, by Hahnemann's reasoning, would make an effective remedy for treating insomnia in minute dosages.)

In 1796 he first published his work in a German medical journal establishing what he called the Law of Similar. He coined the name "homeopathy" (*homoios* in Greek means similar, *pathos* means suffering) to reflect this foundational belief.

According to Dana Ulman, a modern homeopath who has devoted his career to popularizing homeopathy, Hahnemann encountered much opposition from the apothecaries over formulating his miniscule-dosed remedies because they could not make sufficient money from selling such small doses. He also insisted on only prescribing one remedy at a time and formulating them in a strange fashion. These things led to much animosity and frustration with the apothecaries, causing Hahnemann to begin dispensing his own remedies. Unfortunately for him, doing so was illegal in Germany at that time. He was subsequently arrested in Leipzig in 1820, found guilty, and forced to move. After moving to Kothen, Germany,

Grand Duke Ferdinand, a supporter of homeopathy, gave Hahnemann a special dispensation to practice and dispense his own remedies.[199]

According to John Ankerberg and John Weldon, MD, the authors of *Can You Trust Your Doctor*,

> *Hahnemann himself claimed to be "inspired" in his homeopathic writings. In a letter to the town clerk of Kothen in 1828, he said he had been "guided by the invisible powers of the Almighty, listening, observing, tuning in to his instructions, paying most earnest heed and religious attention to this inspiration."*[200]

He also made the same claim, although worded more boldly, in the French edition of the *Organon*. *This book was written **under the dictation** of the Supreme Being.*[201] (emphasis mine). As we shall see through other quotes from Hahnemann's writings, he did not believe this "inspiration" and "dictation" came from the God of the Bible. Who can say if these daring claims of spiritual inspiration were true, but similar ones were made by the founders of several other branches of energy medicine. This alone should bring pause.

After many years in Kothen, Hahnemann moved again and found great acceptance practicing homeopathy in Paris until the time of his death in 1843. His legacy has waxed and waned in popularity throughout the world for the last two hundred years.

Provings

As mentioned, Hahnemann and his followers conducted tests, or "provings," whereby they administered all manner of natural substances to healthy individuals and kept detailed records of the symptoms observed. These accounts were later published in *Materia Medica* (Latin for "materials of medicine"), which are lengthy reference books that homeopaths use as guides to match a patient's symptoms with a corresponding remedy. The following account from *Materia Medica Pura* reveals the type of obscure symptoms recorded for the herb *matricaria chamomilla. Vertigo...Dull...aching pain in the head...Violent desire for coffee...Grumbling and creeping in the upper teeth...Great aversion to the wind...Burning pain in the hand...Quarrelsome, vexatious dreams...heat and redness of the right cheek...*[202] The supposed symptoms of chamomile go on for thirteen pages!

The belief that chamomile could cause thirteen pages of symptoms, and that it can, therefore, be used to treat effectively any ailment listed within those pages has raised many questions as to the validity of these "provings." How, for example, were those conducting the provings able to control the exposure of the one being tested to other substances for weeks following the consumption of chamomile? Did the procedures adhere to a scientific methodology? Since the determination of what remedy to use in homeopathic treatment is solely based on provings, determining their validity and reliability is important. In 2007 a team published a systematic review to address these questions. The abstract begins by saying,

> *The quality of information gathered from homeopathic pathogenetic trials (HPTs), also known as 'provings', is fundamental to homeopathy. We systematically reviewed HPTs published in six languages (English, German, Spanish, French, Portuguese and Dutch) from 1945 to 1995, to assess their quality in terms of the validity of the information they provide.*[203]

Their conclusions state, *The HPTs were generally of low methodological quality... Improvement of the method and reporting of results of HPTs are* required.[204]

The authors of *Can You Trust Your Doctor?* discuss Hahnemann's provings in their meticulously researched, fifty-page chapter on homeopathy.

> ***However, these provings have not been reproduced.*** *In a significant lecture series by Oliver Wendell Holmes, M.D., who was a highly respected anatomy professor for 35 years at Harvard Medical School, he described how a renowned doctor and professor of medicine in Paris and others* ***attempted for a year to reproduce Hahnemann's provings but without success.*** *He goes on to give*

specific examples of others through history who found that Cinchona bark did not produce the negative symptoms that Hahnemann claimed to experience and on which all of homeopathy was founded.[205] (emphasis mine)

Making a remedy through dilutions & shaking

Understanding how homeopathic remedies are made and the philosophies that dictate their formulation is paramount for the Christian to understand when considering its use. As an example of this process, consider the previously mentioned homeopathic remedy for insomnia—coffee. *Coffea cruda* is made from a dilution of coffee beans. One drop of coffee bean extract is placed in a vial with nine drops of water. Then, one drop is removed from the first vial and placed in another with nine drops of water. That process continues sixty times. However, an important detail of the dilutions includes the mixture being vigorously shaken after each drop is placed into a new vial of water.

One might wonder why such a laborious process is used. Why not just put one drop of extract in an enormous vat of water? Although I will later discuss the spiritual reasons driving Hahnemann's methodology, the foremost mouthpiece for homeopathy, Dana Ulman and also his colleague Stephen Cummings, discuss why this dilution practice continues,

Homeopaths have found that the medicines do not work if they are simply diluted repeatedly without vigorous shaking or if they are just diluted in vast amounts of liquid. Nor do the medicines work if they are only vigorously shaken. It is the combined process of dilution and vigorous shaking that makes the medicine effective...[206]

If it is true that these remedies only work if they are diluted and shaken ("dynamized" or "potentized" as homeopaths call it), the question should be asked as to why? If there is no scientific explanation and the remedies do produce results, then there is cause for concern that the answer is spiritual in nature. The National Council Against Health Fraud (NCAHF) position paper on homeopathy from 2020 speaks of the failure of science to explain homeopathic remedies and therefore, how homeopathy has, by and large, changed their rhetoric to the public to emphasize the Law of Similar instead of potentization.

Potentization - dynamization is also the weakest point of homeopathy. In the 19th century it was still hoped science would confirm some healing force in the homeopathically prepared medicines. This has not happened, and at present the importance of homeopathically dynamized medicines has been quietly replaced by the principle 'Similia Similibus Curentur.' The description of the dynamization - potentization process is for the initiated, revealed in courses and schools for homeopaths. For the lay public it is the Law of Similar which is being presented as homeopathy.[207]

Hahnemann stipulated that dilutions were done in factors of ten (represented by the letter X) or one hundred (represented by the letter C). If a remedy is prepared by a scale of one hundred, then one drop of the extract is added to ninety-nine drops of water. Most homeopathic remedies are formulated at dilution rates that far exceed the laws of chemistry based on Avogadro's number, which states that a limit exists to the dilution rate, at which point the original substance is lost completely.[lxvii] This proven limit means that once a homeopathic potency reaches 12C or 24X it no longer contains a single molecule of the original substance. Today, many products of 30C or more are marketed.[208]

To put this in perspective, Stephen Barrett, MD recounts how Robert L. Park, PhD, a leading physicist and director of The American Physical Society, explained,

...since the least amount of a substance in a solution is one molecule, a 30C solution would have to have at least one molecule of the original substance dissolved in a minimum of 1,000,000,000,000,000,000,000,000,000,000,000,000,000,000,

---

[lxvii] More specifically, Avogadro showed that there is a large but finite and specific number of atoms or molecules in a mole of substance.

000,000,000,000,000 molecules of water. This would require a container more than 30,000,000,000 times the size of the Earth.[209]

For those of us who zone-out upon seeing so many numbers, let me offer instead an illustration offered by Dr. Browning in his article *Modern Homeopathy: Its Absurdities and Inconsistencies*:

Weigh out a grain of any substance; it can be held on the point of a penknife. To make the third "potency" the grain must be dissolved in one hundred pints of fluid. This is equal to about half an ordinary barrel. If the grain were dissolved in our city reservoir, the water drawn from our faucets would equal about the sixth "potency." If it were dropped into some lake, about two miles in circumference, the water would equal in strength the ninth "potency." Sprinkle the grain on the bosom of "old ocean" and the waters of the seas would become medicine of about the twelfth "potency." How are we to carry the illustration further? It is unnecessary. It will be sufficient to remark that if the whole grain were to be made up into the thirtieth "potency" it would require more liquid in volume than the bulk of the visible universe.[210]

In light of this, consider one of the most popular homeopathic remedies, *Oscillococcinum*, a **200C** product "for the relief of colds and flu-like symptoms." It is particularly noteworthy in its extreme excesses of Avogadro's number! Barrett writes,

Its "active ingredient" is prepared by incubating small amounts of a freshly killed duck's liver and heart for 40 days. The resultant solution is then filtered, freeze-dried, rehydrated, repeatedly diluted, and impregnated into sugar granules. If a single molecule of the duck's heart or liver were to survive the dilution, its concentration would be 1 in 100^{200}. This huge number, which has 400 zeroes, is vastly greater than the estimated number of molecules in the universe (about one googol, which is a 1 followed by 100 zeroes). In its February 17, 1997, issue, U.S. News & World Report noted that only

one duck per year is needed to manufacture the product, which had
total sales of $20 million in 1996. The magazine dubbed that unlucky
bird "the $20-million duck."[211]

Homeopathic consultation

Another remarkable facet of Hahnemann's homeopathy includes the
homeopathic consultation. Like several other aspects of homeopathy, the
approach is thorough and lengthy. Hahnemann taught that *treating the*
whole person means being guided by the unique aspects of his or her
physical and mental life, and, in homeopathy, by the peculiar symptoms
that he or she manifests.[212] To determine this complete picture of the
patient, the homeopath must spend a considerable amount of time
questioning the particulars of symptoms, thoughts, and behaviors.
Hahnemann further instructed: *He begins a fresh line [of questioning] with*
every new circumstance mentioned by the patient or his friends...[213]

According to Hahnemann, to do this the homeopath should question
the patient about seemingly obscure and unrelated habits and feelings,
such as how one prefers to sleep or whether they like walking barefoot and
how the person feels before a storm or when their collar is unbuttoned.[214]
Homeopath Dr. Jacques Michaud also adds that *dreams are a mysterious*
but important aspect of the personality...The information we draw from
them is sometimes precise enough to indicate a remedy.[215]

According to the volumes of reference books describing homeopathic
provings, there are often a thousand or more potential remedies to choose
from, but the homeopath must select the one most suited to that individual.
This goal guides the homeopath's unique and detailed line of questioning.
For many individuals who feel their physical condition has not been
addressed adequately by the brief appointments typically found in
traditional medicine, the lengthy homeopathic consultation seems
validating.

Occult influences

Earlier, I mentioned that Hahnemann claimed divine inspiration for
homeopathy, but judge for yourself by his own writings what manner of

spiritual influences shaped his thinking. For example, one of his biographers writes:

> *He took offense at the arch-enthusiast Jesus of Nazareth, who did not lead the enlightened on the straight way to wisdom but who wanted to struggle with publicans and sinners on a difficult path toward the establishment of the kingdom of God...The man of sorrows who took the darkness of the world on Himself was an offense to the lover of etheric wisdom [Hahnemann].*[216] (emphasis mine)

Samuel Hahnemann dined from a smorgasbord of spiritually concerning teachers and influences including mystic and heretic Emanuel Swedenborg, Confucious, astrology, and Freemasonry. Consider the following quote from Samuel Pheifer, MD, who writes about these influences in the book, *Healing at Any Price?*

> *On Confucius, Hahnemann himself writes in a letter: "This is where you can read divine wisdom, without [e.g., Christian] miracle-myths and superstition. I regard it as an important sign of our times that Confucius is now available for us to read. Soon I will embrace him in the kingdom of blissful spirits, the benefactor of humanity, who has shown us the straight path to wisdom and to God, already 650 years before the arch-enthusiast..." The reverence for Eastern thought was not just Hahnemann's personal hobby, but rather the fundamental philosophy behind the preparation of homeopathic remedies.*[217] (emphasis mine)

Dr. Pheifer also writes of the testimony given by a leading Swiss homeopath, Adolf Voegeli, who described his interactions with Hahnemann,

> *When I asked him about the cosmic energy which was supposedly working through homeopathy, he explained: "You know, I believe in the power of the zodiac." Voegeli underscores that the effect of high*

potencies in homeopathy is of a "spiritual nature." His best explanation is supplied by the hinduistic Sankhya philosophy. According to it man not only has his physical body but also an ethereal body with a special system of energetic channels. It is this ethereal body that co-ordinates the immunological functions and enhances the wound-healing process. And it is here that homeopathy is active.[218]

Additionally, according to H.J. Bopp, MD, author of *Homeopathy, We know that he was a member of a Lodge of Free Masons.*[219] Dr. Pfeifer also concurs and gives more detail. *As a young man Hahnemann had become a member of the Free Masons...It is no surprise that Hahnemann, as a member of the lodge, disparagingly called Jesus an 'arch-enthusiast.'*[220] He placed the logo for Freemasonry, "Aude Sapere" (dare to be wise) on the title page of *The Organon of Medicine*, his primary text for homeopathy.

Hahnemann also wrote in detail in the *Organon* about other spiritual philosophies that influenced the practices of homeopathy:

I find it yet necessary to allude here to animal magnetism, as it is termed, or rather Mesmerism...It is a marvelous priceless gift of God...by means of which the strong will of a well-intentioned person upon a sick one by contact and even without this and even at some distance, can bring the vital energy of the healthy mesmerizer endowed with this power into another person dynamically...The above mentioned methods of practicing mesmerism depend upon an influx of more or less vital force into the patient...[221]

Vital force or energy

After learning of the many occultic influences in Hahnemann's life, it is not surprising to discover in his writings the pagan idea he calls *vital force*. The same idea has many names such as *chi, prana, subtle energy, orgone,* or the *Innate.* Regardless of the particular name given, all forms of energy-based medicine insist that an imbalance of energy in the body creates illness. That Hahnemann concurred can be read in the fifth and sixth editions of the *Organon*, which contain much discussion of vital force. He wrote:

> *The diseases of man are not caused by any[material] substance...any disease-matter, but...they are **solely spirit-like** (dynamic) derangements of the spirit-like power (the vital principle) that animates the human body. **Homeopathy knows that a cure can only take place by the reaction of the vital force against the rightly chosen remedy that has been ingested.***

> *Thus, the **true healing art is...to affect an alteration in...energetic automatic vital force**...whereby the vital force is liberated and enabled to return to the normal standard of health and to its proper function...Homeopathy teaches us how to affect this.*[222] (emphasis mine)

The spiritual reasons for shaking a remedy.

As stated earlier, homeopaths insist that a remedy must be vigorously shaken in between each dilution or else it will be ineffectual. Hahnemann wrote in the *Organon* his reasoning behind the practice of shaking a remedy. He first likens the process to how an iron bar or a steel rod can be rubbed strongly to magnetize them. He goes on to say, *...similarly by the trituration of a medicinal substance and the succussion of its solution (dynamization, potentization) the medicinal forces lying hidden in it are developed and uncovered more and more, **and the material is itself spiritualized** ....*[223] (emphasis mine)

Dr. Richard Grossinger, author of *Planet Medicine: From Stone Age Shamanism to Post-Industrial Healing* also writes of Hahnemann's reasoning behind shaking a remedy.

> *Then he tried shaking the vials very hard at each dilution. It is uncertain what caused him to try this, and there is no one explanation in Hahnemann's known studies, although many different*

*hermeticisms, including alchemy, urged creative interaction with substances. Later ethnographic literature shows that **primitive peoples prepare medicines by pounding, grinding, ...scraping ...punching [etc.]...--all to wake the spirits in the medicine or bring spirits to attach themselves to it. African [witch] doctors have claimed that medicines contain no power in themselves but gain it from [this] dynamic contact. The well-read Hahnemann may have been aware of some of this lore.*[224]* (emphasis mine)*

The "laws" of homeopathy

To further consider the permeating spiritual influences and basis for homeopathy, let us look more closely at the "laws" Hahnemann originated and promoted. According to the Oxford English Dictionary, a scientific law is a *statement, based on repeated experiments or observations, that describe or predict a range of natural phenomena.* A law can be disproven by future evidence, which science has sufficiently done following Hahnemann's creation of the laws of homeopathy. Nonetheless, homeopathy persists in its insistence that some yet undiscovered explanation will prove his laws.

Understanding these four laws, which continue to undergird the practices of homeopathy, is critical. Homeopath and founder of the Resonance School of Homeopathy, Robert Field, summarizes the appropriate mindset behind understanding these laws. *When mankind embraces our spirituality and recognizes the divinity within each of us, the change will take place... It is best if we remember that homeopathy is spiritual medicine and let it flourish naturally.*[225]

The Law of Similar

Hahnemann defined his Law of Similar as . . . *disease is combatted by a medicine . . . capable of creating in the healthy body symptoms most similar to those of the . . . disease.*[226] To hear a homeopath explain this law (otherwise known as *like cures like*), sounds reasonable at first glance. The foremost spokesperson for homeopathy, Dana Ulman, offers several convincing examples for comparison between homeopathy and conventional medicine. (If you recall from a previous chapter, pseudoscience always attempts to tie a proven scientific truth to an unproven aspect of their practice in order to give their practice legitimacy. False comparisons characterize pseudoscience.)

> *Conventional medicine also uses homeopathic-like therapy in choosing radiation to treat people with cancer (radiation causes cancer), digitalis for heart conditions (digitalis creates heart conditions), and Ritalin for hyperactive children (Ritalin is an amphetamine-like drug which normally causes hyperactivity). Other examples are the use of nitroglycerine for heart conditions, gold salts for arthritic conditions, and colchicine for gout.*[227]

Ulman also points to the use of vaccinations, which use minute amounts of a disease-causing agent to stimulate the immune system to build up future resistance to the disease. Although these comparisons may appear at first glance to be comparing apples with apples, they are definitely not! For example, vaccinations and all of the medicines listed by Ulman in the previous quote actually have measurable amounts of the drug present, whereas homeopathic remedies typically do not have a single molecule of the original substance. Furthermore, each of the drugs he mentioned went through extensive clinical testing and have been proven to do what they claim to do. This is not the case with homeopathic remedies. And so, these significant differences indicate Ulman's comparisons are actually apples and oranges; and therefore, unworthy examples as proof of the Law of Similar.

Instead, William W. Browning, MD, AB, LL.B., offers more accurate comparisons in his article, "Modern Homeopathy: Its Absurdities and Inconsistencies." *Opium will control pain. Quinine will reduce fever. Alcohol and ammonia will relieve faintness. Now if "similia" be a law, opium ought to cause pain in the healthy; quinine, fever; alcohol, faintness, etc.; but this is not the case.*

Hahnemann indicates that the cornerstone of homeopathy, The Law of Similar, came from his experience with Cinchona and the countless provings that followed. Although he is credited with popularizing this teaching, his ideas were not formed in a vacuum. *As early as 400 years B.C., Hippocrates, the father of medicine, made the observation that some diseases are best treated by similars.*[228] (emphasis mine) These ideas also come from a monistic view that is the basis of many ancient practices. The 2020 position paper of the NCAHF on homeopathy discusses monism and gives familiar examples of its beliefs that *like is like, like makes like, and like cures like...e.g., eating the heart of a lion for courage... idolatry in which carving a likeness of a god actually produces the god... snakeroot being good for snakebite, because of their resemblance.*[229]

Hahnemann's law revived the very wording and reasoning behind those beliefs from the well-known 15th century physician and alchemist, Paracelsus, also known as the "Prince of Quacks."[230] He called it *the sole law of cure.* In his *Doctrine of Signatures,* Paracelsus repeated the monistic philosophy when he *declared that herbs would cure conditions or anatomical parts they resembled.*[231]

Because the Law of Similar is the foundation upon which all homeopathy rests, determining whether the house has been built upon rock or sand should be a one goal for evaluating homeopathy. According to Dr. Browning, *In describing the operation of the law of "similia," Hahnemann tells us that nature, unaided, cannot throw off disease; that medicines are, therefore, essential.*[232] However, to take more of what is making one sick, cannot make one better. This reality will be confirmed when we look into the abundant clinical research that has been done on homeopathic remedies. *The homeopathic Law of Similia... is unsupported by the basic sciences of physiology, pharmacology, and pathology.*[233]

The Law of Infinitesimals or minimum dose

Because Hahnemann's logic regarding like-curing-like had obvious flaws, he compensated with the second law—the Law of Infinitesimals. Rather than giving small amounts of a substance that makes one sick to make one better, he instead determined that a no-medicine medicine was necessary, and so was born the Law of Infinitesimals or minimum dose. It is believed that *any homeopathic medicine is made more powerful the more one shakes and dilutes it.*[234] Hahnemann wrote in the *Organon,*

Modern wiseacres have even sneered at the thirtieth potency...[but] we obtain, even in the fiftieth potency, medicines of the most penetrating efficacy...[235]

According to physicist, Robert Park, PhD,

Hahnemann could not have known that in his preparations he was, in fact, exceeding the dilution limit. Although he was contemporary with the physicist Amadeo Avogadro (1776-1856), Hahnemann's Organon...was published in 1810, one year before Avogadro advanced his famous hypothesis and many years before other physicists actually determined Avogadro's number.[236]

Even if Hahnemann knew of the prevailing theory, which would invalidate his work, the revelation mattered little because he *believed that the vigorous shaking or pulverizing with each step of dilution leaves behind a "spirit-like" essence—"no longer perceptible to the senses"— which cures by reviving the body's "vital force."*[237] Homeopathic remedies, according to Hahnemann, were spiritual remedies for a spiritual condition.

Some subsequent homeopaths were not so keen on dismissing science, and they, therefore, promote a false belief that "water has memory." In 1988, the French scientist, Benveniste, who worked at the prestigious INSERM institute, published some astounding claims in the highly regarded science journal, *Nature*. He purported to have proved that *high dilutions of substances in water left a "memory," providing a rationale for homeopathy's Law of Infinitesimals. Nature* included in their publication *the caveat that the findings were unbelievable, and that the work was financed by a large homeopathic drug manufacturer.*[238] Clearly, the theory that "water could remember" required further investigation, so a team from *Nature* magazine and James Randi[lxviii] went to observe

---

[lxviii] Randi is a magician who likes to disprove the unbelievable. He has issued a million-dollar challenge to anyone who can biologically prove homeopathy, and so he had a particular interest in whether Benveniste could prove his claim while others witnessed his experiments.

Benveniste repeat his experiments. Not surprisingly, his lab procedures did not include *proper blind methodology,* [and] *he was unable to reproduce his original results.*[239] Benveniste has since been suspended and has received *two "Ig Nobel" prizes, the most recent one for digitally recording the biological activity of a homeopathic solution, sending it over the Internet as an attached document, and transferring it to another water sample at the destination!)*[240] The experiments on which Benveniste based his claim that water has memory were again unsuccessfully repeated by a British team on BBC television.[241] Again, this is how science works. If something is true scientifically, it is repeatable.

Consider for a moment, the ramifications if water did indeed have memory. How could one safely drink water? Would not all municipal water that has been filtered from waste be a public safety concern? Even if one went to the purest spring on the planet, would it not have water that contained the memory of innumerable natural toxins from the polluted rainwater that filtered down into the aquifer? Thank the LORD, that water does not have memory, and neither does a homeopathic dilution.

The Law of Single Remedy

The next law is one that many modern homeopaths choose to ignore because of its impracticality. According to Dana Ulman, The Law of Single Remedy dictates that only one homeopathic dilution should be used at a time *to address the totality of symptoms primarily according to the chief complaint. Hahnemann referred to those practitioners who used more than a single medicine as "pseudo-homeopaths" and other less kind things.* [242] The symptoms indicate the single, appropriate remedy but not in the sense of focusing on an individual ailment but the collective whole.

For the homeopath to determine the one remedy from the thousand-odd possibilities detailed in the seven, roughly seven-hundred-page, volumes of the *Materia Medica* require a thorough understanding of the patient and a mind-boggling depth of knowledge. Even then, a process of trial and error often ensues. *The conscientious homeopath selects his or her curative from 2,500 base substances: plants, minerals, chemicals, animals, and insects. He or she then chooses among at least 30 degrees of dilution and finally among 20 different pill forms—over one million possible combinations.*[243]

Furthermore, another modern homeopath Robert Field writes that *for as many people who suffer that named disease, there are equally as many remedies for them as a person. We must not forget that it is the organism that the vital force is animating. It is responsible for all expressions of life, dis-ease, and healing. It all comes from the spiritual vital force.*[244]

The difficulties presented by the Law of Single Remedy have caused many a homeopath to disregard their founder's teaching on this point. Some combine multiple remedies into one. Others have chosen to uphold this law but have found the use of divining tools such as pendulums, muscle testing, and radionic devices to be necessary assets for circumventing the time required in accurately selecting the right remedy.[245]

The Law of Spiritual Cause

Six editions of the *Organon* exist. The last two contain much teaching about the vital force being the only cause of disease and the spiritual reasoning behind dynamization. Perhaps the stronger spiritual teachings resulted from the advances in medicine and scientific understanding throughout his career that seriously jeopardized homeopathy's credibility. Perhaps this awareness caused Hahnemann to realize new explanations were required. Whatever the reason, the Law of Spiritual Cause was firmly promoted by Hahnemann. As you have read from numerous quotes in his writings, Hahnemann staunchly taught, *The diseases of man are not caused by any[material] substance...any disease-matter, but...they are* **solely spirit-like** *(dynamic) derangements of the spirit-like power (the vital principle) that animates the human body.*[246]

Although not all homeopaths hold to the Law of Spiritual Cause, many of the vocal proponents of homeopathy do. Consider what Herbert Robert, a homeopath and author of *Art of Cure by Homeopathy* writes,

If therefore, this force, this energy, actuates or permeates all forms and degrees of life..., we may reasonably assume that vital force is

the most fundamental of all conditions of the universe, and that the laws governing the vital force in the individual are correlated with the laws which govern all vital force, all forms of energy, wherever or however expressed...[247]

Some proponents seek to legitimize homeopathy by combining it with modern medicine. Homeopath Robert Field, founder of the Resonance School of Homeopathy, however, makes a strong argument against this.

A pattern I see happening in the world of homeopathy is an attempt to legitimize homeopathy and make it mainstream. This would be nice if homeopathy fit that model of medicine. Unfortunately, it does not... Some people in the homeopathic community want to have homeopathy included along-side of allopathy. This will most likely never work. **The fundamental premise is very different... It is best if we remember that homeopathy is spiritual medicine and let it flourish naturally.**[248] (emphasis mine)

Scientific studies on homeopathy

The task of researching the scientific evidence relating to homeopathy is overwhelming as it requires sifting through the methodology and conclusions from a plethora of clinical studies throughout 200 years of history. It requires patience and persistence to dig deep into the studies that proponents herald as trophies of evidence proving homeopathy. It turns out that misrepresentation or outright deception characterize these ill-gotten trophies. Consider four such studies that follow. All four have now been discounted; yet, in spite of this, these studies are still cited by proponents as compelling evidence.

One such study originally published results from a study on rats, which tested whether a homeopathic remedy using poison oak (Rhus Tox [RT]) worked to reduce inflammation and pain. The study was declared by advocates as proof for homeopathy but was retracted eight months later by Springer Nature journal. Upon looking further into the study, the publisher discovered numerous problems that discounted the favorable results originally reported.[249]

In another case, a year after triumphantly publishing positive conclusions from a meta-analysis another retraction was issued. The article, "Is homeopathy effective for attention deficit and hyperactivity disorder? A meta-analysis," appeared in June of 2022 in *Pediatric Research*, a Springer Nature title. The original conclusion of the paper boldly claimed that *individualized homeopathy showed a clinically relevant and statistically robust effect in the treatment of ADHD.*[250] The review considered six individual studies.

It was discovered that significant bias for homeopathy was shown by manipulation of the subjects chosen for the homeopathic treatment group and misrepresentation of the data. "Based on the above deficiencies following thorough review, the Editor-in-Chief has substantial concerns regarding the validity of the results presented in this article."[251]

A third study was conducted in 1986 and initially purported that Asthma was improved by the homeopathic remedy known as *Dumcap*—a combination dilution made with *nux vomica* (strychnine), arsenic album (arsenic trioxide), *Blatta onentalis* (cockroach extract), and *stramoni folic* (stramonium). Professor Alyn Morice, who is Head of Respiratory Medicine at HYMS, based at the University of Hull, also runs the Hull Respiratory Clinical Trials Unit, specializing in the treatment of asthma and COPD. After the professor initially reported that *Dumcap* was effective in improving symptoms of asthma in a group of students, an analysis was performed of the *Dumcap* used in the clinical trial. Morice then reported a shocking truth. The product used in the study was adulterated with therapeutic levels of the anti-asthma, steroidal drugs prednisolone and betamethasone.[252] (These additional drugs were not listed on the label.) No wonder the product worked!

A fourth study published in 2022 tested the effectiveness of homeopathy as an add-on treatment for small-cell lung cancer. This one caught my attention because it appeared to check off all the boxes for legitimacy— randomized, placebo-controlled, double-blind, three-arm, multicenter, phase III study. In the clinical study world, it does not get much better than that! The conclusions reported would cause anyone to stand up and take notice:

> *QoL [quality of life] improved significantly in the homeopathy group compared with placebo. In addition, survival was significantly longer in the homeopathy group versus placebo and control...The study suggests that homeopathy positively influences not only QoL but also survival.*[253]

Wow! Now that is impressive! However, as I continued to read the abstract and considered the multiple charts and graphs, things did not seem to add up, but then again, such evaluations are not my area of expertise. Nonetheless, my questions did cause me to look further, and alas, I discovered the following official "expression of concern" issued months later by the publisher of the study. *In August 2022, the journal editors received credible information from the Austrian Agency for Research Integrity about potential data falsification and data manipulation in this article.*[254]

As my research continued, I found greater clarification from an update posted on the blog of Edzard Ernst, MD, PhD. He is a researcher and trained homeopath with too many other titles to mention them all. In the article he completes the story as to why the "expression of concern" was issued and why a retraction should ensue. Both Austrian and German agencies appealed to the Medical Institute of Vienna with credible evidence of data manipulation in the lung cancer study. They asked the Institute to consider a review of the study and to look further into the matter, which they did. After much time, their conclusions were as follows: *The committee concludes that there are **numerous breaches of scientific integrity in the Study**, as reported in the Publication. Several of the results can only be explained by **data manipulation or falsification**. The Publication is not a fair representation of the Study.*[255] (emphasis mine)

I highlight those studies as a subset of the numerous ones like them that are falsely promoted as truth. One cannot simply assume the claims of evidence for homeopathy are justifiable or that what is initially reported will hold up to later scrutiny. Those four examples continue to be falsely promoted as legitimate evidence of homeopathy's validity, yet, they are questionable at best and intentionally fraudulent at worst.

Systematic reviews of clinical studies

Because thousands of clinical studies have been done on homeopathic remedies, several systematic reviews have been conducted by various agencies in order to collectively analyze those results more effectively. One such review was performed in 2015 by the National Health & Medical Research Council of the Australian Government (NHMRC). After reviewing around two hundred studies, the agency published a forty-page report that stated the following conclusions:

- *Based on all the evidence considered, there were no health conditions for which there was reliable evidence that homeopathy was effective.*
- *No good-quality, well-designed studies with enough participants for a meaningful result reported either that homeopathy caused greater health improvements than placebo or caused health improvements equal to those of another treatment.*
- *Homeopathy should not be used to treat conditions that are chronic, serious, or could become serious.*[256]

In May of 2023, another systematic review was done to evaluate clinical studies that were conducted to test the effect of homeopathic treatment on patients undergoing cancer treatment. The studies considered spanned over two hundred years (1800-2020) and analyzed whether homeopathy brought physical or mental improvement during oncological treatment. They concluded: *For homeopathy, there is neither a scientifically based hypothesis of its mode of action nor conclusive evidence from clinical studies in cancer care.*[257]

Although there are numerous reviews of clinical studies that I could share, I will conclude with a notable one that summarizes them all because it is a systematic review of systematic reviews. This one is also unique, in that, it was done by the trained homeopath mentioned previously with his long list of impressive qualifications—Edzard Ernst. It is worth mentioning that he was also awarded the 2015 John Maddox Prize "for his long commitment to applying scientific methodologies in research into complementary and alternative medicines." With his significant knowledge and expertise in the field, the conclusions he came to are worthy of notice. After thoroughly analyzing seventeen other systematic reviews/meta-analysis, Ernst states:

> ...*the hypothesis that any given homeopathic remedy leads to clinical effects that are relevantly different from placebo or superior to other control interventions for any medical condition, **is not supported by evidence from systematic reviews**. Until more compelling results are available, homeopathy cannot be viewed as an evidence-based form of therapy.*[258] (emphasis mine)

Like it or not, the "laws" of homeopathy contradict proven laws of chemistry, physics, and biology so the conclusions of those clinical studies should not be surprising. In the words of David Gorski, MD, PhD and managing editor for "Science-Based Medicine," *We have already trusted in the scientific method that tells us that, for homeopathy to work, several laws of physics would have to be not just wrong, but spectacularly wrong.*[259] In light of this, homeopathy has the burden of proof in establishing its validity through the scientific method. Sadly, time and time again, one discovers that any apparent positive outcomes are merely deceptions. As Thomas Paine (1737-1809) asked, *Is it more probable that nature should go out of her course or that a man should tell a lie?*[260]

Evaluating homeopathy—How does it "work?"

Some may ask, why does it matter that scientific study has failed to prove homeopathy as long as it works? As I have discussed in previous chapters, determining HOW these practices work reveals significant insight into the true nature of it. If something is measurable according to the scientific process, then we know that it is "working" according to laws within the physical realm—*the fixed order of heaven and earth*.[lxix] Even quantum mechanics operates consistently and measurably in the physical realm. Therefore, if something does not hold up to scientific scrutiny, yet appears impactful, we have to ask, "why?". I began this chapter with real anecdotes of homeopathy working. The National Center for Homeopathy has a website to collect stories of people who have had positive experiences with homeopathy so that others might be encouraged to also use it. If homeopathy has yet to be proven in two hundred years, in spite of thousands of clinical studies being done, how can so many people emphatically declare; "It works!"?

Dr. Edzard Ernst, offers the following perspective that is also held by many knowledgeable doctors:

> *Yet as a clinician almost 30 years ago, I was impressed with the results achieved by homeopathy. Many of my patients seemed to improve dramatically after receiving homeopathic treatment. How was this possible? ...Experience is real, of course, but it does not establish causality. If observational data show improvements while clinical trials tell us that homeopathic remedies are placebos, the conclusion that fits all of these facts comfortably is straightforward: patients get better, not because of the homeopathic remedy but because of a placebo-effect and the lengthy consultation with a compassionate clinician. This conclusion is not just logical, it is also supported by data. Homeopaths from Southampton recently demonstrated that the consultation not the remedy is the element that improves clinical outcomes of patients after seeing a homeopath.*[261]

I have previously discussed the legitimate and powerful placebo effect. Ernst suggests, with evidence to back up his conclusion, that the lengthy and compassionate nature of homeopathic consultation produces

---

[lxix] Jeremiah 33:25

a placebo effect in the patient. However, this explanation fails to consider the many who never actually consult with a homeopath but instead experience results after deciding independently which products to take. In these cases, a simple belief in the effectiveness of the products could also produce the placebo effect. Placebo effects can be powerful, of course, but the potential benefit of relieving symptoms with placebos should be weighed against the harm that can result from relying upon—and wasting money on—ineffective products.

Another physical realm explanation for how they work has been suggested, which is the normal recuperative ability of the body. For instance, in my experience with *Oscillo*, the homeopathic flu remedy, we may not have truly had influenza but some similar infection that we would have recovered from in two or three days regardless of what we did. In the example at the start of this chapter of the sudden end to pain from a bee sting, it may have been coincidence that the pain stopped after my friend ingested the remedy. As a beekeeper myself, who has been stung numerous times, the pain of honeybee stings often subsides abruptly after a few minutes. When dealing with any symptom or illness, people often attribute recovery to something they did, when in reality spontaneous remission occurred.

Because the FDA does not regulate homeopathic remedies, the rate or frequency of adulterated products is unknown. We do know, however, that it does happen, as came to light in the study of the asthma remedy *Dumcap*. When a homeopathic remedy has an actual drug added to it, the effectiveness will likely be the result of the added drug. The danger, of course, increases when you know nothing of what you are actually taking and how it may interact with other things you ingest.

Evaluating homeopathy—Is it dangerous?

I would suggest one final explanation for how homeopathy works— witchcraft. I realize that such wording is strong but consider what we know. The foundational premises of homeopathy are occultic. Two pagan beliefs form bookends to a permeating demonic philosophy undergirding homeopathy—from a belief in an energy imbalance (*vital force*) being the root of one's illness to the intentional methodology in creating a spiritual remedy to restore that balance. It is known by all in homeopathy that most of the remedies do not contain a single molecule of the original substance and yet are believed to be made potent by a pagan process of dilution and shaking.

Before I knew anything about homeopathy, I became suspicious of demonic influences simply because of the anecdotes I heard. Many responses to these remedies are dramatic and instantaneous. How can this be? Unless you are being given intravenous drugs, the results of medications, even powerful ones, take time to have an effect. How, I ask, can a no-medicine medicine work so powerfully and quickly? Yes, the placebo effect could certainly be the answer and may often be the answer, but the alternative is that there are spiritual forces at work.

As Ankerberg and Weldon write, *Does not the history of animism prove that spirits often seek to work behind material objects such as idols, Tarot cards, dowsing rods, and many other items? Then could they not also work behind homeopathic medicines?*[262] Hahnemann himself concluded that homeopathy must produce spiritual medicines, not physical ones.

Some may believe that a Christian can "redeem" homeopathy and still benefit from its use. As previously sited, the non-Christian homeopath Robert Field speaks of the fact that homeopathy cannot be separated from its origins. *A pattern I see happening in the world of homeopathy is an attempt to legitimize homeopathy and make it mainstream. This would be nice if homeopathy fit that model of medicine. Unfortunately, it does not.*[263]

As I have maintained throughout this book, if something is inherently evil, it cannot be redeemed. If you divorce the spiritual influences from homeopathy, you no longer have homeopathy. The two are inseparable. Consider what Christian physician, Dr. Bopp said in his book *Homeopathy*,

> *There are to be sure some honorable and conscientious ones seeking to utilize a homeopathy detached from its obscure practices. Yet, the occult influence, by nature hidden, disguised, often dissimulated behind a para scientific theory, does not disappear and does not*

happen to be rendered harmless by the mere fact of a superficial approach contenting itself simply with denying its existence. Homeopathy is dangerous. It is quite contrary to the teaching of the Word of God. It willingly favors healing through substances made dynamic, that is to say, charged with occult forces. Homeopathic treatment is the fruit of a philosophy and religion that are at the same time Hinduistic, pantheistic, and esoteric.[264]

Ankerberg and Weldon write in *Can You Trust Your Doctor?* of the danger in flirting with the occult and the price Hahnemann himself paid for doing so.

Although Hahnemann founded a form of medicine that became popular and continues to this day, his own life was fraught with endless personal tragedy, as though the devil was determined to take his due. His children lived in terrible poverty...One son died shortly after birth; another, who was mentally ill, left one day and never returned. Three of his daughters' marriages ended in divorce; two daughters were murdered in a mysterious way. Another daughter died at birth. Another died when she was thirty. His only remaining son deserted his wife and child. Over the years Hahnemann's character and personality had changed in strange ways. A. Fritsche, one of his biographers, observes: "Hahnemann had to empty the cup of demonism with which his father had endowed him"[265]

Dr. Bopp similarly shares his serious concerns about homeopathy born out of his clinical experience: *"The occult influence in homeopathy is transmitted to the individual, bringing him consciously or unconsciously under demonic influence...It is significant frequently to find nervous depression in families using homeopathic treatments"*[266]

I could also write of the numerous illnesses and death caused by adulterated remedies or of the tragic death of children due to parents who failed to seek true medical treatment for infections because they put their hope in homeopathy.[lxx] The devil does not care how destruction is achieved, only that it is. Many who use homeopathy do so out of a false belief that its remedies are natural and that homeopathy treats the root cause of disease rather than symptoms. However, neither is true. If one believes that the root cause of disease is an imbalance in energy and therefore a spiritually empowered remedy (witchcraft) can alone restore that balance, then homeopathy is the answer. However, for the child of God, 1 Thessalonians 5:22 gives clear instruction: ***Abstain from every form of evil.***[lxxi]

[lxx] Child dies from brain infection that began as an ear infection. https://fstdt.com/4RZ5 and *Death by homeopathy—Contaminated products* https://edzardernst.com/2023/09/death-by-homeopathy-2/ Ernst, Edzard
[lxxi] If you have homeopathic products in your home, I urge you to destroy them, just as I also recommend doing with any paraphernalia associated with energy-based practices.

CHAPTER 13

Discernment in Alternative Health
11 Red Flags

But solid food is for the mature, for those who have their powers
of discernment trained by constant practice to distinguish good from evil.
Hebrews 5:14

After repenting from muscle testing and energy medicine, I rightfully questioned my ability to discern anything. I did not want to ever fall prey again to Satan's wiles and, therefore, needed to understand how to gain discernment for the future. Many have expressed similar concerns to me. While looking for passages that might give insight into the topic, I became intrigued by Hebrews 5:14 and began to study the original Greek of each word.

For context I will include Verse 13 as well. It says, ***Anyone who lives on milk, being still an infant, is not acquainted with the teaching about righteousness. But solid food is for the mature, who by constant use have trained themselves to distinguish good from evil.*** (NIV)

Those two verses contrast infants in the faith who lack proper knowledge or skill in the teachings on righteousness with those who are mature in the faith who consume the solid food of deep doctrine. Although these verses seem awkward in the King James Version, compared to our typical way of speaking, it does provide a more literal translation of the original Greek, and so I will restate the previous verse using the KJV. I Please focus on the description given of someone who is a mature Christian. The four underlined key words allow us to better understand the profound truths revealed about mature discernment. ...*even those who by reason of use have their senses exercised to discern both good and evil* (KJV).

1. **Reason of use**—Greek *hexis*: means, "habit, practice" (Strongs #1838)
2. **Senses**—Greek *aisthétérion*: means, "organ of perception, (perceive, discern through the senses) emphasizing the result of sensory experience (sensation) – i.e., moral feeling to know what is right or wrong in God's eyes" (Strongs #145)
3. **Trained**—Greek *gumnazó*: means, "to exercise naked, to train as with an ancient Greek athlete in a sporting event; (figuratively) to train with one's full effort, i.e., with complete physical, emotional force like when working out intensely in a gymnasium." (Strongs #1128)
4. **To distinguish**—Greek *diakrisis*: means, "a judgment i.e., a discernment (conclusion) which distinguishes "look-alikes," i.e., things that appear to be the same." (Strongs #1253)

Apparently, general discernment does not come as a sudden, spiritual opening of the eyes, but through great effort and practice. Indeed, it is a hallmark of the mature believer who feeds deeply on the Word of God. Although it seems that good and evil are such opposites that they should be easily distinguishable, this passage suggests otherwise. We should not find this surprising since the embodiment of evil itself, Satan, masquerades as an angel of light.[lxxii] Therefore, we need discernment to make a right judgment when good and evil appear deceptively similar. According to Verse 14, to do so requires much practice in training one's senses.

Feelings can be deceptive, and so learning to perceive or discern through our senses takes practice and training. As I have said before, the

---

[lxxii] 2 Corinthians 11:14

Bible tells us that the Holy Spirit brings life and peace. A sense of peace is tangibly felt, and, likewise, the lack of it can also be felt. Unless you learn to take notice of this sense of peace, or lack thereof, you can easily ignore the subtle leading of the Holy Spirit. Learning to recognize this as you seek to discern good from evil is like building strength in your spiritual muscles. Remember, though, all of this "practice" and "training" is in the context of ingesting "solid food." If you start your search for discernment apart the Bible, you will fail to come to a proper judgment.

So let me apply these things to discernment in health care. Suppose you are seeing a practitioner who recommends that you purchase and wear devices that purport to block electromagnetic frequencies (EMFs). You are unsure about the recommendation, so you begin to research online and perhaps talk to friends to find out what they know about the devices. Although such a course may seem a wise approach, you have already mis-stepped.

Instead, start with seeking God for wisdom and leading on the matter BEFORE you research anything. After all, God may have an opinion beyond the inherent moral considerations of owning such devices. He is also concerned with what is best for you, practically, and He will make such things known to you if you just stop and seek Him. Do you notice any sense of unease when you think or pray about purchasing the devices? (Make certain that you are in the Word!) After a time of prayer, if you wish, ask questions of your spouse and friends. (Married ladies, remember that God has given your husband to have spiritual responsibility for you and your household, so pay careful attention to his thoughts.[lxxiii]) Prayerfully begin to research, all the while asking for God's leading and taking special notice of your senses.

In the beginning of training your spiritual muscles of discernment, you may question what you are sensing— "Is it just me or does my peace (or lack thereof) really indicate the Holy Spirit's leading?" You may suspect the answer but need verification. That is okay. Just keep prayerfully seeking the answer, and God will provide the needed insight in time. Having done these things, your spiritual muscles will be a little

---

[lxxiii] Ephesians 5:22-33

stronger the next time, and you will recognize His leading sooner. Over time, you will have more confidence in your ability to make a right judgment. Never forget that all of this must be in the light of time spent daily in God's Word. I cannot emphasize that enough!

Recently, I had the opportunity to speak with a woman who contacted me with questions following her repentance from muscle testing. Through her sharing with me the events that led her to an eventual turning from sin, I was reminded of the schemes of Satan. This woman, whom I will call Eve, described how her accountability partner reached out one day to express her conviction that Eve should no longer see her practitioner who muscle tested. Eve agreed to pray about it. Shortly thereafter, she received word that the appointments and many of the supplements would now be covered under a workman's comp claim she had. This apparent "open door" wrongly solidified Eve's certainty that God was behind her seeing the practitioner. Years later, God used a dream, followed by the same accountability partner and another friend independently expressing their concerns to open Eve's eyes. She now recognizes that the earlier "open door" was not from the Lord and effectively served the devil's purpose to further ensnare her.

The Bible tells us of a similar test involving what appeared to be an open door. In 1 Samuel 24, we are told of how David and his men were hiding in caves as King Saul sought to find and kill David before he could become king. The story makes it clear that God had rejected Saul and chosen David as the replacement. A surprising incident occurred in which Saul went to relieve himself in the very cave where David was hiding. David's men urge him to seize this unlikely opportunity to kill Saul as being from God. However, David responds to this "open door" argument with the truth he already knew: *The Lord forbid that I should do this thing to my lord, the Lord's anointed, to put out my hand against him, seeing he is the Lord's anointed.*[lxxiv] Sometimes, God does provide an open door as an answer to prayers for direction, but if the open door contradicts His Word, rest assured, it most certainly is a test. [Also see 1 Kings 13:1-32]

[lxxiv] 1 Samuel 24:6

Most Christians are aware of the strong biblical warnings against divination and witchcraft and abhor the thought of ever being party to such wickedness.[lxxv] Through the ages, however, the cunning deceiver has continually morphed the appearance of divination and witchcraft so as to ensnare the unsuspecting. Part of building your spiritual powers of discernment is knowing what to look for in order to make a right judgment. The remainder of the chapter will describe eleven things to be on the lookout for when considering a particular type of alternative or energetic medicine.[lxxvi] To emphasize its importance, number one in the list restates what I have already said.

1. Do you have a sense of unease (lack peace) when you think about the practice?

Many people who have contacted me about these practices indicate that, although they did not know why, they had a sense that something did not seem right about the alternative practice they were considering or using. As Christians, we have the indwelling Holy Spirit to guide us into truth and to convict us of sin. His presence brings life and peace. If these are missing, then it is good to consider why.

2. Does the practice acquire information through secret knowledge?

Meriam Websters Dictionary defines divination as *the art or practice that seeks to foresee or foretell future events or discover hidden knowledge usually by the interpretation of omens or by the aid of supernatural powers.* Beware of alternative practices that claim the body can reveal knowledge about itself, often even knowledge that typical scientific tests fail to show or that contradicts traditional testing. A belief that one can gain hidden knowledge from the body comes from the religious underpinnings of these practices—that God is in all things. Therefore, your body is its own separate entity that, as a god, can communicate

---

[lxxv] Deuteronomy 18:10&14, 2 Chron.33:6, Lev. 19:26, & many others
[lxxvi] The following red flags are largely taken from *Life to the Body—Biblical Principles for Health & Healing*, by Marci Julin.

energetically. These pantheistic ideas are rampant in eastern and new age religions and the health practices that developed from them.

Besides the inherent physical danger of possibly treating a condition that does not exist, there is a spiritual danger to participating with demons. Satan wishes to steal, kill, and destroy. If any health practice relies on some form of divination, such as pendulums, medical mediums, frequency machines, or muscle testing, it provides a foothold for the one whose end-goal is to destroy you and your family.

Sadly, I have heard from many Christians that they use muscle testing as a way to make their every decision. The availability of this method as a replacement for the Holy Spirit's guidance clearly reveals it as divination. If the Holy Spirit worked in such ways, God would have instructed us about this in His Word.

3.   Have the results of alternative testing been verified through traditionally accepted methods (blood tests, x-rays, etc.) or do the alternative methods contradict traditional results?

Practitioners who use muscle testing or other divination techniques to diagnose conditions are quick to dismiss traditional results in favor of their own because they believe "the body doesn't lie." They guide their patients into unverified, expensive, and all-consuming protocols based on unproven testing that often leads to downward spiraling health. However, because patients have enough "good days" to encourage them, they stay the course and never truly get better. Verify any supposed diagnosis and improvements with traditionally accepted tests. Such testing may prove financially costly but aids in determining what could be only a temporary placebo benefit or a spiritually deceptive snare rather than a lasting physical improvement.

4. Does the method used for testing or treatment ever occur through a surrogate, the telephone, or by a machine that has not been scientifically proven to consistently achieve results?

Much insight into someone's health can be gleaned through conversation and physical examination. However, if a practitioner claims to be able to definitively test and know what illness or allergy exists over the phone or by testing the energy of one person through another (surrogate), beware. Because these things are not scientifically possible, the only explanations for such "results" are either chance or unclean spirits, neither of which are likely to provide viable health solutions. The idea of a transference of energy (electric frequencies) is false, whereas the transference of spiritual power is real.

5. Is mysterious gifting required to perform the alternative practice or does the presence of certain people interfere with the effectiveness of the diagnoses or treatment? (i.e. a spouse must leave the room)

To use muscle testing as an example, the physical explanation of how muscle testing works indicates that anyone should be capable of performing it, however; that is not the case. Many Christians cannot. My husband could test me but no one else. Furthermore, like with myself and my son, some people become remarkably "gifted" at it. Such oddities are readily explained in the spirit realm but not in the physical realm.

If the test or practice cannot be performed in the presence of certain individuals, beware. I have been told by numerous Christians that their spouse was told to leave the room because their "energy" interfered with the ability to perform the test or treatment. This is easily explained by the Holy Spirit's presence rather than "energy." Furthermore, God placed the husband as the spiritual head of the home—the protector and responsible party for the family's spiritual well-being. Be particularly wary if his specific presence interferes with the efficacy of an alternative practice.

6. Are the methods consistent with historically Satanic practices, eastern religions, or associated with the New Age?

The Bible warns Christians to be aware of the Enemy's schemes.[lxxvii] Satan's tactics change in appearance throughout time, but they follow recognizable patterns or characteristics. Paul warns that *the coming of the*

[lxxvii] 2 Corinthians 2:11 *so that we would not be outwitted by Satan; for we are not ignorant of his designs.*

lawless one will be in accordance with the work of Satan displayed in all kinds of counterfeit miracles, signs and wonders, and in every sort of evil that deceives.[lxxviii] What might such counterfeit miracles look like?

From the story of Job, we know that the devil can physically harm an individual. It stands to reason, therefore, that specific symptoms caused by Satan's forces might be remedied in one of two ways: Either God orders Satan to back-off or Satan does it of his own accord. Think of it as the removal of a splinter from your hand. The hand is made better, not because of a miracle but because of the splinter's sudden absence.

In the "healing" of my thyroid, it is a reasonable possibility that, similar to Job's case of boils, Satan had been the cause of my trouble all along, and the only action necessary to affect my "healing" was to remove whatever he was doing to suppress my thyroid. Doing so at the moment of my first NAET treatment created a perception that NAET had healed me.

Paul also warns that *for even Satan disguises himself as an angel of light. So it is no surprise if his servants, also, disguise themselves as servants of righteousness. Their end will correspond to their deeds.*[lxxix] Over and over again, people tell me that they became ensnared with alternative practices because a Christian did it. If Satan can convince a servant of righteousness to become involved through counterfeit miracles, then he can effectively infiltrate the Christian camp. Perhaps this was his motivation in creating a counterfeit miracle to cure my thyroid.

Another consistent trait of Satan's power to affect people physically is through muscle strength or weakness.[lxxx] As I said before, I became uniquely "gifted" at muscle testing. I could make a muscular man's arm go as weak as a baby's arm with the slightest downward pressure while he held one substance, even though he was easily able to stay strong while holding another. Accounting for this muscle weakness is critical.

One additional consideration involves taking notice of the practice's beginnings. Although many Christians conveniently dismiss the pagan, occultic, or New Age origins of a practice, this is a mistake. If the founder

---

[lxxviii] 2 Thessalonians 2:9-10 NIV
[lxxix] 2 Corinthians 11:14-15
[lxxx] Biblical examples of this include Mark 5:1-3, Mark 9:22.

claims to have gained his or her insight, knowledge, or skill through occult sources such as channeling, automatic writing, or visions and dreams, then what follows is the result of demonic influence. This does not mean there is no truth in the practices, for a scheme of the devil is to mix truth with deception. Just because those who later follow play down occultic origins, does not change the original source of information. Also, take note if the founder claims to have studied or learned from Native American, indigenous, or tribal peoples. The spirituality of these groups makes no claims to following the Christian God. It can also be eye-opening to read what is said about a practice by those who make no claim to Christianity.

7. Do the practices produce "bondage" in people?

Satan desires to ensnare people and bring them into his bondage. Beware of any alternative practice that produces an ever-increasing need for itself. Before I became involved with muscle testing, I used acupuncture for a number of months. It was remarkable how much improvement came immediately from the treatments but how short lived the relief was. It was like a drug that kept me going back over and over again for relief. This formation of dependence is bondage and an important trait to notice.

8. Do the explanations for how it works use any of the following buzzwords: energy, quantum physics, chi, chakras, the subconscious, inner child, tapping, frequency, or talk of the body as though it is a separate entity-- "the body knows how to fix itself, the body doesn't lie," etc.?

Just as any field has a "lingo" that goes with it, so too does energy medicine. That wording can clue one in to recognize areas of concern. When trying to determine the validity of a particular practice, machine, therapy, or substance, notice whether or not certain buzzwords are used in its explanation.

9. Anything that uses muscle testing in any form is divination and is, therefore, forbidden for the Christian.

Numerous examples abound of substances or modalities that might or might not be intrinsically demonic but are made so by adding muscle testing to their practice. An association with AK should not be discounted. Additionally, simply asking a practitioner who uses muscle testing not to muscle test you is not advisable either. Many experienced in muscle testing do not need to make physical contact with the patient but divine the answers automatically. Such demonic empowerment will likely impact the practitioner's recommendations without your knowing it. Lastly, other forms of divination (i.e., pendulums, medical mediums) in combination with a health practice are forbidden by God.

10. Over time, does the general progression of symptoms worsen, even though there may be individual improvements? Are the symptoms that develop strange, include suicidal thoughts, or is there great fighting and strife in your home?

Through the hearing of stories from hundreds of individuals before and after repenting from involvement with energy medicine, I have noticed that a hallmark of demonically based symptoms is a suddenness of onset combined with an intensity that cannot be accounted for through normal physical responses. I have also noticed that symptoms often take on an unusual nature for which traditional medicine finds no explanation. Unexplained weakness is common, as well as neurological symptoms or extreme vertigo that cannot be explained. Extreme sensitivities to electricity and mold are commonplace in those who get involved with divination-based health practices. Practitioners frequently diagnose Lyme Disease, parasites, mold toxicity, and thyroid conditions even though standard testing (if it is even done) shows no such condition.

For some of those particular disorders, enough online information exists about the inadequacies of standard testing to make a diagnosis that contradicts the test results seem believable. Satan can easily hide his torments in this way and distract people through endless "treatments" that have nothing to do with the true source of suffering. If demons are causing the symptoms in the first place, Satan has full control over when and to what degree the symptoms will exhibit. All he has to do is back off a torment that he controls in coordination with a test or treatment that he also controls in order to string someone along by giving them some "good" days.

Because Satan's goal is to destroy, pay particular attention to the presence of suicidal thoughts or debilitating fear/anxiety develop following its use. I personally know of two individuals who committed suicide following their use of energy medicine. Another common problem not to ignore is unusual levels of strife in the home that begin or escalate after involvement with a particular health practice.

Last, take notice if a reaction to a supplement, remedy, or treatment brings immediate and significant reactions, good or bad. That is not to say that every immediate or significant reaction indicates demonic power is producing it—a severe, true allergy could also be the cause. However, if the significant reaction is atypical to accepted medical symptoms, then questions should be asked. For example, if one has seasonal allergies, the expected symptoms include sinus problems, sneezing, watery eyes, and perhaps a fever. What is not expected is collapsing because of muscle weakness, stomach cramping, hallucinations, depression, unusual pain, severe anxiety, tantrums, and so on. Be careful of concluding that bizarre symptoms really are a normal reaction based on the experiences of others who also participate in energy-based health modalities or have occult ties. They too could very well be deceived.

Alternative practitioners and testimonials online are quick to dismiss the ever-increasing "bad days" as being a Jarisch-Herxheimer Reaction (JHR), otherwise known as a *Herx* reaction. A true JHR is caused by the immune system reacting to the rapid die-off of harmful spirochete bacteria in response to antibiotics.[lxxxi] Symptoms include chills, fever, skin rashes, hypertension, myalgia, and various organ malfunctions. It typically resolves itself in 24 hours.[267] Alternative health practitioners often wrongly blame JHR for strong and lasting reactions in detoxifying patients in an attempt to reassure their patients that the suffering indicates the therapy is working.

[lxxxi] Spirochetal infections include syphilis, Lyme disease, leptospirosis, and relapsing fever.

Many years ago, when I was endlessly taking supplements in an attempt to detoxify from numerous things, I was miserable day in and day out. This went on for many months without noticeable improvement, but I was assured by the practitioner and online research that this was normal. I have spoken to many who have experienced the same for months and years on end as they have sought to detoxify. They press on believing the symptoms indicate good is being accomplished even though they feel terrible. This constant state of misery is not a JHR. What truly causes the symptoms, I do not know for sure. It may be that the supplements being taken are poisoning the individual or it may be demonic torment. If this is you, I urge you to prayerfully reconsider the path you are pursuing.

11. Have you developed symptoms characterized as Lyme Disease, EMF or mold sensitivity, heavy metal poisoning, parasites, dizziness, or brain fog but have not, through traditionally accepted testing, been shown to have these conditions?

In a previous chapter, I wrote of how Abrams, the founder of Radionics, typically diagnosed individuals through his machine with one or more of three conditions: syphilis, tuberculosis, and cancer. Similarly, I have observed that there are a handful of likely "diagnoses" made through alternative practices. Although I cannot see or hear the spirit world, when one has had as many conversations as I have had with those coming out of energy medicine, a malicious, strategic pattern seems to emerge in the frequent diagnoses of a handful of illnesses. Practitioners frequently diagnose Lyme Disease, parasites, mold toxicity, and thyroid conditions even though standard testing (if it is even done) shows no such condition.

Each of these symptoms or conditions can be real conditions. However, the alternative medicine realm strongly promotes the hypothesis that traditional testing frequently fails to diagnose these conditions. Whether or not the traditional diagnostics for these conditions are unreliable, these are illnesses that are easily counterfeited. By calling into question traditional testing, the door is opened to assumptions and unreliable forms of testing. I have no desire to debate whether or not the claims about traditional testing are true. I merely wish to point out that the devil is in the counterfeit business and that these symptoms and conditions are easily counterfeited and remarkably prevalent in those who frequently use energy-based practices. This handful of conditions are easily mimicked by demonic torment and therefore controlled or escalated according to the devil's desire. Satan can easily hide his torments in this way and distract people through endless "treatments" that have nothing to do with the true source of suffering.

If you are seeking discernment regarding a particular treatment, practice, practitioner, etc., and find that these questionable symptoms and assumed diagnoses have been made, I would urge you to pause for a time of seeking the wisdom God promises to those who ask.

Modern witchcraft

When I picture a witchdoctor, I envision a native in New Guinea with a bone through his nose and only a loin cloth to cover his flesh. In the missionary stories of my youth, witchdoctors gave potions to the tribal people that were concocted by interactions with the spirit world. Certainly, no Christian would knowingly take such a potion, and yet, without their knowledge, many do exactly that.

If the power to muscle test is indeed the result of divination, then taking any substance that is arrived at by such methods is witchcraft or sorcery. The substances themselves may or may not be helpful, but when they are chosen under demonic influence, taking them is participating with demons. Not only is this dangerous; it is forbidden in the Bible. Attempting to attach God's holy name to such practices through prayer is to misuse His name. Paul explains the faulty logic of trying to follow God while participating with demons in 1 Corinthians 10:20-22.

I do not want you to be participants with demons. You cannot drink the cup of the Lord and the cup of demons. You cannot partake of the table of the Lord and the table of demons. Shall we provoke the Lord to jealousy? Are we stronger than he?

As we seek to make a right judgment between good and evil, may we be as mature Christians who diligently train our spiritual muscles of discernment in the context of much time spent in the truth of God's Word.

CHAPTER 14

Top 3 Arguments & Questions Answered

They did not destroy the peoples, as the LORD commanded them; But mingled themselves with the nations, and learned their works: And they served their idols; which became a snare unto them   Psalm 106:34-36

1. Can Christians redeem the world's practices, and can anything be used for good or evil?

Some wish to defend their continued use of questionable health practices by claiming the Bible teaches the Christian can and should redeem what Satan has stolen. Others approach their defense from a different angle by claiming that anything can be used for good or for evil; it all depends on how you use it. Since both arguments require the same response from Scripture, I will address both simultaneously.

Alternative health practices cover a spectrum regarding the perceptibility of their spiritual influences. Some are blatantly demonic, such as Reiki or medical mediums. The majority, however, masquerade as science, using enough pseudo-scientific buzz words to sound believable. Some Christians deem health modalities that fall outside of traditional medicine, including chiropractic, homeopathy, and acupuncture, to be spiritually safe, even though they originate from pagan, occultic, or New Age belief systems. They discount the concerning origins, but should they? Many report that they attempt to "Christianize" the practices through the addition of prayer, Scripture, and Jesus' name, just to be on the safe side. Surely, if there is any cause for concern, praying first makes it alright. Or does it? I want to address this particular argument with an abundance of Scripture because it is God's Word, not mine, that refutes the lies of the devil.

Can a believer redeem (make acceptable in God's eyes) pagan, occultic, or New Age practices? The answer is simple: No. If something is inherently evil, it is off-limits for the Christian. Period. For example, one cannot transform adultery from sin into something acceptable in the eyes of God by praying before fornicating. Furthermore, committing adultery with another Christian would not reduce the offensiveness of this act God has declared to be sin. Such thinking is ludicrous!

As with adultery, the Bible speaks unequivocally regarding witchcraft, sorcery, mediums, and divination, calling those who practice such things detestable. (The KJV translates the word *detestable* as an abomination.) For example, Deuteronomy 18:9-13 says,

> **When you enter the land the Lord your God is giving you, _do not
> learn to imitate_ the detestable ways of the nations there. Let no one
> be found among you who...practices divination or sorcery,
> interprets omens, engages in witchcraft, or casts spells, or who is a
> medium or spiritist or who consults the dead. _Anyone who does
> these things is detestable to the Lord;_ because of these same
> detestable practices the Lord your God will drive out those nations
> before you. You must be blameless before the Lord your God.**
> (Emphasis mine)

Moses gave those firm instructions from God after the Israelites left Egypt behind and were making their way toward the Promised Land. God intended for His set-apart people to take possession of a land where numerous pagan nations resided. The detestable sins of these nations had reached such a climax that their complete destruction was warranted. Upon entering the land, God did not institute a plan of redeeming what could be saved out of the land but instead told Joshua to tell the people; *keep yourselves from the accursed thing, lest ye make yourselves accursed, when ye take of the accursed thing, and make the camp of Israel a curse, and trouble it.*[lxxxii] Bad things corrupt people and bring trouble upon them and, therefore, cannot be redeemed.

Rather than heeding the warnings from Moses, the Israelites imitated the abominable practices of the former inhabitants. Hundreds of years later, the prophet Isaiah told of God's response to their rebellious hearts: *For you have rejected your people, the house of Jacob, because they are full of things from the east and of fortune-tellers like the Philistines.*[lxxxiii] Sadly, these Eastern sins have continued to be a snare to God's people through the ages.

We must distinguish between the neutral and the inherently evil. Consider herbs for a moment: They are natural substances that are neither good nor evil. They are neutral. If you make a cup of tea by combining various herbs, you have committed no sin. If you research clinical studies and learn that peppermint can be used successfully to reduce fever, and therefore, you drink it for that purpose, you have committed no sin. However, if demonic power is harnessed to determine which herb to consume or to formulate a combination of herbs to be used medicinally, that is witchcraft. Witchcraft is inherently evil and cannot be redeemed. It is detestable to God.

Neither can something that God has declared evil (i.e., divination, sorcery, and consulting the dead) be redeemed or made acceptable by prayer or attaching God's name to it. In fact, to do so is to profane the name of God. Sin is sin! The problem is not in HOW you do it but that you do it at all. It is not at all like an alcoholic drink or a gun that can be used properly or improperly. To quote my husband, "The Christian can redeem football but not sorcery."

I have heard 1 Corinthians 8, used out of context, to defend the idea that a Christian can safely participate in questionable health modalities. In that passage, Paul gives instructions to the early church on how to deal with the common practice of eating food sacrificed to idols. The apostle

---

[lxxxii] Joshua 6:18 KJV
[lxxxiii] Isaiah 2:6

discusses the freedom of the believer in Christ and the reality that an idol is not truly a god but a lifeless object.

Paul then goes on to raise concerns about eating such food in front of someone who is weak in the faith but, at this point, never forbids eating food sacrificed to idols. One might, therefore, wrongly conclude at the end of Chapter 8 that consuming food sacrificed to idols is perfectly fine. What really matters is how it is done. This false principle is then used to justify participation in pagan, energy-based health practices. Anything can be used for good or evil, right? It all depends on how you do it! In isolation from the rest of Scripture, such a conclusion might be warranted.

But wait just a minute! This must not be what Paul was saying because that conclusion runs contrary to several other biblical passages. For example, in Acts 15:19-20, Peter announces the apostles' unified decision regarding things that the new Gentile believers should avoid. He says, ***Therefore, my judgment is that we should not trouble those of the Gentiles who turn to God but should write to them to abstain from the things polluted by idols.*** How interesting! Idols, which are nothing in themselves, can pollute other things (such as food sacrificed to them) and should be avoided. The same instruction was repeated in Acts 21:25. In the book of Revelation, churches of Pergamum and Thyatira are both summarily rebuked for eating food sacrificed to idols.[lxxxiv]

Although it might appear that Paul concluded the matter in 1 Corinthians 8, he circles back to the topic again in Chapter 10 to further clarify the matter of eating foods sacrificed on pagan altars. This time he comes at it from a different and surprising angle. He speaks of the communion table the believer partakes of through the body of Christ. He then goes on to say the following in Verses 18-22.

> *Consider the people of Israel: are not those who eat the sacrifices participants in the altar? What do I imply then? That food offered to idols is anything, or that an idol is anything? No, I imply that what pagans sacrifice they offer to demons and not to God. **I do not want you to be participants with demons. You cannot drink the cup***

[lxxxiv] Revelation 2:14 & 20

of the Lord and the cup of demons. You cannot partake of the table of the Lord and the table of demons. Shall we provoke the Lord to jealousy? Are we stronger than he? (Emphasis mine)

Paul continues his thought in the next chapter by giving instructions on taking communion. He strongly warns believers to examine themselves before participating in the table of the Lord because many who have taken it an unworthy manner have been judged by God with death.[lxxxv] When one considers the entire context of Paul's discussion on food sacrificed to idols, the conclusion becomes clear. One *cannot drink the cup of the Lord and the cup of demons*. God does not allow for "redeeming" practices associated with demons.

Also consider the book of Haggai, which opens with a call to contemplate why it is that the Israelites' actions provided them no fulfillment or satisfaction. He asks why God's blessing had been withheld from every area of His people's lives? We learn that the people wrongly concluded that they could participate in the sinful practices of the pagans around them and yet be made clean through their additional participation in the practices of God. Sound familiar? The prophet responds by drawing attention to the details of the ceremonial law that the priests followed. In 2:11-14, Haggai says,

Thus says the Lord of hosts: Ask the priests about the law: 'If someone carries holy meat in the fold of his garment and touches with his fold bread or stew or wine or oil or any kind of food, does it become holy?'" The priests answered and said, "No." Then Haggai said, "If someone who is unclean by contact with a dead body touches any of these, does it become unclean?" The priests answered and said, "It does become unclean." Then Haggai answered and said, "So is it with this people, and with this nation before me, declares the Lord, and so with every work of their hands. And what they offer there is unclean.

[lxxxv] 1 Corinthians 11:27-34

The point the prophet makes is clear: One cannot make something clean that is already unclean; however, something unclean will always defile what was previously clean. Think of how a drop of feces in a bowl of pudding would defile the entire bowl. Would you eat the pudding?

In case any further doubt remains about the feasibility of "redeeming" evil, consider three more passages:

- Jeremiah 7:8-10 & 15-16

  Behold, you trust in deceptive words to no avail. Will you steal, murder, commit adultery, swear falsely, make offerings to Baal, and go after other gods that you have not known, and then come and stand before me in this house, which is called by my name, and say, 'We are delivered!'—only to go on doing all these abominations? And I will cast you out of my sight, as I cast out all your kinsmen, all the offspring of Ephraim. As for you, do not pray for this people, or lift up a cry or prayer for them, and do not intercede with me, for I will not hear you.

- *Leviticus 18:2-5*

  Speak to the people of Israel and say to them, I am the Lord your God. You shall not do as they do in the land of Egypt, where you lived, and you shall not do as they do in the land of Canaan, to which I am bringing you. You shall not walk in their statutes. You shall follow my rules and keep my statutes and walk in them. I am the Lord your God. You shall therefore keep my statutes and my rules; if a person does them, he shall live by them: I am the Lord.

- *Leviticus 20:6-8*

  If a person turns to mediums and necromancers, whoring after them, I will set my face against that person and will cut him off from among his people. Consecrate yourselves, therefore, and be holy, for I am the Lord your God. Keep my statutes and do them; I am the Lord who sanctifies you.

Since Scripture clearly teaches that evil practices cannot be redeemed, the question that is critical is whether energy medicine is inherently evil and therefore, unredeemable? As I have described in previous chapters, muscle testing to gain knowledge is divination and therefore, unredeemable. Using muscle testing to create supplements by determining formulations or dosages is witchcraft/sorcery and therefore, also an abomination. Finally, using New Age or occult based practices for health (energy medicine) is witchcraft/sorcery and, therefore, an offense to the LORD God.

The enemy frequently uses subtly to ensnare people through alternative practices, and so, often, the difficulty lies in discerning whether a particular health modality falls into the physical realm or the spiritual realm. Ignorance does not remove culpability, so I urge you to back off from participation with any modalities of which you are unsure to allow for a time of prayer, research, and waiting on the Lord. James 1:5 promises that God will give wisdom to any who ask. Listen for the Holy Spirit's leading, even if all you hear is a sense of unease. A lack of peace is an answer, as the Holy Spirit will give life and peace,[lxxxvi] if the practice is of Him. As we have seen laid out in God's Word, the consequences for participation in sorcery or divination of any sort is not a trifling matter.

2. Lots of Christians practice energy medicine, so it must be okay!

A tremendous number of those who reach out to me about muscle testing were first introduced to that practice by another person claiming to be a Christian. This alarming reality causes some to ask whether energy medicine is truly wrong. Can so many professing Christians be deceived?

The apostle Paul writes in 2 Corinthians 11:3-4 of his fear that false teachers will lead the *elect* astray by *a different gospel, another Jesus,* and

---

[lxxxvi] Romans 8:6

the acceptance of *a different spirit* from the one they previously accepted. Clearly, then, Christians can be and are capable of being deceived and deceiving others. Sometimes, Satan does this through a wolf in sheep's clothing,[lxxxvii] and at other times he uses a sincere believer who has fallen into sin.

The Bible warns us in 2 Thessalonians 2:3-12 that in the last days many will be led astray by Satan's energy.[lxxxviii] In fact, it says that God Himself allows the devil to use his energy to provide a convincing delusion that will lead many astray. Why would God permit this? According to Verses 11-12, it is to reveal those who do not love the truth and should be condemned.

Throughout the history of the Bible, false prophets and teachers arose to lead God's people astray. One such example is detailed in 1 Kings 13. It tells an unusual story of a prophet of God being enticed to disobey God's direct instruction by a fellow prophet. One prophet had been told specifically not to eat or drink during his sojourn in Bethel where God had sent him to prophesy to the wicked king Jeroboam. An old prophet living in Bethel heard about the visiting prophet and invited him for a meal. Oddly, after hearing the visiting prophet's restatement of God's direct instruction to him not to eat or drink in Bethel, the old man lied, claiming to have received a contrary message from an angel of the Lord.

Convinced by the fellow prophet that God's original message had been rescinded, the visiting prophet happily joined the old man in his home for a meal. But, while eating, the old, deceptive prophet heard a true message from God, harshly rebuking the visiting prophet for disobeying God's instruction. As punishment for that disobedience, a lion attacked and killed him when he resumed his journey home. If only the visiting prophet had trusted the Word of God rather than an individual.

The New Testament relays numerous instances of followers of Jesus being deceived and deceiving others to their peril. Ananias led his wife Saphira into deception, and both were struck dead. By Satan's influence,

---

[lxxxvii] John 10:12

[lxxxviii] The Greek word *enérgeia* means spiritual power to accomplish work and is only used in reference to God's power (energy) and to Satan's.

Peter famously attempted to lead Jesus away from the Father's will and had to be rebuked. The letters to the churches repeatedly sound a warning to not be deceived by those walking in sin or teaching false doctrines. Many professing a belief in Jesus as their Savior have been and will be deceived and go on to deceive others.

Sadly, I was one of those who led many into deception by my zeal for muscle testing and NAET. During that time of sin, I truly loved the LORD with all of my heart. Like many others who have since reached out to me, I simply desired to serve God by helping others but was, nonetheless, in error. Blindly following others can prove dangerous. Even the sincerest in the faith are just mortals, prone to sin and deception. Our authority must always be the infallible Scriptures and not those who profess to know them.

3. Every good & perfect gift is from God, and since energy medicine brings good sometimes, it must be from God.

What qualifies a gift as good? Is it good because it is something we want? Can a gift be good when we do not want it? Is it good if it satisfies us at the start but not in the end? These questions deserve consideration in a discussion of this next argument people make in favor of muscle testing and energy-based health practices.

The familiar passage that some love to quote in defense of AK is found in James 1:17. *Every good and perfect gift is from above, coming down from the Father of the heavenly lights, who does not change like shifting shadows* (NIV). The argument I once used, and have heard repeated by others, states that since some people have noteworthy and positive experiences with energy medicine, this must indicate that such medicine is from God. After all, every good gift comes from Him. Is this a correct conclusion? To answer, we must first consider what God defines as a "good gift."

To rightly divide the Word, we must always look at the context of the passage and interpret Scripture by Scripture, not by our own thoughts. The context of Verse 17 is rather interesting and not at all what one might expect. Right out of the gate, James begins Chapter 1 with: *Count it all joy, my brothers, when you meet trials of various kinds, for you know that the testing of your faith produces steadfastness. And let steadfastness have its full effect, that you may be perfect and complete, lacking in nothing* (vs. 2-4). Considering the nature of a good gift, we see that, by God's definition, a trial, which we do not want, can truly be a good gift. How? It brings steadfastness, completeness, and leaves us lacking nothing.

James continues his thought in the next verse by discussing another gift from God. He says that God will gladly give wisdom to those who ask. Unlike trials, we can get behind the idea that wisdom is a gift. However, as James continues his discussion of various gifts, he once again turns things upside down in Verse 9: The *lowly brother should boast in his exaltation*, unlike the rich who will perish in their selfish pursuits. Humility is a gift if it leads one to eternal rather than earthly glory. The final example given in this chapter listing God's good but unexpected "gifts" includes bearing up under temptation. Why? Because that one will warrant the crown of life in eternity.

After James finishes his description of good gifts, he warns, ***<u>Do not be deceived</u>, my beloved brothers. Every good gift and every perfect gift is from above...*** (vs.16-17a). Having considered the context, we can now understand why James would feel the need to tell us not to be deceived about the nature of good gifts. Many deceptive gifts may come our way: a pleasurable rendezvous with an attractive individual other than our spouse; a chocolate cake that tastes amazing but leaves our clothes too tight; a fun night on the town that leaves us retching all night. You get the idea.

A few sessions into my NAET treatments, my thyroid suddenly began working. It seemed a miracle and a "good gift" for sure! It was because of that experience and the verse about good and perfect gifts (taken out of context) that I concluded muscle testing and NAET was from God. However, as I detailed in the retelling of my story in an earlier chapter, that experience brought much harm to myself and others through me. I had been deceived by the master deceiver.

I have heard countless stories of individuals who had one remarkable improvement from muscle testing only to eventually realize that the general trajectory of their health was declining. I have heard others who never had a remarkable improvement but only slight and temporary improvements or "good days." Still others have had disastrous experiences from which recovery was difficult. Regardless of the initial experience, many have ended up in financial ruin, broken marriages, children with frightening demonic experiences, or other forms of torment. If something begins good but leads to destruction, it is not a gift from God.

The Gospels describe a time of testing that Jesus endured at the start of His ministry. After forty days without food, Satan showed up to tempt the Savior at his weakest and most vulnerable state and even quoted Scripture out of context to do it. Make no mistake, the temptations of food, power, and status were real. If the Messiah had accepted any one of these deceptive "gifts," the fate of the world would have changed forever. Thankfully, Jesus knew that truly good gifts from the Father required of Him a time of suffering and waiting, and so He resisted the temptations. Jesus wisely responded to the devil's misuse of Scripture by countering with verses that put things into the correct context. Oh, the power of the Word of God!

Brothers and sisters do not be deceived. If a gift is from the Father, it is always good at the end.

Part 2

What Now?
Moving Forward with
Hope

CHAPTER 15

From Bondage to Freedom

So if the Son sets you free, you will be free indeed. John 8:36

When one has pinned all hope for wellness, healing, or, in the case of a practitioner, even the means of financial provision on the sinful practices of energy medicine, the road following repentance can seem confusing and frightening. Perhaps, you can relate to others who have expressed grief over their sin and confusion over how to move forward. One man said it this way: *I wanted to write you because I feel the Lord has used you to drop a nuclear bomb in my lap, and now I feel very stuck BUT with a much more open mind toward the Lord's leading.* Another wrote, *my wife and I stumbled across your article about* NAET *and we are so confused...we have spent tens of thousands of dollars on* NAET *treatments for seven years...Needless to say, we need help processing.* One woman said, *I too have struggled with years of chronic illness which led me to muscle testing, and I started feeling uncomfortable with it a few weeks ago. I was wondering if you offer counseling sessions as I'm now trying to understand how to heal without it.*

If you find yourself full of questions about what to do now or are anxious and overwhelmed by the road ahead, then the next several chapters should be helpful. I will share the same biblical and practical counsel that I have communicated with hundreds of people coming out of energy medicine. Walk with me, step by step, along the path of repentance and freedom in Christ. Like any journey, some sections are easier than others, but referencing these chapters along the way can offer assurance that you are on the right path.

Repentance

As with any trip, upon discovering one is heading in the wrong direction, the individual must first stop, then evaluate, and finally, change course. In spiritual terms, this is called repentance. If you now recognize your sin, simply stop your former practices and confess your sin to God. God already knows but desires that you admit your wrongdoing to Him. 1 John 1:9 promises that if you do so, you will be forgiven and cleansed from all unrighteousness.

A passage from James 4 has much to say that applies to repentance and gaining freedom from evil. It will provide the framework for my writing in this chapter. It says,

> *Submit yourselves therefore to God. Resist the devil, and he will flee from you. Draw near to God, and he will draw near to you. Cleanse your hands, you sinners, and purify your hearts, you double-minded. Be wretched and mourn and weep. Let your laughter be turned to mourning and your joy to gloom. Humble yourselves before the Lord, and he will exalt you* (vs. 7-13).

Some who come to recognize the sin of their involvement with energy medicine are quick to accept God's forgiveness and feel little, if any, guilt for their sin. If you feel no sorrow (grief) over a sin that God considers an abomination, then perhaps the first order of business is to pray that God will allow you to see His perspective of your past sin. As you can clearly see, the verses in James picture one who is broken over his sin. Sadness over sin indicates a heart change. Think of a time when someone apologized to you with a nonchalant attitude. Did their lack of remorse not convey an absence of concern or awareness over the hurt their actions caused you?

The apostle Paul said, *godly sorrow brings repentance that leads to salvation and leaves no regret.*[lxxxix] In the days to come, your resolve will likely be tested, but godly sorrow over sin will hold you fast. Yes, a deep awareness of your past transgressions will also leave you greatly humbled but with no regrets as to changing course.

Others, however, find themselves devastated by the crushing weight of the guilt of their sin. The purpose, however, of God-given sorrow is to bring humble repentance that brings deliverance rather than shame. Yes, we are guilty, but the blood of Jesus cleanses us completely so that we can boldly come before a holy God. Psalm 32:1-2 describes the great blessing of complete forgiveness. *Blessed is the one whose transgressions are forgiven, whose sins are covered. Blessed is the one whose sin the LORD does not count against them and in whose spirit is no deceit* (NIV).

Following my awareness that I had participated in divination through muscle testing and also led many others into that sin, I was consumed with shame and a certainty that God could never again use me for His Kingdom. I remember clearly being on a walk, which normally provided a sweet time of prayer, but on this day, all that went through my mind were harsh messages of failure. After a time of berating myself, the precious voice of the Holy Spirit began to call to my mind the truth of God's Word, which countered the condemnation of the evil one. Scripture after Scripture came to mind of God cleansing me from all iniquity, and finally, I had to choose to whom I would listen. *For whenever our heart condemns us, God is greater than our heart, and he knows everything.*[xc]

I then considered the saints of old: Abraham lied twice, and in so doing placed his wife in the arms of others for his own security, yet God made him the father of all who would believe. King David committed adultery and murder, and yet God established His throne forever. Rahab was a prostitute, yet by faith, became a part of the lineage of the Messiah. Peter denied Jesus three times, yet through him, God established His church.

[lxxxix] 2 Corinthians 7:10 NIV
[xc] 1 John 3:20

Paul persecuted the church, and yet through him God gave us much of the New Testament and spread the Gospel to the world. The blood of Jesus cleansed each one by faith. If God could forgive them and use each one mightily for His kingdom, then His grace toward you and me is no different. As Jesus said to the woman caught in adultery, and I believe now says to you and me: ***Neither do I condemn you; go, and from now on sin no more.***[xci]

Be certain of your salvation.

When people reach out to me to talk on the phone about questions regarding their past involvement with energy medicine, I, in turn, almost always ask them an unexpected question. "If you died today and stood before God, and He asked you why He should let you into heaven; what would you say?" The question generally takes people by surprise but is not asked without good reason. If you have been involved in demonic activity, then you have opened a door to spiritual forces that must be firmly closed. However, the Bible makes it clear that there is only one who has authority over Satan, and that is Jesus. The Son of God imparts His authority only to those who believe in His name as the only means to salvation from the penalty of sin. Scripture indicates that to seek to stand against Satan's forces without first being in right standing with God is dangerous.

A story is told in Acts 19 of men who were not true believers who sought to imitate the disciples by casting out demons. The results were disastrous. Verses 15-16 say,

> ***One day the evil spirit answered them, "Jesus I know, and Paul I know about, but who are you?" Then the man who had the evil spirit jumped on them and overpowered them all. He gave them such a beating that they ran out of the house naked and bleeding*** (NIV).

If you lack certainty that you will go to heaven when you die, then I implore you to carefully consider the Gospel (good news) before

---

[xci] John 8:11

proceeding. Please stop and read Appendix G to know how you might know for certain that you are saved.

Closing the door

Once you are certain of your salvation through grace, it is time to follow the simple, two-step plan spelled out in James 4:7 to stand against the evil one: *Submit yourselves therefore to God. Resist the devil, and he will flee from you.*

1. Submit yourself to God in confession & repentance

Before you take your stand against Satan, James says you must submit to God, which simply put, means to place yourself under His authority. As described earlier, confess your sin, and tell God of your desire to repent. Ask for his protection and authority over demons. If your children are old enough to understand, and they have also been involved, then explain to them, in simple terms, why you are repenting. Even though they were involved at your direction, they may personally need to repent as well. From the example of my own son and the stories of others, it is apparent that children are very susceptible to Satan's influence and often easy targets. Make sure they are age-appropriately included in your family's repentance.

2. Resist the devil out loud in the name of Jesus.

It is clear from numerous passages in Acts and the Gospels that the rebuking of evil spirits was done out loud.[xcii] It is also clear from the New Testament that it is only the name of Jesus that has any authority over Satan. It is Christ's presence indwelling a believer that allows the individual to have authority over demons. If you are a believer, you do not need a priest, deliverance group, or another individual to resist the devil

---

[xcii] i.e., Luke 4:35 / Luke 10:17 / Acts 19:13-16

for you. James 4:7 instructs you to personally resist and promises that Satan WILL flee.

I have heard some teach that you must call the unclean spirits by name to rebuke them (i.e., spirit of divination, spirit of fear, etc.), but this is not necessary judging from almost every instance in the Bible, whether it was Jesus or His followers.[xciii] Married women, if your husband has also been involved and is a believer in Christ, I encourage you to discuss this with him and ask him, as the biblically mandated head of his family, to lead you all in resisting Satan. Regardless of who speaks, say something like the following out loud:

- First to God, pray, "Almighty God, I know that I have sinned against you by participating with divination and witchcraft. (Be specific here as it pertains to the things you were involved with and the Holy Spirit's personal conviction.) Thank you for forgiving me and cleansing me of all my sin. Empower me now to stand against the devil in Jesus' name. Thank you, Father."
- Then to Satan's forces, speak out loud: "All spirits who serve Satan, in the name of Jesus you have no authority over me or my household. We are covered with the blood of Jesus. In the name of Jesus, you must leave this house and leave us alone."

If your child(ren) are too young to understand and might be frightened by all of this, I would recommend that they not be listening when you *resist the devil*. However, you do not want to leave them vulnerable to the evil one's attack. Consider waiting until they are sleeping soundly and then, softly speak something like the following while in their room:

- First to God, pray, "Almighty God, I know that you have given me this child to raise in your ways, but I instead led them into sin. Please forgive me and help me now to stand against the devil so that he will have no grounds to touch my child. Thank you, Father."

16:18, Matthew 17:18, Luke 13:12

- Then to Satan's forces, say: "In the name of Jesus, no demon may have authority over my child. In the name of Jesus, you must leave this house and leave _____ (your child's name) alone."

When Seth and I concluded that we had sinned by our involvement with muscle testing and energy medicine, Seth spoke something similar to what I have outlined. We had never previously done such a thing before, and it seemed strange to do so. However, when Seth first told Satan to get lost, terror gripped me that was unlike anything I have ever before or since experienced. I began to scream and held my chest in pain. Seth immediately rebuked the devil again in the name of Jesus, and, just like that, the fear was gone.

I have often heard people recount lengthy and dramatic episodes of doing "battle" with demons where a group of people work together to bring "deliverance." That, however, is not what the Bible depicts. In the passages already discussed such as James 4 and Ephesians 6, as well as numerous examples in the Gospels and book of Acts, a single person spoke with firmness but not with a big, lengthy show.

It calls to mind the story of Elijah and the prophets of Baal on Mt. Carmel found in 1 Kings 18. The false prophets called on their god for many hours as they danced around, hooped-and-hollered, cut themselves, etc. but nothing happened. Elijah, on the other hand, prayed a simple prayer acknowledging God's power and asked Him to work. I know that story is not specifically about resisting the devil, but it does highlight the contrast between God's and Satan's ways of doing things. Either God has power over demons, or He does not. Either He gives that power to us, or He does not. In Scripture, it is not a show or drawn-out "battle".

3. Eliminate ALL paraphernalia & literature from those practices regardless of the cost.

Immediately following the momentary, profound fear, I felt a compelling desire to rid the house of anything and everything related to energy medicine. Without hesitation, all three of us went through the house gathering up books and paraphernalia. We threw it all into the large trash can outside. However, I began to feel as though voices were calling to me to rescue those items from the trash. The temptation to do so was almost overwhelming, so I asked Seth to get rid of them for good. Once he did so, peace finally filled my heart.

Referring back to the passage in James, we see the command to *cleanse your hands, you sinners, and purify your hearts, you double-minded.* What do you suppose this might look like? Surely, it is to rid oneself of all traces of impurity with single-minded devotion. I urge you to eliminate objects like crystals, pendulums, yoga DVDs, computer files or literature, frequency machines or devices, or anything gained through a health practice that used muscle testing, including supplements purchased from practitioners who use muscle testing or that were purchased elsewhere as a result of the leading of muscle testing. Why? Because, if those supplements were chosen under the influence of demonic power, then they are the result of witchcraft and may give demons the opportunity to afflict you.

New converts in the early church set a strong precedent for completely destroying paraphernalia from demonic practices, despite the tremendous financial costs. Acts 19:18-20 says,

> *Many of those who believed now came and openly confessed what they had done. A number who had practiced sorcery brought their scrolls together and burned them publicly. When they calculated the value of the scrolls, the total came to fifty thousand drachmas. In this way the word of the Lord spread widely and grew in power.*

As I have said, many people have contacted me through my website indicating that they have decided to repent of their involvement with muscle testing, and they report that they have followed James 4:7 to do so. Sadly, though, some have stopped short of completely eliminating every trace of paraphernalia. I understand that it is very hard to give up things that cost a lot of money. However, that is exactly the model we see in Scripture. To hold on to items associated with evil gives the devil a continued foothold in your life and a ground to stand on for temptation.

Ephesians 4:27 instructs us to **give no opportunity to the devil.** If you can burn the items, do so. If you have items that could be sold, please do not do so or you will be profiting from someone else's participation with demons. Instead, follow the example of the early church and do not count the cost![xciv]

Stand and stand again

It can be surprisingly difficult for some to break free of these practices. For me, the temptation to muscle test plagued my mind for many days to come. It made no sense! I knew the truth without question, but I missed the former practices terribly. I especially struggled as a mother when my son was sick, and I could no longer muscle test to divine what was wrong and how to make him well. Honestly, I missed the power and control I once felt through those practices. I had much to learn about how to walk according to the Holy Spirit. Others have told me that they personally or one of their family members got very sick and the temptation to return became overpowering. Whatever may come in the days ahead, be prepared to stand on the day of testing, which is why James' instruction immediately following the teaching to resist the devil is crucial: **Draw near to God, and he will draw near to you.**

Keep in mind that for some time now, your sin has separated you from close fellowship with your Savior and Lord. Hebrews 12:14 says, **without holiness no one will see the Lord**, and Isaiah 59:2 says, **But your iniquities have separated you from your God; your sins have hidden his face from you, so that he will not hear** (NIV). I urge you to now seek Him with all of your heart. Read His Word daily as if your life depends on it. Hunger and thirst for truth and righteousness! If you want to be able to stand in the days of testing that will come, draw near to God now. Be wary if you begin to find yourself thinking thoughts justifying your former sin. Make sure you inundate yourself with the Word of God in the days ahead so that you can stand on the truth therein.

[xciv] In her testimony at the end of the book, "Meg from Pennsylvania" gives further biblical reasons for completely eliminating every trace of these practices.

The story in the Gospels of the temptation of Jesus provides insight into the way Satan works and the proper response to his attempts to ensnare.[xcv] The devil used Scripture out of context to tempt Jesus in three different ways. Jesus, in return, quoted Scripture that put things in the correct context. The evil one does not give up easily and attacks when we are at our weakest! Three times and in three different ways the devil tempted our Savior after forty days of fasting. Can you imagine how weak and hungry he was? Jesus had to rebuke the devil during multiple, separate enticements before being left alone.

Luke 4:13 concludes the story by saying, *And when the devil had ended every temptation, he departed from him until an opportune time*. So, even after Satan retreated, he only did so until he could find another opportunity. From this we gain valuable insight. We may need to take a stand in Jesus' name more than once before the devil leaves us alone. God promises that Satan will flee, only continue to stand! We see this same instruction in the famous Ephesians 6 passage on the armor of God. In those verses depicting spiritual warfare (as some like to call it), Paul repeats the words *stand* and *withstand* five times. Not once does he say to fight.

God, not Satan, is to be feared. The Almighty has already done the work in conquering the enemy. We need only to submit to Jehovah in righteous obedience and stand against the evil one. THEN, Satan WILL flee! Do not be afraid. The God who spoke the universe into being loves you and has already fought the battle for you and won the victory. Stand in his power! Your deliverance is at hand.

Confessing to others you have wronged

The final step of my repentance was perhaps the most difficult. I had sinned against many others by inadvertently introducing them to demonic practices. God impressed upon me the importance of confessing my sin to these individuals and asking their forgiveness. Matthew 5:23-24 says, *so if you are offering your gift at the altar and there remember that your*

[xcv] Matthew 4:1-11, Luke 4:1-13

brother has something against you, leave your gift there before the altar and go. First be reconciled to your brother, and then come and offer your gift. I knew that I had wronged many brothers and sisters and needed humility and wisdom to be reconciled. Perhaps the same is true for you.

The final verse in the James 4 passage says to *humble yourselves before the Lord,* and truly God requires this difficult step in repenting from energy-based practices if you have wronged others by your participation. Many factors must be taken into consideration before proceeding. For instance, are the individuals you wronged believers? Are you a practitioner who has signed a contract about how you deal with clients currently or in the future? Are the wronged individuals close friends and family members or people you only know casually? I urge you to spend time in prayer for these people and how God would have you to reach out to them.

Personally, I decided, after prayer and discussing the matter with Seth, to speak in person or on the phone to certain ones, to send a letter to the majority, and to pray for one individual I no longer had a way to contact. The approach I recommend and that I followed was to simply tell the story behind the change in perspective and the reasons for concluding those practices are demonic. Then, to ask them for forgiveness.

As is to be expected, I received a myriad of responses. Some thanked me for letting them know, while others disregarded my reasons for repenting. Regardless, I knew that I had done what honored the Lord by humbly reaching out to them. Sin always has consequences, and tragically, mine included the realization that I had wreaked havoc in the lives of some. I continued to pray for these individuals for years to come. I urge you to do the same.

Former practitioners have a unique and difficult time knowing whether to reach out to former clients. Some have shared with me that, after much prayer for wisdom, they determined it was unethical to reach out directly to those they had wronged because of contracts they had previously signed. Instead, they began to pray diligently for their former clients and asked God to provide opportunities to somehow share with them. God answered their prayers in surprising ways. Other practitioners, who ran their own practice, explained their change of heart to clients and transformed their businesses.

Reaching others who are deceived

Following repentance, many wish to share the truth with others they know who are also deceived by energy medicine but do not know the best way to do so. The best advice I can give is to pray for wisdom to know how God would have you to reach out to them and also that they might receive the truth. If there is someone you personally led into this sin, then humbly reaching out to them with your own story gives you the perfect way to also share other sources for information. I have a couple of videos on my YouTube channel, blog articles on HeartandMindMinistries.com, and this book that could be beneficial in sharing with others.

However, the more difficult scenario is in sharing with a close friend or family member who is ensnared and defensive. What then? I urge you to remember that this is a spiritual matter. You and I do not have the power to change hearts, no matter how persuasive we might be. You can say all of the right things and get the wrong result or vice versa. God alone brings repentance! We are simply to be obedient in sharing the truth as He leads.

Many who become involved in energy medicine do so because of significant health challenges who have suffered much. For these individuals, the thought of losing the practices that have provided some measure of comfort or hope is unacceptable. If you reach out to someone in this situation, please do so with great kindness, humility, gentleness, and no judgment in your heart towards them. Do not be like the biblical friends of Job who battered him with lengthy speeches and condemnation when he was barely hanging on to his will to live. Resources that offer a hopeful alternative can be especially helpful to these hurting souls. Believers are called to be intercessors, a royal priesthood, so fulfil that role for your friend or family member. Let God do the work of opening their eyes and changing their hearts.

Many who reach out to me do so because a friend had the courage to share my article, video, or books with them. Others have told me that they initially rejected the truth shared by a friend but, sometime later, God brought them to repentance. Be patient with others who are ensnared and pray diligently for them. Consider the wise instruction found in 2 Timothy 2:24-26.

And the Lord's servant must not be quarrelsome but kind to everyone, able to teach, patiently enduring evil, correcting his opponents with gentleness. God may perhaps grant them repentance leading to a knowledge of the truth, and they may come to their senses and escape from the snare of the devil, after being captured by him to do his will.

Praise be to God in granting you repentance and allowing you to come to your senses and to escape the devil's snare! For some, the veer off the path of life and down the rocky trail of energy medicine has been brief, and therefore, the return trip is simple. For others who have journeyed farther down that dangerous trail, the return to God's path proves difficult. If this is you, cast aside all of the garbage accumulated, and fix your eyes on Jesus as your guide. Do not take your eyes off Him as He leads you back to the path of life.

CHAPTER 16

Supplements, Oils, & Herbs

Is there no balm in Gilead? Is there no physician there? Why then has the health of the daughter of my people not been restored? Jeremiah 8:22

The number one question people ask me following their repentance from energy-based practices, is what to do about supplements. Generally, the longer one has been seeing a muscle testing practitioner, the more supplements they consume daily. I am no longer shocked when someone reports that they take more than seventy a day. Whether you take five or seventy-five, you are likely questioning what to do moving forward.

When one contemplates the subject of supplements, herbs, and oils, many avenues for discussion arise. Others more qualified than I have written lengthy books addressing the fascinating topic of the medicinal use of herbs and oils. Numerous experts have also expounded on the potential dangers of the unregulated supplement industry. Another hot topic some vehemently expound upon includes the apparent nutritional needs created by depleted food sources, which ostensibly make supplements a necessity. Obviously, I cannot cover such a vast topic in one chapter, so I will instead limit my focus to the spiritual considerations that arise with supplement use. To that end, I will address how to steer clear of witchcraft in the use of natural products. Additionally, I will discuss a biblical approach to supplement use, as well as some practical recommendations.

Witchcraft

Much confusion exists about what witchcraft actually means. Many have heard that the Greek word used in the New Testament for sorcery/witchcraft is *pharmakeia,* from which we get the English words "pharmacy" and "pharmaceuticals." From that knowledge, some wrongly conclude that all medications are, therefore, sorcery. This belief is especially popular among Christians who prefer alternative to traditional medicine.

Most are aware of the fact that language constantly morphs as people adapt old words for new purposes. For example, "*hussy* comes from the word *housewife* (with several sound changes, clearly) and used to refer to the mistress of a household, not the disreputable woman it refers to today."[268] You might also recall that earlier in this book, I discussed the morphology of the word "energy" from the Greek *enérgeia,* which referred only to spiritual power to accomplish work but was later adopted by physicists for an entirely different purpose. Because of this shifting nature of language, it is incorrect to say that because modern words like pharmacy and pharmaceuticals originate from the root *pharmakeia* that all drugs are sorcery.

The original meaning and use of the Greek word *pharmakeia,* indicated *the use of medicine, drugs, or spells* used in *magic, sorcery, or enchantment.*[xcvi] When applied to health, sorcery/witchcraft involves things used medicinally that were created specifically through the practice of magical arts. Many things can be said about modern drugs, but one cannot say they are created through magical arts. There are only two verses where the word witchcraft is used in the New Testament, and in both instances, the writer combines witchcraft with idolatry (the worship of

---

[xcvi] Strongs Concordance #5331

false gods).[xcvii] Both practices involved demons and were forbidden. This is not the case with modern pharmaceuticals.[xcviii]

Although the creation of traditional drugs, to my knowledge, does not involve witchcraft, alternative medicine frequently relies on sorcery in numerous ways. The two most commonly employed include the utilization of muscle testing to formulate supplement recipes, and the ritualistic shaking of a dilution done in an attempt to impart spiritual energy, as is done in the development of homeopathic remedies. Other methods of employing sorcery in the creation of supplements includes attaching special frequencies to substances or supposedly speaking or writing a remedy into existence as with "paper remedies." (Likely, that is far from a complete list, as I am continually learning of new methods the evil one devises to deceive people.)

Although divination and witchcraft (sorcery) both rely on demonic power, there is a distinction between the two, which is why Deuteronomy 18:10 lists them separately when naming numerous demonic practices. Divination involves determining and disseminating hidden knowledge, and witchcraft/sorcery creates spells or medicinal substances. Using muscle testing, a pendulum, or some other divining tool to determine a diagnosis or treatment plan is divination. Additionally, it is divination if demonic power is used to gain knowledge of what supplements, herbs, or oils should be used and at what dosages. However, when a recipe for formulating those substances is created according to demonic leading through the aforementioned practices, this is practicing witchcraft. What turns a peppermint leaf from a simple herb with medicinal benefits into sorcery? Is it not the involvement of unclean spirits?

If you do a search online for videos on essential oils, you will quickly encounter many encouragements to use muscle testing to formulate your own combination oils. This is witchcraft! Some supplement companies openly admit to using muscle testing in the creation of their products.

[xcvii] Galatians 5:20 & Revelation 18:23

[xcviii] By stating that pharmaceuticals are not witchcraft, I am not suggesting their use is necessarily appropriate or safe. There are many factors to consider, and I recommend prayers for wisdom in making those decisions.

Some sell muscle testing kits to use for testing their products more easily. To use or ingest products that come from demonic influence is to open a door to evil. God forbids all magical arts and calls those who participate with them an abomination.[xcix] I urge you to repent and eliminate any products that came from a company or practitioner involved in sorcery.

Should I take supplements?

Let us suppose that you burn or in some other way rid your home of every product from your sorcery-based practitioner or company, your next question will likely be how to find a new, safe supplier. But before offering practical suggestions on finding a new source for supplements, I ask you to first consider what caused you to determine your need for each supplement. Was the "need" based on muscle testing or some other spiritually questionable method? If so, then continuing to follow that counsel gives the devil a continued hold on your health. Or perhaps upon analyzing your interest in taking that product, you realize it was based on some nebulous idea of what you believe to be good for your health. Online research and word of mouth have great power to generate fear that can motivate one to become their own doctor. Ask yourself if God was left out of the decision, whatever the motivation.

The Almighty desires that we seek Him in all things, but especially for our health. He alone is the Creator and Sustainer of life, so surely the Great I AM knows what is best for every physical condition. I encourage you to pause and spend time praying about each supplement you take or are considering taking. Initially, pray and immerse yourself in the Word rather than research. Then, give the Father time to respond through the gentle prompting of the Holy Spirit. Wait on the LORD.

Many have asked me whether to stop taking their supplements during this time of seeking the Lord. I am neither a doctor nor God; therefore, I would not presume to advise anyone for or against doing so. After initially praying about what to do, some I know have chosen to stop all of their supplements cold turkey and then waited for specific direction while

---

[xcix] Deuteronomy 18:9-12

seeking God further on the matter. Expecting to awaken with symptoms out of control, these individuals have reported to me their shock to discover either improvement or no change for better or worse. Some individuals, on the other hand, told me they initially only chose to stop the supplements used due to the guidance of muscle testing and then sought wisdom from God on the rest. How God will lead you I cannot say.

I am guessing, however, that you have likely spent much time and money doing things your own way regarding your health. Therefore, your repentance may not just include turning from divination and witchcraft but also turning from making your health an idol. This is discussed more in the coming pages, but for now, consider asking God to help you surrender your health decisions to His leading. I know this may be a terrifying prospect but remember that God loves you and knows every fiber of your being. He will not ask you to stop taking something that He knows you truly need. Conversely, neither does God desire to have you squander the resources He has given you on something unnecessary or even detrimental to your health.

A biblical view of supplements

Many have asked me whether I take any supplements. Yes, I do take a couple of products daily, although only after feeling at peace on the matter following prayer. I also use certain herbs and vitamins when colds and short-term illnesses strike. I base these decisions on the freedom I see in Scripture to do so.

So, what does the Bible have to say on the matter? I have read articles from professing Christians about the biblical support for using herbs and essential oils with the passages cited clearly taken out of context. For example, they quote Revelation 22:2, which speaks of the Tree of Life that will be found in the New Jerusalem during the millennial reign of Christ. Conveniently ignoring the incredible uniqueness of this single tree, the last part of the verse is quoted, which says, *The leaves of the tree were for the healing of the nations.* Clearly, this is not a good passage to reference in making a case that God endorses herbs for healing.

Another misused passage in the defense of making and using essential oils comes from Exodus 30:22-33 where the priests are instructed to make an anointing oil from a secret recipe of spices mixed with oil. Once again, context is crucial! Verse 32 stipulates that *it shall not be poured on the body of an ordinary person* and that any who tried to make or use this oil for personal use were to be cut off from God's people. In other words, the only place in Scripture where oils are combined is not for medicinal or private use but for the priests to use in consecrating the people and articles found in the tabernacle/temple. Plain olive oil, on the other hand, represented God's blessing and had many biblical uses.

In actuality, there are only a small handful of biblical references to medicines (remedies) and physicians. Keep in mind that until modern medicine, the remedies available all came from natural substances. This does not mean that modern medicine is evil or taboo just because it was not spoken of in the Bible, any more than planes, trains, and automobiles (of which God's Word is also silent) are evil. Instead, principles gleaned from the few Scriptures mentioning "balms" and "remedies" can be applied to any product with intended medicinal application.

God frequently used the prophet Jeremiah to speak to the Jews of how they had turned from their God and pursued sin in many forms. In Jeremiah 8 and 9, the prophet speaks of the physical illnesses they had developed despite availing themselves of the famous doctors and remedies available in the area known as Gilead. The Israelites were perplexed by their inability to get well. Jeremiah asked and answered some key questions that remain applicable today.

> *Is there no balm in Gilead? Is there no physician there? Why then is there no healing for the wound of my people?...Therefore this is what the LORD Almighty says: "See, I will refine and test them, for what else can I do because of the sin of my people?* (Jeremiah 8:22 & 9:7 NIV)

Jeremiah did not forbid or condemn the use of healing balms or physicians but instead indicated that God blocked the effectiveness of those means because of unrepentant sin. Because God used their illnesses as a method of testing and refinement, He did not allow healing to come from any method they employed.

We see this same principle played out in the story of an Old Testament king who developed a debilitating illness. Over a period of years, the generally godly King Asa, failed the test of seeking God's direction during illness, and the result was death. Although the passage makes no mention of medicinal remedies, one can safely assume his "physicians" employed many treatments. 2 Chronicles 16:12-13 says,

> *Asa was afflicted with a disease in his feet. Though his disease was severe, even in his illness he did not seek help from the Lord, but only from the physicians. Then in the forty-first year of his reign Asa died and rested with his ancestors* (NIV).

Again, in this instance, no commentary is made forbidding medical treatment. The passage instead speaks of seeking God's direction while dealing with illness. The story of another king in similar circumstances points to the same lesson. Unlike King Asa, when King Hezekiah became deathly ill, he sought the prophet Isaiah for God's guidance. Initially, God announced through Isaiah that the king would indeed die, but then Hezekiah humbly cried out to God. As a result, God instructed the king through the prophet on a specific remedy to use that would aid in his complete healing from the disease.

God could have simply healed the repentant king without further ado, but instead, a poultice brought healing over a period of time. We know the recovery took time because God gave Hezekiah a dramatic sign to encourage the king that healing would come eventually.[c] From these passages we see the biblical importance of seeking God when dealing with plaguing symptoms. We also see that God can either block or make the way for healing. These simple yet profound principles may lie at the root of why so many of God's children never recover from their illnesses no matter how much money and effort they expend.

---

[c] The story is found in 2 Kings 20:1-11 and Isaiah 38:1-22.

Replacing food with supplements

Part of the argument made for the necessity of supplements involves a belief in the lack of nutritional potency found in modern food sources. Surely, a strong argument can be made for this depletion when one considers the practices of modern farming, but does that mean supplements should fill the supposed gap? Although meat, sugars, and dairy are often vilified, many today opine on the supposed evils of bread in particular. Depending on the source or individual, the emphasis may be placed on gluten, carbohydrates, the inferiority of wheat or some other supposed failing of this historically accepted, life-sustaining substance. In recent years, countless individuals have concluded that supplements provide better nutrition than foods such as bread. But the question by one who seeks God on matters of health should be, what does God's Word say?

While the passages specific to remedies or physicians are few, the Bible speaks abundantly on food. God makes it clear in numerous passages that He desires food to be satisfying to His children and a sign of His blessing. Just one example of this comes from Psalm 103 where David calls us to praise God for specific benefits from God. Verse 5 says, *Who satisfieth thy mouth with good things; so that thy youth is renewed like the eagle's* (KJV).

God often spoke through the prophet Isaiah regarding the removal of the LORD's intended blessing to the Jews because of their sin. Carefully consider the words of Isaiah 55:2. *Why do you spend your money for that which is not bread, and your labor for that which does not satisfy? Listen diligently to me, and eat what is good, and delight yourselves in rich food.* Certainly, supplements do not satisfy, and yet people spend enormous sums on them while denying themselves the intended blessing of God—rich, satisfying food. Surely something is amiss.

If we look now to the New Testament, we discover a lengthy discussion of the many forms of deception that Satan will work in the last days. 1 Timothy 4 begins with the following words: *The Spirit clearly says that in later times some will abandon the faith and follow deceiving spirits and things taught by demons. Such teachings come through hypocritical liars, whose consciences have been seared as with a hot iron.* What will these "things taught by demons" include? *They forbid people to marry and order them to abstain from certain foods.* Sound familiar?

The passage goes on in interesting detail to give God's commentary on the forbidden foods by saying,

> *God created* [them] *to be received with thanksgiving by those who believe and who know the truth. For everything God created is good, and nothing is to be rejected if it is received with thanksgiving, because it is consecrated by the word of God and prayer.*[ci]

How interesting it is that this is written specifically with regard to the days leading up to Christ's return and the tribulation. Did God not know that modern farming practices might strip the land of nutritional sustenance? Did the Almighty's foreknowledge not include a perfect grasp on the many shortcomings of the modern food supply? So, then, what is His instruction to us? Is it to load up on supplements? No, it is instead to receive all food with thanksgiving because God created good food that is consecrated (set apart) by God's own word and our prayers. Wow! Meditate on that truth.

God intricately designed the human body to require a host of vitamins, minerals, acids, fats, proteins, enzymes, and so on, and they all work in concert with each other to perform complicated biochemical processes. Although a study of the complexities of nutrition may be fascinating, in reality, God made it very simple for humans. Everything God created is good!

Unsubstantiated fear of food that God has called good is from Satan and should be dealt with as such. When someone has a negative, physical reaction (pain, digestive distress, headaches, etc.) in response to a particular food, that person can understandably become afraid to eat it. If one dwells on that reaction to food, and/or it happens a second time,

---

[ci] The entire passage quoted in the previous verses comes from 1 Timothy 4:1-5 (NIV).

something scientists call *brain plasticity* comes into play and can increase the likelihood of further occurrences.

In a fascinating book on neuroscience by Norman Doidge, MD, called *The Brain That Changes Itself*, he explains how every thought we have forms synaptic connections in the brain. Synapses are the gaps between the neurons and require various neurotransmitters to bridge the gaps. Because neurons and synapses work as pathways for information, the brain is constantly forming new pathways or strengthening existing ones upon which information might travel more efficiently. The more times we think a particular thought, the stronger those connections become, and the more likely it is that we will think that thought again.

Frequently, this powerful association between food and physical discomfort is not the result of a true allergy or a particular disease but the plastic brain responding to fear. As neurologists say, "Neurons that wire together, fire together." Science has proven that thoughts and emotions directly trigger the autonomic nervous system, thereby stimulating the digestive system. Therefore, negative thoughts and emotions while eating will have a tremendous impact on the body's response to food.

This was the case with me. Although I did have true allergies to a handful of foods (based on blood allergy testing), over time more and more foods made me feel sick. I eventually got to the place where just putting any food or liquid in my mouth would send my stomach into spasm and painfully swell up like a balloon about to burst. It took me years to discover that I somehow needed to change the nerve pathways in my brain so that I no longer considered food to be the enemy. Since the Bible speaks of being transformed by the renewing of our minds by truth, I decided to try a particular tactic that worked beautifully.

I wrote 1 Timothy 4:4-5 on a notecard and would read it as part of my prayer of blessing before I ate anything. Again, it says, ***For everything God created is good, and nothing is to be rejected if it is received with thanksgiving, because it is consecrated by the word of God and prayer.*** I would then go on to pray something like this, "Lord, thank you that this food you have given me IS good, and I trust you to make it a blessing to my body."

Over the course of that first couple of weeks of praying those verses, my physical reactions to food diminished until they largely disappeared. When they occasionally reappear, I remind myself of God's truth and make sure not to take too much notice. I know that an occasional reaction to food is completely normal, but now I also know that the brain can respond to those reactions with unwanted, powerful associations. Taking such thoughts captive has yielded great dividends for me. So, before you conclude that the supplements you consume are necessary because you cannot eat this or that food group, spend some time considering if you too have traded God's intended blessing for what does not satisfy.

Researching supplements

If, after seeking the Lord for wisdom on your supplements, you deem it appropriate to move forward on researching and purchasing some, how do you go about it? As you well know, countless doctors and individuals claim expertise on nutrition and supplements. I recommend you skip over all such recommendations. Instead, search for double blind, clinical studies that have been done on the supplement you are considering. You only want to know if that product has been scientifically proven effective for your particular situation. Such studies rule out old wives' tales, word of mouth, biases, and ulterior motives. Additionally, so much can be gleaned from these studies, including dosages, duration of treatment, side effects, and degree of effectiveness.

I recommend the following type of online search: *Do clinical studies on* _____ (fill in the blank with the product of interest) *show it to be effective in treating* _____ (fill in the blank with the symptom of interest). For example, "Do clinical studies on D Mannose show it to be effective for treating urinary tract infections?" Then, scan through the details of the study(ies) to learn all kinds of helpful information. I encourage you to disregard websites that claim "studies show" this or that to be effective because the studies referred to may or may not be up to the rigors of double blind, clinical studies. Often such claims are wholly fictitious or interpreted to come to a desired conclusion. Rarely do websites cite the source for the study backing up their claims, but if they do, make sure to check it thoroughly and not just assume it is valid or even that the study actually exists.

I realize that reading clinical studies can be intimidating, but you can always jump to the conclusion section at the end to determine if you wish to read further. Generally, the abstracts for clinical studies are available on PubMed and also include links at the end to similar studies that have been done on that supplement or condition.

Weeding out bad supplement companies

In light of numerous companies utilizing muscle testing in the formation of their products, I recommend further investigation. Go to the company's website to look for anything that promotes an energy-based philosophy. This information often appears on pages discussing the company's origins or philosophy. Also, read the product descriptions to see if any of their jargon raises red flags. Remember, if you are praying for God's guidance in all of this, He will draw your attention appropriately. This is another opportunity to flex those spiritual muscles of discernment and take notice of the lack of or presence of peace in your heart.

Finally, you may want to also take the step of contacting the company to ask them directly if they employ muscle testing in any aspect of their product development or the company as a whole. I have done this on a few occasions. Once, the employee reported back to me that he took my question to their board for discussion before answering definitively. Other times, I have received no response, and since I was skeptical based on the website, I chose to take my business elsewhere. One former nutritionist, who formerly utilized muscle testing in her practice, told me that one popular supplement company does not directly use muscle testing in product development but does sell "testing kits" for their supplements to make them easier for practitioners to muscle test with their clients.

Some readers might wonder why I make an issue over purchasing products from a company that might or might not be involved in witchcraft. First, 1 Corinthians 10:20-22 warns Christians against secondhand participation with demons by consuming food associated with pagan practices. Second, wherever possible, it is good practice for

Christians to avoid using their money to support businesses that participate with demons. Third, unclean spirits are both intelligent and mobile. As such, it seems likely that they attach themselves to objects (i.e., certain crystals, Ouija board, pendulum, etc.) in anticipation of the objects' use. If demons indeed do so, possessing those objects opens a door for evil in your home.

Consider what can be learned by comparing our dilemma over whether to purchase products from companies involved in demonic practices with the New Testament one of eating meat previously sacrificed to idols. In Revelation 2:14 & 20 the churches of Pergamum and Thyatira are rebuked for eating such meat. In a long discourse in 1 Corinthians 8-11, the apostle Paul also cautions against knowingly eating food sacrificed to idols for various reasons. However, he also instructs Christians who are eating dinner with unsaved neighbors to not ask the origins of the meat being served. In such cases, one's conscience should be at peace.

That mindset may be applicable to how we should approach supplement purchases. If you know the company or practitioner you purchase products from is involved in demonic practices, do not use their products. Perform due diligence in researching a company and praying for direction so that you do not personally support companies who practice what God has forbidden. Having done these things and made the best decision you can make, let your conscience be at rest.

Cautionary tales

On a few occasions since the LORD healed me fromthirteen diagnosed health conditions, I have failed to follow my own advice regarding first seeking God about supplement consumption. One such time occurred after many years of peaceful health, when I entered the dreaded time of menopause. Like many women in that phase of life, hormonal fluctuations began to wreak havoc on my mood and health. With little thought and certainly no time of prayer over the decision, I purchased and began taking a supplement claiming to boost fading hormones in menopause. Surely natural hormone balancing through herbs was an appropriate course of action. It seemed such a simple matter. To my dismay, the estrogen boosting herbs began to recreate the female problems the good LORD had healed me from a decade earlier. Oh my! Repentant, I finally began a time of seeking my heavenly Father for the wisdom that He alone held about what was best for my body during that change of life.

On another occasion, my husband came down with a bad cold while we were traveling. Our anniversary falls a few days before Christmas, and we had gone to visit my parents before heading out for our yearly anniversary trip. To my great disappointment, Seth fell sick. Coughing and sneezing did not fit into my expectations for a romantic getaway. Never fear, I thought; I would just load him up on Vitamin C and B-complex, which I happened to have with me. I failed to consider that he was not used to taking B vitamins, especially at high doses, and that suddenly doing so would trigger an immediate and massive detoxification episode. As a result, my poor husband spent the next 24 hours with not just a bad cold but debilitating flu-like symptoms and diarrhea. My remorse did little to ease his misery, but I was humbly reminded of the power of supplements and my need to pray first rather than act on my limited knowledge.

I share these personal mistakes to highlight a common misconception. While it is true that God gave us brains so that we can assimilate information and make decisions to the best of our abilities, the Bible reveals a loving Father who desires that His children look to Him for guidance in every aspect of their daily lives. Proverbs 3:5-6 says, ***Trust in the Lord with all your heart, and do not lean on your own understanding. In all your ways acknowledge him, and he will make straight your paths.*** Does it really say NOT to lean on our own understanding? Yes, it truly does. It is pride that causes us to think that we know best and do not need the Holy Spirit's special leading. Our knowledge, no matter how well-informed, pales in comparison to the infinite knowledge and wisdom of the Father.

The alure of divination is to feel like we have insight into the workings of the human body that can guide us in knowing what to do for our health. Knowledge is power, and through muscle testing, we are led to believe that we have an instantaneous answer that is definitive. We do not have to wait for traditional lab work or imaging results. We do not have to wait for weeks or months to make our case to traditional doctors who may not help a bit. And, perhaps without even consciously recognizing this motivation, we do not want to go through the uncomfortable process of seeking and waiting on God for His promised wisdom. Instead, the temptation is to determine, through muscle testing, what is wrong and exactly how much to take of the revealed supplement. Yes, divination seems so much easier!

However, out of love for His treasured people God has forbidden divination and witchcraft because the devil seeks our destruction not our good. Look to the Father. The sovereign LORD knows what is best for your body and has made you a beautiful promise: *If any of you lacks wisdom, let him ask God, who gives generously to all without reproach, and it will be given him.*[cii]

[cii] James 1:5

CHAPTER 17

A Biblical Perspective of Health

*Do not be wise in your own eyes; fear the LORD and shun evil.
This will bring health to your body and nourishment to your
bones.* Proverbs 3:7-8

When God first impressed upon me to write a series of blog articles speaking out against muscle testing, I pleaded with Him not to require this of me. Two reasons existed for my resistance. One centered around the shame I felt at the time over having fallen prey to deception, but the other reason caused even greater angst. I knew the despair that often comes when dealing endlessly with poor health, and the dire need for hope. Muscle testing lures with the illusion of hope. Even though I knew, without a doubt, those practices were wrong, I hated to be the bearer of bad news without simultaneously offering hope to those who were suffering. Despite my arguments as to how God's plan required tweaking, the Holy Spirit's conviction did not relent, so I wrote the articles.

Following their publication, I intensified my biblical studies on health so that I might write a book about the true hope for healing revealed in God's Word. Sadly, few know and understand the abundance of teaching found in Scripture on health, illness, and healing. Instead, most of Christendom consumes a secular perspective of health and merely adds a side dish of prayer just in case God is inclined to intervene. Having studied, in-depth, every passage in the Bible that references health, illness, and healing, I can assure you that a biblical perspective of health often runs counter to the mere biological understanding to which medicine points. I cannot possibly summarize all of the studies that my book, *Life to the Body—Biblical Principles for Health & Healing*, contains, but I will provide an overview in this chapter.

If you desire hope that will not disappoint, you must begin with the life-giving Word. The Psalms speak repeatedly of this truth: ***He sent out his word and healed them, and delivered them from their destruction,***[ciii] and ***Your testimonies are righteous forever; give me understanding that I may live.***[civ] But, what in His Word must we understand to live? Is it a special diet, as some teach or much, much more? The book of Proverbs speaks repeatedly of a "path of life" that the wise will follow—***She does not ponder the path of life; her ways wander, and she does not know it.***[cv] And, ***The path of life leads upward for the prudent, that he may turn away from Sheol beneath.***[cvi] Those who long for hope that will not fail must carefully consider this "path of life" described in the Scriptures.

There is a path of life.

I am a list person who loves the sense of accomplishment that comes when I can cross through completed tasks; however, the biblical path of life does not work that way. Just as Christianity is a relationship with the Savior, so also the path of life flows out of that relationship. Psalm 16:11 says, ***You have made known to me the path of life. You will fill me with joy in your presence.*** In knowing God, we discover the source of life. King Solomon speaks at length in Proverbs chapters three through six of the path of life being a continuous journey with God's truth as the roadmap. As you read the following verses, notice the multiple references to four critical elements that lead one to refreshment, healing, and life. I have

---

[ciii] Psalm 107:20
[civ] Psalm 119:144
[cv] Proverbs 5:6
[cvi] Proverbs 15:24

highlighted the references to these four elements: peace, the heart, wisdom to obey, and discipline for disobedience.[cvii]

> *My son, do not forget my teaching, but let your heart keep my commandments, for length of days and years of life and peace they will add to you.... Trust in the Lord with all your heart, and do not lean on your own understanding. In all your ways acknowledge him, and he will make straight your paths. Be not wise in your own eyes; fear the Lord and turn away from evil. It will be healing to your flesh and refreshment to your bones...*
>
> *My son, do not despise the Lord's discipline or be weary of his reproof, for the Lord reproves him whom he loves, as a father the son in whom he delights. Blessed is the one who finds wisdom, and the one who gets understanding...Long life is in her right hand; in her left hand are riches and honor. Her ways are ways of pleasantness, and all her paths are peace. She is a tree of life to those who lay hold of her; those who hold her fast are called blessed.*
>
> *Let them* [wisdom] *not escape from your sight; keep them within your heart. For they are life to those who find them, and healing to all their flesh. Keep your heart with all vigilance, for from it flow the springs of life.* (Proverbs 3:1-2, 5-8, 11-13, 16-18 4:21-23, emphasis mine)

When you unpack those verses, you gain many insights that are generally ignored, and a rough framework for a biblical perspective of health emerges. First, obedience to God's wise instruction brings life. Now, some would say that this is simply because God knows best, and sin has consequences that can affect health. For example, getting drunk on wine will affect your health negatively or being a glutton leads to obesity, which causes a myriad of health problems. This perspective is absolutely true but falls short because it portrays God as passive in matters of health.

[cvii] I have taken a selection of verses out of a lengthy passage to give the big picture in a condensed form. However, reading Proverbs 3-6 in its entirety is recommended.

Pause for a moment to reread those verses from Proverbs. Do they not clearly portray God as actively involved in the health of His children? Just as the LORD does not watch from a distance while letting His children stumble around in the process of sanctification, neither is He a casual observer in matters of health. His influence is not a side-dish but the whole buffet! Scripture repeatedly bears this out.

Those verses also strongly connect peace with health. The wise will remember that *all her paths are peace.* Analyzing the entirety of biblical passages on health, illness, and healing reveals a fascinating picture of how God has directly tied physical well-being to peace in one's heart with God, man, and self. This should not be surprising, considering He is the God of Peace.[cviii]

The third key element the three chapters from Proverbs draw our attention to is that God made the heart the wellspring of life! When you look at the original languages of the Bible, you discover a staggering number of uses of the word heart (roughly nine hundred) compared with almost complete silence about the head, mind, or brain. In fact, most of the time when you read the word mind in Scripture, the original language does not reference the mind at all. Instead, it is either soul, spirit, heart, or a generic word for the center of everything (the inward part). When I discovered the significant biblical emphasis on the heart, I spent many hours reading every one of the nine hundred passages using that word, as well as every use of spirit and soul. What I learned in my studies explains why Solomon advised his son to *keep your heart with all vigilance, for from it flow the springs of life* (4:23).

Once you begin to pay attention to these elements in the Bible, you will notice them throughout its whole and a biblical view of health shines through.

[cviii] Romans 5:13, 16:20, 1 Corinthians 14:33, 2 Corinthians 13:11, & others.

The common versus biblical view of health

The following chart depicts how Christians typically view the influences on health, with all things physical having the greatest impact.[cix]

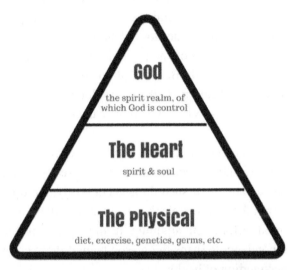

Common Perspective of Health

chart created by Marci Julin--HeartandMindMinistries.com

Because people commonly assume that everything in the physical realm affects health to the greatest degree, their seemingly logical reasoning goes like this: If something affects me in the physical realm, the solution must also be found through physical means. So, medical intervention, diet, exercise, etc. become the sole focus. The thought is that I just need to eat right, exercise enough, and eliminate germs, stress, and toxic influences. Then, I will be healthy! Physical realm problems equal physical realm solutions. It is thought to be as simple as that!

Continuing upward in this pyramid diagram, we see that it is generally thought that the heart impacts health to a lesser degree than the

---

[cix] I have taken much of the information shared in this chapter from my book, *Life to the Body—Biblical Principles for Health & Healing*. If you desire to gain a deeper understanding of a biblical perspective of health, you will find that book a tremendous asset.

physical realm. For instance, psychology recognizes things like trauma, depression, or a broken heart will detrimentally influence anatomy. Also, in recognition of the negative effect of such things on health, numerous energy-based practices have sprung up in an attempt to bring healing.

Finally, the top of the pyramid acknowledges that, as a Christian, we also believe God can supersede normal biological processes and bring miraculous healing. The top of the pyramid gives assent to the LORD's sovereign control over health. Because of this belief, prayer meetings are filled with requests for healing. Sadly, God seldom answers those prayers, which begs the question—Why? We know Yahweh is good, so there must be a reason.

With more resources, modalities, and knowledge available now than ever before, one would expect health to have greatly increased among those who take advantage of such things. Tragically, the opposite is true. A staggering number of people have spent countless thousands and expended untold efforts on attaining healing only to find increased suffering and bondage. Perhaps the reason behind these conundrums lies in a false understanding of health.

When one investigates the biblical portrayal of health, one discovers a complete reversal in the top and bottom layers of the chart. God and the spirit realm, acting in submission to His will, have the greatest impact, with the heart following closely in importance. All the physical components, whether diet, exercise, germs, or genetics, only influence health to the degree that God and the heart allow. Yes, we live in a sin-cursed world and are subject to the impact of physical elements. Have you noticed, though, that a variety of responses occur among people exposed to the same germ or illness? The assumption, of course, is that immune systems vary, or that genetic factors account for the disparity. Perhaps, more often than ever imagined, the reasons fall outside mere biological controls.

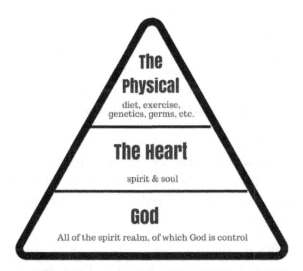

A Biblical Perspective of Health

chart created by Marci Julin--HeartandMindMinistries.com

Consider just a few of the passages that establish that God, not things in the physical realm, largely determines health. As Paul said, *For physical training is of some value, but godliness has value for all things.*[cx] Romans 8:13 says, *For if you live according to the flesh you will die, but if by the Spirit you put to death the deeds of the body, you will live.* Do we want life and peace? Then, we must allow the Holy Spirit, not the flesh, to govern our hearts. Romans 8:6 says; *The mind governed by the flesh is death, but the mind governed by the Spirit is life and peace.*

The apostle Paul said in Acts 17:28 that *in him we live and move and have our being.* Meditate on that truth for a time! It is God, the Creator and sustainer of life, that empowers you to live, move, and exist rather than the things you assume hold sway. That is how godliness has value for ALL things. Because God has the power to bless or block the way to health, and the heart gives or hinders life, everything in the physical realm can be effective or ineffective and beneficial or detrimental, depending on factors outside of that limited realm. Understanding and applying this

---

[cx] 1 Timothy 4:8

knowledge brings a complete paradigm shift in how one approaches illness.

Also recognized by the bottom tier of the pyramid diagram is the biblical teaching that the spirit realm, regulated by the sovereign LORD, often influences health. Ephesians 6:11-12 reminds us that the seemingly physical struggle we face is actually a spiritual one.

> *Put on the full armor of God, so that you can take your stand against the devil's schemes. For our struggle is not against flesh and blood, but against the rulers, against the authorities, against the powers of this dark world and against the spiritual forces of evil in the heavenly realms.*

Consider also the following biblical list of physical conditions that are directly attributed to unclean spirits: Job had boils from head to toe.[cxi] Children had seizures.[cxii] A man was mute,[cxiii] and a woman was crippled for eighteen years.[cxiv] Acts 5:16 speaks of the *sick and those tormented by evil spirits* being *healed,* and 19:12 also says that *their illnesses were cured, and the evil spirits left them.* Therefore, the Bible clearly contradicts the assumption that all physical symptoms are from physical causes.

A heart at peace

As I read through the entire Bible in three months while highlighting and recording every passage that referenced health, illness, or healing, I noticed a striking picture of the God of Peace actively controlling health through the heart (soul and spirit) based on one's state of peace with God, others, and oneself. Let us consider each one separately. The most prominent in the Bible concerns the impact on health when peace with God is lacking, so let us begin there.

[cxi] Job 2:4-7
[cxii] Matthew 17:15-18
[cxiii] Matthew 9:32-33
[cxiv] Luke 13:10-16

When Christians walk in rebellion towards God or have a pattern of sin that grieves the Holy Spirit, they are not at peace with the Father. Because He desires fellowship with His children and sin prevents that, God may bring discipline through illness. Consider, for example, Isaiah 1:4b-6, which says,

They have forsaken the Lord, they have despised the Holy One of Israel, they are utterly estranged. Why will you still be struck down? Why will you continue to rebel? The whole head is sick, and the whole heart faint. From the sole of the foot even to the head, there is no soundness in it, but bruises and sores and raw wounds; they are not pressed out or bound up or softened with oil.

Although numerous passages can be found in the Bible that demonstrate God's use of illness as a means of loving discipline for sinful children, I chose that one because it also makes a key point. When illness is due to discipline for sin, typical means of eliminating distressing symptoms will fail to bring lasting relief. In Old Testament times, oil was used to bring healing to wounds, but verse 6 describes the ineffectiveness of those normal treatments because God's discipline for unrepentant sin was at work. Why would the Father allow healing when His child still walks in disobedience?

According to Romans 8, to walk according to the flesh brings death, but to walk according to the Spirit brings life and peace. When I have unexplained and lingering symptoms and cannot seem to break out of the cycle of walking according to the flesh, I find it very helpful to fast.[cxv] By purposefully denying the flesh, I silence the clamor of fleshly demands that I might better hear the Spirit's gentle voice. He may reveal sin so that I might repent, thereby restoring peace with God, myself, and others. Even if God's discipline for sin is not the cause of the illness, turning the focus from the misery of the flesh to the Spirit who gives life is exceedingly valuable. God will not despise a broken and contrite heart.[cxvi]

[cxv] For more information on fasting, see Appendix G.
[cxvi] Psalm 51:7

If the Holy Spirit brings conviction, the promises in Scripture that true repentance leads to healing from illness provides great hope. Jesus' suffering at the cross conquered the curse of the flesh (death) making provision through sanctification so that we can be healed. The work has been done. Provision has been made.[cxvii] Ezekiel 18:30-32 speaks of this.

> *"Therefore, I will judge you, O house of Israel, every one according to his ways, declares the Lord God. Repent and turn from all your transgressions, lest iniquity be your ruin. Cast away from you all the transgressions that you have committed and make yourselves a new heart and a new spirit! Why will you die, O house of Israel? For I have no pleasure in the death of anyone, declares the Lord God; so turn, and live."*

The prophet Jeremiah also spoke of this when he wrote,

> *But my people do not know the requirements of the LORD...Since they have rejected the word of the LORD, what kind of wisdom do they have?*
>
> *For they have healed the wound of my people slightly, saying "Peace, peace," when there is no peace... (KJV) We hoped for peace but no good has come, for a time of healing but there is only terror.*
>
> *Is there no balm in Gilead? Is there no physician there? Why then is there no healing for the wound of my people?...Therefore, this is what the LORD Almighty says: "See, I will refine and test them, for what else can I do because of the sin of my people?* (Jeremiah 8:7, 9,11-12, 15, 22 & 9:7 NIV)

[cxvii] I go into great detail in my book *Life to the Body—Biblical Principles for Health & Healing* to present the biblical case for healing for those who wish to learn more on that specific topic.

Peace with yourself

Love your neighbor as yourself.[cxviii] In only five words Jesus summarized the teaching of much of the New Testament. The verse coming before that simple command speaks of loving the Lord with every part of our being. It is then, out of the Father's love that we can love both ourselves and others. The converse of that simple command indicates that if you hate yourself, you will certainly be unable to love others. Are you consumed with self-loathing because of guilt, shame, or anger towards yourself? If so, then your heart lacks peace and disease can obtain a foothold. Proverbs 18:14 says, *A man's spirit will endure sickness, but a crushed spirit who can bear?*

We see the same truth in Proverbs where Solomon contrasts the negative impact of heartache and discouragement. *A happy heart makes the face cheerful, but heartache crushes the spirit. All the days of the oppressed are wretched, but the cheerful heart has a continual feast.*[cxix] Again, we see this spoken of in Proverbs. *A cheerful heart is good medicine, but a crushed spirit dries up the bones.* That simple verse contains so much truth, which unfortunately is lost in translation. The literal meaning of the Hebrew phrase, "good medicine," is actually "a cure." Therefore, a more literal translation would be, *A cheerful heart is a cure, but a crushed spirit dries up the bones*. A biblical perspective of health recognizes the importance of a heart that is at peace with oneself.

Peace with others

Last, perhaps you are holding on to anger, unforgiveness, and bitterness towards someone who has wronged you. According to the Bible, that lack of peace towards others will quench your well-spring of life—the heart, and illness can take hold. Proverbs 14:30 says, *A heart at peace gives life to the body but envy rots the bones.* (NIV) Colossians 3:12-16b reminds us in greater detail of the need to demonstrate love and to be at peace with others.

[cxviii] Luke 10:27
[cxix] Proverbs 15:13 & 15

Put on then, as God's chosen ones, holy and beloved, compassionate hearts, kindness, humility, meekness, and patience, bearing with one another and, if one has a complaint against another, forgiving each other; as the Lord has forgiven you, so you also must forgive. And above all these put on love, which binds everything together in perfect harmony. And let the peace of Christ rule in your hearts, to which indeed you were called in one body. And be thankful. Let the word of Christ dwell in you richly...

I do not know about you, but this is where I stumble so often. I do not want to overlook an offense or love those who reject me or forgive wrongs that wound me deeply. In fact, I cannot do it, and neither can you! Only when we allow the love of Christ dwelling in us to shape our thoughts, desires, and actions can we glorify the Father in our day-to-day life. Peace with others encompasses who we are intended to be in Christ and the very plan of God to glorify Himself through us. *We know that we have passed from death to life because we love each other. Anyone who does not love remains in death*.[cxx]

Some alternative practices seek to replace obedience to God's ways with a modality of biofeedback, such as tapping, while speaking what you wish to be true. Supposedly, this retrains the brain. Such practices are godless and completely absent from Scripture. According to Scripture, the brain is not the problem; the heart is. We do not make something true by speaking it, and we cannot convince our hearts of a lie by "tapping it in." Reliance on such behaviors produces bondage, not freedom. No amount of tapping will ever bring peace towards yourself or others. Instead, Romans 12:2 instructs, *Do not be conformed to this world, but be transformed by the renewal of your mind, that by testing you may discern what is the will of God, what is good and acceptable and perfect.* It is the Word that transforms and renews.

[cxx] 1 John 3:14-15

By faith, we trust the living Word and walk in obedience to what He says. For example, when dealing with unforgiveness, the Bible says, *If your brother sins against you, go and tell him his fault, between you and him alone. If he listens to you, you have gained your brother.*[cxxi] And, *if one has a complaint against another, forgiving each other; as the Lord has forgiven you, so you also must forgive.*[cxxii] When acted upon, these and many other such instructions about how to deal with hurt and brokenness bring healing because of the love of God working and moving in your heart.

If you lack peace in your heart towards others, you also undoubtedly suffer from health issues or will before long. Having, myself, suffered childhood abuse and then trauma as an adult, I understand the incredible difficulty of being at peace with oneself and others. Praise be to God that He promises to heal the brokenhearted and bind up their wounds! Just remember, wound care takes time. The Lord and His Word are faithful. As you *stand praying, forgive.*[cxxiii] Ask the Lord to totally replace any hurt, anger, and bitter poison crowding your soul with the love the Father has lavished on you. Then, you too will see God glorified through your healing.

Faith required

The examples of healing in the Bible all indicate that the individual must have faith to be healed. Jesus praised the Canaanite woman for her great faith and in response, healed her daughter.[cxxiv] When a man whose son was demon-possessed asked if Jesus could heal him, the response was, *"'If you can'?" said Jesus. "Everything is possible for one who believes." Immediately the boy's father exclaimed, "I do believe; help me overcome my unbelief!"*[cxxv] Many times Jesus followed his healings

---

[cxxi] Matthew 18:15
[cxxii] Colossians 3:13
[cxxiii] Mark 11:25 KJV
[cxxiv] Matthew 15:22-28
[cxxv] Mark 9:22-24

with the statement, ***your faith has healed you.***[cxxvi] So, faith or trust that God can heal is required, but many put the cart before the horse. God brings healing according to His Word, which says that peace with God, oneself, and others comes first. If you seek to know the Father through His Word with the same fervor with which you previously sought medical answers, the results will astound you. The LORD is faithful!

I am frequently contacted by people who have heard my teaching on the biblical principles of health. With great joy, I listen to these individuals describe to me the realization that their hearts have not been at peace in some area, but how they have now chosen to turn their focus to seeking after God and following His ways. It thrills my soul to learn how God brings them healing in time. Such changes do not occur overnight. Many questions, blunders, and struggles along the way are inevitable. The fear of missing something or not doing things just right can consume the thoughts of those who want to be right with the Lord. If this is you, remember that the heart of God is that His people would seek Him with all their hearts. Is that your desire? If so, keep on! Do not stop! Your heavenly Father is greatly pleased. He will hear and answer your prayer for healing. ***He who promised is faithful.***[cxxvii] Go in peace.

[cxxvi] Matthew 9:22, Mark 10:52, Luke 8:48 & 18:42
[cxxvii] Hebrews 10:23

CHAPTER 18

Moving Forward in the Light

the people dwelling in darkness have seen a great light, and for those dwelling in the region and shadow of death, on them a light has dawned.
Matthew 4:16

A heart at peace gives life to the body...[cxxviii] For most who have walked in the dark for a time, coming into the light initially brings confusion and uncertainty, not peace. Just as our physical eyes resist sudden brightness with temporary squinting, blurriness, and adjustment, so do our spiritual eyes. Oh, but once one has acclimated to the light, what peace comes in the seeing!

Perhaps you have come into the light and now see the deception for what it is, but you find yourself fearful, full of questions, and uncertain about the future. Let me say to you: If you are in Christ, you and your family will be okay! Consider the words of Zecheriah about the Lord Jesus, *because of the tender mercy of our God, whereby the sunrise shall visit us from on high to give light to those who sit in darkness and in the shadow of death, to guide our feet into the way of peace.*[cxxix] God's desire is that you come into the light because that is where He will walk with you in the way of peace…one step at a time.

[cxxviii] Proverbs 14:30 (NIV)
[cxxix] Luke 1:78-79

I remember well the disorientation I felt upon coming into the light of truth regarding my former involvement with energy-based practices, and I have heard from hundreds of others who have experienced the same. The devil rages against the light and will likely mount a full-scale attack to draw you back into the darkness of deceit and sin. This may begin by provoking questions or doubts about what you have concluded—***Did God really say…***[cxxx] To counter this, I have devoted the last section of this book to the real testimonies of many others who have concluded the same and come into the light. You and I are not alone!

Another form of attack may involve the continuation of disturbing symptoms or an onslaught of new ones that leave you desperate for help and desiring to return to your former manner of dealing with illness. After all, even Job despaired when God allowed the devil to test him with physical suffering. But even in Job's despair, what was his response? ***Though he slay me, I will hope in him.***[cxxxi] I beg of you—Do not return to the darkness of your former ways. Put your hope in the God who loves you but is allowing you to be tested. Stand firm. This time of testing will pass, and you, in great joy, will walk the path of peace.

Let me offer you three very practical recommendations for the days ahead. Continue to clean house. Establish new ways of dealing with health concerns. And last, seek, with all of your heart, the LORD Almighty through His Word.

Continue to clean house

Have you ever noticed when you clean house that the brighter the light in the room, the more dirt is revealed? My kitchen has large, east facing windows that bathe the room in light every morning. At first light, I am frequently shocked at the revelation of crumbs and debris littering the floor and counters. Surely, I had wiped down every surface the night before, and yet, the bright light of day makes known all that was missed.

[cxxx] Genesis 3:1 (NIV)
[cxxxi] Job 13:15

Similarly, you have come into the light, and the Holy Spirit will now begin to reveal other areas of deception and sin requiring repentance. Your previous sin had grieved the Spirit and you lacked ears to hear, but now things are changing. Throw back the curtains and welcome the light so that you might continue to clear away the cobwebs and grime. How? Pray daily that God will make known to you any areas of deception and sin in your life and that He will give you a heart of willingness to repent when He does. Then act on what the Lord reveals.

Part of this process may involve taking a second look at the philosophies of health that you have believed and followed. For example, ask some of the following questions: Are the things I have believed about my health true? Which of these supplements should I really be taking? Are certain foods truly bad for me? Am I in bondage to anything other than the loving Savior? While I have pursued answers to my health, have I neglected the state of my heart—peace with God, with others, and myself?

For those working in the healthcare industry, you will probably need to spend time prayerfully scrutinizing the things you have been taught in light of Scripture. For example, Will the body really heal itself if you give it what it needs? What protocols are energy-based and need to be discarded? What "science" have you been taught that is really pseudoscience? What practices or approaches can I use with clients that reflect evidence-based medicine and biblical principles? Consider starting a notebook so that you can write individual questions such as those at the top of separate pages. Make corresponding notes on the appropriate page as you begin to sort through your training and analyze what is true and what is deception.

Whether you are a practitioner or not, hold each question up to the Father and ask for the wisdom that He promises to abundantly give when asked. Consider the words of this promise from James and the exhortation that follows.

If any of you lacks wisdom, let him ask God, who gives generously to all without reproach, and it will be given him. But let him ask in faith, with no doubting, for the one who doubts is like a wave of the sea that is driven and tossed by the wind. For that person must not suppose that he will receive anything from the Lord; he is a double-minded man, unstable in all his ways. (1:5-8).

Remember that often the guidance of the Holy Spirit is as subtle as the presence of peace or the lack thereof. Sometimes, He brings confirmation through other means AFTER one acts in obedience. If you feel like a wave of the sea, driven and tossed back and forth in your thinking about the matter, then, you probably have your answer—That substance, practice, or belief is not what the God of peace knows is best for you. Do not doubt but act upon the wisdom God has provided.

One area of cleaning house that you may not think of but that I have often found coincides with participation in demonically based health practices is false religious beliefs. Throughout the letters to the churches found in the New Testament, the apostles equate false teachers with demonic activity. False beliefs undermine truth and provide open doors to the evil one.

But false prophets also arose among the people, just as there will be false teachers among you, who will secretly bring in destructive heresies, even denying the Master who bought them, bringing upon themselves swift destruction. And many will follow their sensuality, and because of them the way of truth will be blasphemed. And in their greed, they will exploit you with false words.[cxxxii]

The hyper-charismatic movement and New Apostolic Reformation (NAR) are rife with heresy. Contemplative prayer and word of faith teachings must also be held up to the lens of Scripture as a whole rather than a few words taken out of context. Yoga and eastern meditation practices, along with breathing exercises may also open doors to the enemy of your soul. Do not suppose that combining prayer and Scripture with them changes their nature and prevents corruption. *Do you not know that a little leaven leavens the whole lump?*[cxxxiii]

[cxxxii] 2Peter 2:1-3
[cxxxiii] 1 Corinthians 5:6

We are told to search out the Scriptures daily for ourselves in order to test what we are taught.[cxxxiv] Although heresy in the church is not within the scope of this book, I mention it because I have encountered so many who were unknowingly involved in both energy medicine and religious deception. A soil depleted of nutrients from the presence of one weed will allow all manner of weeds to thrive. Root out deception of all kinds.

Establish new ways of dealing with health concerns.

We live in a sin-cursed world where deterioration, germs, and defective genetics wreak havoc on our bodies. This is unavoidable. You and those you love will get sick. In the past, you have approached those challenges and struggles as you deemed best with the knowledge you had at the time. Before entering alternative health care, perhaps you suffered much at the hands of traditional doctors. Now, you are uncertain about what to do when problems arise. Although I previously covered this topic in the chapters on supplements and a biblical perspective of health, so much more could be said. I strongly recommend my book, *Life to the Body—Biblical Principles for Health & Healing*, for really understanding a biblical approach to health and as a source of encouragement as you strike out on the path of peace.

To reiterate—if you or your family have a medical emergency, DO NOT hesitate to seek medical help. For everything else, rather than first doing an online search, pray. Take time to ask for God's wisdom and direction BEFORE scheduling an appointment, taking something, or acting upon your fear. You will be astounded at how He will faithfully lead you.

I truly understand the profound fear that seeing a traditional doctor can evoke in one who has been harmed by past tests and medicines or made to feel ridiculous and misunderstood. I remember the first time I had to go to the doctor after repenting of muscle testing. I spent time in prayer before scheduling the appointment and sensed God's leading to do so. Nonetheless, as the day drew near, I found myself talking to my husband

---

[cxxxiv] Acts 17:11

about why I should cancel the appointment. He pointed out my fear to me and encouraged me to stay the course. The truth was that I was terrified, but God used this to again teach me to put my hope in Him and to be obedient to His leading in my life.

As discussed previously, there are many options, both traditional and natural, through which God may bring you help and healing. Ask Him! He may, however, reveal a need for you to deal with sin or issues of the heart. Be aware that fear can be a consuming force, driving us to make rash decisions. In such times, remember the words of Paul: *For you did not receive the spirit of slavery to fall back into fear, but you have received the Spirit of adoption as sons, by whom we cry, "Abba! Father!"* Abide in Him!

With all of your heart, seek God through His Word.

When we are sick or in pain, we just want it to go away. A magic bullet would be perfect! If that is not possible, then we want a list of what to do so that completing X, Y, and Z guarantees we will be better. I understand that thinking all too well. Unfortunately, that rarely happens because God frequently uses pain and illness to sanctify us. Sanctification happens while we walk with Him. Most likely you have spent vast amounts of time and money focused on your health. If you are honest, you might recognize that you have made health an idol. Your heavenly Father is a jealous God. Surrender this idol to Him and turn all of that time and focus towards knowing Him. *But seek first the kingdom of God and his righteousness, and all these things will be added to you.*[cxxxv]

Many who reach out to me have allowed me the privilege of staying in touch with them as they walk out of the deception and sin of involvement with energy medicine. A handful of those chose to determinedly seek God with all of their hearts by getting into the Word. They did not choose to merely find replacements for their former ensnarement but instead completely changed their focus. You will read

---

[cxxxv] Matthew 6:33

about a few of those in the testimony section. One stands out in my mind whose testimony is not at the end, but I will instead share her story here.

Jane is a young, ambitious woman who created a successful business as a nutrition consultant.[cxxxvi] While doing phone consultations with clients, she relied on muscle testing to determine "appropriate" recommendations. She had previously learned muscle testing in an attempt to deal with her own chronic stomach issues and other health struggles. Upon repentance, she had difficult decisions to make moving forward. Her business could not continue as it had without muscle testing, and she did not know what she would do about her own health. We discussed her many questions and concerns at great length. One year after that conversation, she contacted me again to update me on what had transpired in her life.

With great joy I listened to her report. Jane had chosen to stop muscle testing and close her business. She immersed herself in the Word daily, not simply listening to others preach and teach but actually reading the Bible for herself in great quantity. She prayed for discernment and studied what she heard from the pulpit in her own private devotions. Remarkably, she completely cut out any involvement with social media so that she did not have that once consuming distraction. She read my book, *When You Can't Trust His Heart—Discovering the Limitless Love of God* and began to allow God alone to heal her brokenness. She read *Life to the Body* and began to let God's Word reshape how she viewed her health.

During the year, she told me that there had been times of confusion and deception that crept in but that as she sought God's wisdom, He faithfully guided her steps and opened her eyes. Where once she had an extremely limited diet and frequent stomach problems, she reported that she now enjoyed eating a diverse diet with only occasional stomach issues similar to what anyone might experience. After a year of learning to walk closely with the Lord, she was thriving and excited to begin a new phase of life. To God be the glory!

God's energy versus Satan's

[cxxxvi] Her name has been changed, but her story is real.

Recently, while listening to the Bible while I worked, a passage from Hebrews 2 caught my attention. It says, *God also bore witness by signs and wonders and various miracles and by gifts of the Holy Spirit distributed according to his will.* (v 4) Those words called to mind 2 Thessalonians 2, a passage I wrote about at great length in the chapter on energy. It says, *The coming of the lawless one is by the activity* [energy] *of Satan with all power and false signs and wonders, and with all wicked deception for those who are perishing.* (vs 9-10)

If you recall, Thessalonians 2 uses the word *enérgeia* multiple times to speak of God's energy to accomplish His purposes, and how God will allow Satan to use his own energy to accomplish the purpose of deceiving people in the "last days." Both God and, by God's allowance, Satan powerfully use signs, wonders, and various methods to convince the world of their witnesses. God's energy bore witness of the Messiah, the Son of God—Jesus Christ. The best that Satan's energy can do, however, is to create false or counterfeit signs and wonders that will deceive the nations and point them to the antichrist.

The counterfeit is a poor substitute for the real deal, but it can be convincing. Energy medicine is full of counterfeits because it comes from the energy of one who is the father of lies. Let us bring such lies into the light and be guilty no longer of trading the truth of God for a lie. Mark 4:21-23 says, *And he said to them, "Is a lamp brought in to be put under a basket, or under a bed, and not on a stand? For nothing is hidden except to be made manifest; nor is anything secret except to come to light. If anyone has ears to hear, let him hear."*

The closing words of 2 Thessalonians 2 make for a fitting benediction, and so I will conclude with Paul's inspired words.

> *So then, brothers, stand firm and hold to the traditions that you were taught by us* [the apostles]*, either by our spoken word or by our letter. Now may our Lord Jesus Christ himself, and God our Father, who loved us and gave us eternal comfort and good hope through grace, comfort your hearts and establish them in every good work and word.* (vs 15-17)

Part 3

Redemptive Testimonies

CHAPTER 19

Real Stories

And you were dead in the trespasses and sins in which you once walked, following the course of this world, following the prince of the power of the air, the spirit that is now at work in the sons of disobedience – among whom we all once lived in the passions of our flesh, carrying out the desires of the body and the mind, and were by nature children of wrath, like the rest of mankind. Ephesians 2:1-3

Each story that you are about to read was written by the individual whose real name precedes it. I hear repeatedly from people that Satan's method for ensnaring them through energy-based practices was word of mouth testimony from fellow brothers and sisters in the Lord. This must change! Following repentance, people often think they are largely alone in coming to those conclusions, but this is not the case. From the time God laid it on my heart to write this book, my desire has been to share the remarkable stories of others who have also repented and found unending grace and provision from God. May you be blessed and encouraged as you read their stories and words of wisdom.[cxxxvii]

[cxxxvii] Although I have not personally verified specific details of these testimonies, I have no cause to doubt that they are accurate.

Lori from Kentucky

After having my second child I started having health issues that were persistent and painful; things I couldn't solve on my own. I was a stay-at-home mom with two toddlers at the time, and I was desperate for relief and answers. Being naturally minded and having removed myself from conventional medicine and pharmaceuticals a decade ago, I entrusted the only like-minded Christian health practitioner (chiropractor) I had in my life at the time to help me. His approach would be to get to the root of my problems in a "precise" way. The approach was called Nutrition Response Therapy (NRT), which I later discovered is a form of energy medicine. This began my two-and-a-half-year involvement, as well as (it grieves me to say) my young kids, who were tested through a surrogate.

There were many warnings and indications that something wasn't right as I went through this "therapy". Even though I sensed my mind was being played with, I didn't pay heed. These indications would eventually become confirmations of the bondage I had to NRT and the evil that was prevalent in my life. Since hindsight is 20/20, I'll share some of the signs that seem obvious to me now but that I disregarded before God brought me to repentance.

After starting NRT, my symptoms got much worse. In a short amount of time, I became nonfunctional due to not being able to use my hands from the spreading of painful skin eruptions. I experienced bizarre findings, new and strange symptoms that didn't make sense to me, presentation of acute infections that would heal and come back weekly. I had insurmountable inner turmoil and self-hatred. I got to the point where I wanted to die. I had increasing anxiety and dependence on my chiropractor and "my body" to give me answers.

I often felt I was becoming a hypochondriac. I felt controlled by my symptoms, food restrictions and wondering if there was something brewing inside me without me consciously being aware of it or that I was developing an eating disorder. My skin issues may have been where it all started, but soon a myriad of other problems was found. As I "healed" of one problem, something else would appear. This eventually became a downward spiral and never-ending rabbit hole into a dark world that resulted in a year's worth of weekly appointments. I didn't know my body anymore, but I became convinced that this "therapy" did since it would prioritize or precisely indicate the body systems to target first, second, and so forth.

I started to get choked and have a hard time swallowing the plethora of supplements that "my body said it needed" through the testing. Rather than considering that I was getting worse because of the treatments, my initial lack of healing (and worsening symptoms) caused me to become increasingly reliant on the muscle testing because of fear of getting even worse. Later on, the sudden healing of some chronic symptoms and heavy metal toxicity continued my reliance on the muscle testing for fear of returning to my prior painful condition.

I began to resist the still, small whispers and the Scripture I had in my heart saying, "don't worry about what you will eat" and "trust me" and "your faith will heal you." I resisted my husband's encouragement to discontinue the practice. My ongoing pursuit of NRT caused much marriage and financial strain.

I mysteriously lost my ability to think and speak clearly. As I "progressed" with NRT and some symptoms disappeared, I started to become more and more frustrated with my brain function. I'd call my kids the wrong names, stumble on my words, stutter, have terrible recall of ordinary objects, lose my thoughts, not know why I walked into the room, say the weirdest things, and afterwards want to smack my forehead for being so foolish. I truly believe it was more than just natural occurrences after having children. It was so much more than mommy brain, which was confirmed in a miraculous recovery of my mind after repenting.

Due to the increasing expense of keeping up with the NRT practice at my chiropractor's office, I went online to fervently search for a way to learn or be trained in self-muscle testing and testing my family. I wholeheartedly believe God was at work. I came across Marci's video, *Why I No Longer Muscle Test* and was initially angered that anyone would speak negatively about this "wonderful" way of "healing" the body. But God...He moved. I felt His presence and I came back to the video after starting and pausing it a couple times. It didn't take long before the Holy Spirit convicted me that my involvement in muscle testing was not aligned with biblical truth and that I was participating in something I shouldn't be near.

The testimonies in the video speaking about the bondage to muscle testing and to the supplements were eerily similar to mine. Also, Christianizing the practice to make it seem more acceptable was something I experienced. This grieved me. I wept. This brought light to the darkness around me, and I felt held by the Holy Spirit. Even writing this makes me tear up and get chills at His everlasting love and willingness to fight for me.

In that moment I sought forgiveness from the Lord and decided to not pursue NRT training or testing at my chiropractor's office any longer. I texted my husband who was at work and told him I needed to stop NRT. That night, we prayed together to renounce the devil and for Jesus to take care of our family and our health. What's miraculous to me is that I slept through the night (which hadn't happened in a long time), and the very next day I woke up joyful and feeling incredibly free! I won't claim to be completely healed because I'm not yet, but that next day I had my mind back! I could think again. I could articulate myself clearer than I had been able to do since beginning NRT. That's the amazing healing power of Jesus!

Marci's other video, *What The Bible Says About Energy Medicine* and her blogs about muscle testing being repackaged divination provided so much evidence and Scriptural support that I was searching for that convinced me even more about the detestable sin muscle testing is. Understanding the origin of energy medicine, the powers that were evident in my life as I went through NRT, and the presence of God I experienced through my discoveries led me to freedom.

What's most impactful (that I mentioned earlier) is the restoration of my mind and brain function after repenting as well as the compassion and love I felt at the moment my eyes became open to deception. I'm not completely healed, but I have noticed significantly less symptoms, not nearly as much worry over food and illnesses, and more joy to be at home, homeschooling my kiddos.

Having said that, though, I don't want to dismiss the anxiety I faced after walking away from Nutrition Response Therapy. It was truly a trying time for me. I had many concerns about what I was going to do next without the former practice and what was going to become of some symptoms that persisted. However, I continued to dig into the Word and pray. Within 7 months of leaving my chiropractor's practice and ending Nutrition Response Therapy a large rash on my back, right behind my heart that had been there for 5 years, healed! God's Word and Marci's book *Life to the Body* have inspired me so much that I have decided to go to Bible School!

If I could give any encouragement to others from what I've learned through my muscle testing experience it's this: (1) seek God first and learn to discern His voice (2) heed the warnings He gives, (3) above all guard your heart and put on the full armor of God daily. We may or may not see healing in the time we want it, but as we lean into Him, become obedient to His Word, and truly repent He will not only lift our faces but show us the next steps. He's never late in His timing. He truly does love His children and fights for us!

Angela, an RN & former practitioner from Florida

My involvement with muscle testing and energy medicine began when I was recruited to work as a LPN in an integrative wellness center. Initially, the center was primarily focused on natural pain relief, physical fitness, and healthy eating. After a couple of years, the practice began to see more and more clients experiencing chronic health issues, and so the focus of the practice shifted. We began implementing many energy/frequency-based modalities including one called Psych-K (Psychological Kinesiology). It claims to address the mental and emotional aspect of healing.

Psych-k claims to rewrite self-limiting and self-sabotaging beliefs in the subconscious mind. We would muscle test the client to supposedly determine if their subconscious mind accepted a new, healthy belief statement. If the arm went weak, the subconscious mind, supposedly, was not in agreement with the new statement, and so we proceed to do what's called a balance. This is key--In order to move forward with a balance, we first had to get permission from what's called the "super consciousness."

I assumed this was God. We would ask *super consciousness* if this was an appropriate balance at that time and would muscle test again just as we did with the goal statement. It was one of my favorite modalities at the time. I really thought I was making a difference and doing God's work. But unfortunately, I was deceived myself and deceiving others by utilizing this modality.

What lead me to repentance was pretty profound. I had a dream where God was speaking to me. I had never before or since that time had such a dream, but in late October 2019, I did. In the dream God said "Angela, Psych-k is a form of divination, and it worships a false God named Param." In the dream I looked at my husband and said, "Pray for my job." Then I woke up. As you can imagine, I was shocked. I wrote down the words, *divination* and *Param,* as I had no idea what either meant. I found nothing online at the time referencing Param, but as I began searching for a connection between divination and Psych-k, I came across Marci's blog and audio lesson sharing how muscle testing was divination. I was absolutely floored!

I'm ashamed to say that even with this revelation, I did not renounce the practice right away, as I was afraid of how this would impact my job. Instead, I put it at the back of my mind for a few months. However, I could not shake the dream, the truth it shed light on, and how I felt it was the Lord calling me out of that practice. In these few months I facilitated a number of Psych-k sessions and with each came a growing conviction that I was seriously going against the will of God. By the last session I had reached my breaking point and afterwards repented and renounced Psych-k. I told my boss of my decision to no longer facilitate those sessions, and she agreed to let me continue working there without doing Psych-k. After the conversation with my boss, I felt very discouraged. I knew I was standing firm in the Lord and following His will, however, thoughts of putting my career in jeopardy and doubts if that was the right decision flooded my mind.

Then, I suddenly felt like the Lord was wanting me to look up the name *Param* once more. This time when I searched, immediately the following popped up from a book called, *Kirshna: The Ultimate Idol* by Dr. Jakhotiya: "Param is described as super consciousness" (p.125). I was absolutely floored by this information! The dream was accurate despite me having no idea what Param or divination was, and God revealed it more fully to me in His perfect timing. I first needed to walk in obedience before He revealed the whole picture to me.

Sadly, even after this new knowledge, I continued to work at my job for 4 more months until I was fired. As a practitioner, it was a struggle for me to risk my employment. I really should have made the decision to leave, but I was focusing on my career and the impact leaving would have on my family's income, instead of focusing on the will of my heavenly Father. I was in error and, in retrospect, believe that this may have led to some significant spiritual and physical attacks as I was willingly walking in disobedience.

To my surprise, 2 weeks after my partial repentance, I suddenly started to experience some alarming symptoms with my health. The new health issues began suddenly with a "anaphylactic like" reaction to a food I had never had an issue with before. I ended up losing consciousness. After I developed several symptoms like food allergies, environmental allergies, hives, vomiting episodes, extreme fatigue, heart palpitations and dizziness. This came as a huge surprise to me because I was, what I considered, to be very healthy. I ate mostly organic foods, I exercised often, and I avoided chemicals in my home and self-care products. Adrenal fatigue also crept in and brought my life to a halt.

Prior to this, I made little time to truly seek the Lord. This smack in the face with my health caused me to reevaluate things. And by God's grace I was given the fire and desire to truly seek Him and His Word. I can't say for certain whether these symptoms were the result of a spiritual attack or of God's loving correction, but during this delicate time, God began to expose the sin in my life, and idols I had made. Health, although very important, for me, was above the Lord. He also exposed my vanity, pride, and selfishness. Although the symptoms were unpleasant, I am extremely grateful for this time God used to strip me down and to begin this process of renewing me in the Spirit.

As God exposed my sin, I felt the heavy conviction of the Holy Spirit as He revealed truth to me. Satan twisted that conviction into a sense of condemnation. I began having thoughts that I would not be forgiven by

God for what I had been involved in. I would wake up in the middle of the night with a sense of terror that somehow, I had committed the unpardonable sin. One morning after a horrible night, my husband looked at me and saw I was in distress. I told him what I had been feeling over the last few weeks. And he said to me "Angela, you can continue to torture yourself if you choose to, but God has already forgiven you," After this pep talk, I began to learn to stand against the Accuser's lies by the truth of God's Word and how to rest in that Word. During this process, I also realized that my feelings are not gospel.

I just want to praise God for all the healing He's allowed in my body. I am almost completely free of all the symptoms I experienced before. What's more is the peace He has given me! Prior to this, I had struggled with mild anxiety almost daily as well as having frequent obsessive thinking patterns. Since being liberated, I do not struggle with either of these any longer.

Yes, there is loss and pain on some scale. More than losing income, I lost the relationships with the clients I had grown to love over the course of 7 years. I also ultimately repented of all the alternative modalities I was trained in after further revelation from the Lord that these were also rooted in either divination or energy medicine, resulting in me not being able to continue my career in the field of holistic health. Yet in Matthew 16:24-26 it says:

> Then Jesus told His disciples, "If anyone wants to come after Me, he must deny himself and take up his cross and follow Me. For whoever wants to save his life will lose it, but whoever loses his life for my sake will find it. What will it profit a man if he gains the whole world, yet forfeits his soul? Or what can a man give in exchange for his soul?

So, I chose to deny myself and follow him. And God proved Himself faithful to me. He showed me that He is the provider, not me. Since being unemployed, through His miraculous provision, we have not lacked anything at all. Jesus is worthy to leave it all behind to follow Him! And as Paul said in 2 Corinthians 4:18: *For our light and momentary troubles are achieving for us an eternal glory that far outweighs them all. So we fix our eyes not on what is seen, but on what is unseen, since what is seen is temporary, but what is unseen is eternal.*

Beth from South Dakota

I recently started with a Christian herbalist who does muscle testing and have had a gut feeling this isn't something I should be a part of. I have several Christian friends who swear by these individuals as they or family members have been greatly helped. I have struggled off and on over the years with my health and when several friends recommended herbalists, I thought it might help me on my journey towards full recovery. But like I said earlier there was always something in my gut saying it doesn't feel right.

Besides having Christian friends recommend this type of healing I have struggled with the fact that sometimes they suggest treatments that are not all that uncommon or unusual. In fact, a friend of mine was given almost the exact same protocol as my family, even though the health issues are different, (which leads me to wonder if all are given the same advice!). The protocol consisted of herbs and foods that I know to be helpful for the body and would make sense to suggest to almost anyone.

Even though I am at peace with my decision, it is difficult to accept the reality of what I had thought to be an acceptable (even Christian) form of healing.

Lee from Florida

I came across Marci Julin's blogs about Muscle Testing as Divination one night in early 2020, as I was seeking to know the truth of the origins of muscle testing. Muscle testing and other forms of energy medicine were introduced into my family when I was 12 years old. My family and I accepted it as a non-spiritual, purely physical phenomenon. For the next 20 years I allowed myself to be tested, diagnosed, and treated with special nutritional supplements via muscle testing, both by professional practitioners as well as by family members. I grew pretty dependent upon it, but as I grew up and moved away, I became involved in it much less frequently.

Even during this time, I recognized the danger of getting obsessed by the practice as I had seen that happen to others. However, I did not suspect any spiritual powers or dangers. When I got married, my wife tried to be open minded toward it, but ultimately rejected the practice because of inconsistencies she noticed. It was when a church friend suggested it sounded like divination that I became concerned and decided to find out what I could about its origins.

That is when I found Marci's blog articles, and I was both intrigued and shocked at how her experience with muscle testing so closely mirrored that of my own. Up to that point I had always thought mine was a unique experience in the realm of muscle testing. What particularly caught my attention was the description of her bondage to myriad, ever-changing sensitivities or "allergies" that had developed as she got deeper into muscle testing. This was so closely on-point with my own experience that it validated her story and concerns about the dark spiritual powers behind it. I have watched this very thing happen to myself and family members. Marci's thoughts about how the enemy can create health crises and then provide the solutions made perfect sense to me in how it can appear to work and keep one in bondage.

I appreciate Marci's dedication to this particular ministry because very few Christians are saying anything about it. I had never wanted to seek any friend or pastor's opinion about the matter because I knew it would sound very strange to them and would probably be uncharted territory for them. Her blogs and videos have helped inform me tremendously. The very evening that I found the blog, I decided to completely cut off all involvement with muscle testing and energy medicine.

Since then, two years ago, I have experienced much more peace about my health. Anxiety attacks that I'd begun having a couple of years prior to that went away. It's not that I now have perfect health, but I have pretty normal health for a dad in his mid-30s with young kids. I work hard, and I get tired; I get seasonal colds, and I do have a few mild but true allergies that stay pretty constant and predictable. The Lord has blessed me greatly since then in my family, work, ministry, and friendships. I feel as if life is moving forward without bondage to fear. There have been times since repenting from muscle testing when I've even experienced doubts about whether the spiritual power and dangers in energy medicine are real, but I keep coming back to the evidence and the bondage that I've personally seen and experienced, and the freedom I now have from it. You really do not need energy medicine and muscle testing in your life and will be much better off without it.

Brittany from New Mexico

I first heard of energetic practices such as homeopathy and muscle testing while reading through comments and posts on health-related Facebook Groups. I have a background in science, so I never took these "woo-woo" practices seriously. One day, I spoke to a Facebook friend about her success healing herself and her two autistic sons using the *Emotion Code.* I thought to myself, "How can a health practitioner diagnose someone over a video call and prompt them to do certain actions with their hands... and suddenly they're healed?" Nevertheless, I was intrigued that she seemed to get better from Lyme using this method. Even so, God in His grace convicted me that this practice wasn't Christian, so I shouldn't get involved (even though I didn't consider myself a born-again Christian back then).

In 2016, my health declined severely after a significant mold exposure in my apartment following the damage from Hurricane Harvey. During this time, I started seeing an ayurvedic doctor who recommended I take up yoga and meditation to manage my stress. I always thought these two practices were a bit strange. Nevertheless, this was a convenient suggestion because I found out I was pregnant and wanted to do everything I could to manage my stress well. I started practicing yoga and meditation every day. I even included chanting mantras and participated in visualization exercises regularly. I thought taking up these practices was a good idea but would come to find out these practices stem from the New Age and are frankly not biblically safe nor sound. Although I perceived some benefits, I believe whatever positive feelings I felt were counterfeit and were induced under the workings of evil spirits. It was as if I supernaturally became more open and receptive to spiritual practices.

Then, I stumbled across Simona Rich's work. She was an ex-New Ager who converted to Christianity and exposed the origins of these types of mystical practices, which have a pagan present and past. I personally think I opened doors to the demonic because I couldn't sleep at all during the third trimester of my pregnancy up until my daughter was 2 months old. I would be awake but having hallucinations that can soon come with a lack of sleep. Interestingly enough, I would attempt to pray to Jesus during those moments, and those disordered thoughts subsided somewhat.

I discovered yoga and meditation had been linked to unexplained psychological disturbances. We should never forget that God isn't the author of confusion but of peace. After my desperate need for relief, I went to a chiropractor, and he recommended I allow him to muscle test me for food intolerances. At the time, I didn't connect the dots—that what the chiropractor recommended was similar to my old friend's experience with *Emotion Code*. He promised to reveal hidden knowledge in order to heal me. The eerie part of this whole ordeal was that the results lined up almost perfectly with lab results I've taken for food sensitivities. I believe subconsciously, the practice of muscle testing began to legitimize itself within my mind.

Soon after that, I consulted with a health coach I trusted, and she claimed homeopathy was the ultimate answer to healing. So, I tried it. It was very cheap and had a low risk of harm in my mind. Interestingly enough, I perceived that I was feeling better while taking my homeopathic "remedies" for a few months. My functional medicine doctor began to pressure me to learn muscle testing using a pendulum. His urgent, almost frantic persistence in getting me to learn this practice didn't sit right with me. Notwithstanding, I pushed my reservations aside under the crushing weight and desperation of wanting to be well. So, I took a muscle testing masterclass from a psychic medium. I then began testing all of my supplements, foods, and even life decisions.

Thankfully, Jesus started slowly removing the scales from my eyes. God led me to Steve Bancarz's book, *The Second Coming of the New Age*. His book exposed the New Age infiltration in Christian churches. I became convicted of the practices I was involved in while reading the book's biblical reference of Deuteronomy 18:9-14. Still, what motivated me to look into these alternative practices, even more, was when I noticed I had suicidal thoughts and thoughts of harming my daughter that would appear out of nowhere right after taking a homeopathic remedy. I later found out the homeopathic remedies I was taking were supposedly intended to balance out your chakras. In fact, the primary remedy I took was said to mend a broken heart through balancing out your heart chakra. How can a homeopathic sugar pill do that? Only God can.

I discovered that many holistic and alternative practices are pagan and pantheistic in nature. There is the New Age, but there is also New Age Medicine. Both of these schools of thought have many people in bondage. Both philosophies promise peace when there is no peace. Many people, Christians included, are deceived into these practices because we hear about people who are frequently healing from using energy medicine. So that means these practices are good, right? Wrong!

After reading through the Old Testament into the new in 2018, the Lord showed me who He was within Scripture, and I accepted Jesus into my life and made a commitment to follow Him. This meant repenting from my sin and allowing His righteousness to mold me into the woman He created me to be. I'm not healed as I'm typing these words, but muscle testing and energy medicine practices didn't make me better and repenting of them didn't make me worse as I feared it would. What changed with repentance from those practices is that those dark thoughts of harming myself or others ended, and I no longer have this gripping low self-worth. I carried the guilt of my sin heavily. I now know the energetic practices I was involved in could never bring true peace or healing. Only God can. Trust God and His goodness in good times and bad. He will fill you with unshakeable joy and peace no matter your circumstances when you put your faith in Him and Him alone.

Amberlea from Virginia

I have always had chronic health issues from as early as I can recall. I had a multitude of intestinal issues throughout childhood and adulthood, skin staph infections, and the most recent was a diagnosed Hailey-Hailey disease, which is a genetic disorder that causes blisters to form on the skin that was passed on to me by my paternal grandfather. My grandfather was a Catholic priest with four secret children, my father being the youngest, and he had the incurable disease, Hailey-Hailey. My grandmother, his secret wife, drank herself to death when my father was 19. My father gave his life to the Lord shortly after her death and married my mother. I am 34 now and when I was 28 years old, I started developing the symptoms of Hailey-Hailey. My skin would split open, become infected, and was excruciatingly painful. This led me to constant supplement taking, crazy diets, and even laser skin therapy. I also at 28 years old developed stomach ulcers that were at times debilitating. This sent me on a quest for healing. My life was consumed by fear, perfectionism, works based salvation (despite being in a healthy evangelical church), and the need to have it all together.

In 2018, I started going on crazy diets, which did relieve some of my issues (intestinal and ulcers), but the Hailey-Hailey was not healed. In December of 2022, I was desperate for answers and set up an appointment to see a Holistic Doctor. The night before going, I had a very demonic dream about the person and was extremely anxious in my spirit, but out of my desperation I ignored it.

On my first visit, something was off, but I ignored it. On the second visit she asked me to take a test where the frequencies and auras would be studied. She called it the biofield. I knew something wasn't right and I began searching on YouTube for information about energy medicine and biofields. After some searching, I came across Marci's video on the dangers of energy medicine. I couldn't believe what I was hearing but it gave me the assurance I needed to run away from it and run fast. I ended up cancelling my contract with this practitioner and was met with some pretty crazy spiritual warfare. I then started listening to all of Marci's videos, bought her books, and began my healing journey.

One day, I sat in my bed and repented for all the sins of my forefathers and all the sins I could think of that maybe led to Hailey-Hailey. I didn't feel anything special at that moment, but I asked God to take it away. I can honestly tell you that since that day, I've never had a Hailey-Hailey flare again. I also started realizing that a lot of my issues were linked to an incorrect view of God based on the emotional abuse from family. I am still working through all of that as there are days and seasons where I revert back to negative and false thinking. How can God love me? He must not be really good? The things I've done are not redeemable. God must be just like my earthly father. It takes time to change wrong thinking, and there are times when I have to go back and refresh.

Despite all of that, I can stand here and tell you that I've had no Hailey-Hailey, no stomach ulcers, no intestinal distress, and no skin infections, since coming to find her videos in 2022. God really used Marci's books to transform my life. Praise the Lord!

Jenny from Colorado

When the Lord brought Marci along my path, I had been battling unexplained health issues for 3 years. My health crashed after the birth of my second baby, and I was desperate to feel well and energetic again. I was struggling with adrenal fatigue, painful eczema covering my hands, terrible hormone imbalance, gut issues, and weight-loss resistance – just to name a few things. I was irritable, stressed, and tired, all while trying to maintain a pulled together image, as a mom of two young boys, running an at-home business. I knew from the onset that stress was a factor. Gradually, God began to show me my health decline was linked to guilt, shame, regret, and hopelessness, but I didn't know how to give those things to Him, so instead I focused on the things I thought were in my control.

I determined that if I could just eat a perfectly clean diet and take the right supplements, my body would heal itself. We spent hundreds of dollars on holistic health practitioners, cleanses/detoxes, supplements, and healing protocols, with little improvement. Because I knew stress was an issue, I started doing yoga at the gym, infrared sauna treatments, and occasional massages. I was using all sorts of essential oils, in an attempt to treat various emotions. I would listen to hours of podcasts, health summits and YouTube videos on health to see what more I could add to my rigorous routine. As I delved into holistic medicine, I was introduced to energy work. Not only was I struggling with my health, my toddler and newborn both had eczema and gut issues of their own.

I had found temporary answers for them through muscle testing and elimination diets, so when I found *Emotion Code*, I thought why not use muscle testing to heal my emotions? I did have some red flags in my spirit, so I searched online for "Christian energy work," thinking that would be safer. That is when I found *Splankna*, which claims to work with the Holy Spirit through muscle testing to determine past traumas and agreements with the enemy that could be linked to health concerns and then releases them through EFT (tapping) and prayer. I went to two sessions, which seemed to help initially.

It was around that time that a friend sent me Marci's blogpost on muscle testing. I reluctantly agreed to check it out. By the grace and mercy of God, the Holy Spirit opened my eyes to how lost I was! When I read Marci's story, so similar to my own, I realized the enemy had deceived me hook, line, and sinker. I broke before the Lord with weeping and repentance. I couldn't believe how deceived I had been!

How did I, a "good Christian girl", get to this point?! In every way, I had been trying to heal myself in my own strength, knowledge, and pride. In the process, getting well had become my idol, and I had fallen prey to the schemes of the enemy. I was willing to try anything in hopes of feeling like myself again. I remember looking in the mirror, thinking, "Who is that person? This isn't me." My eyes looked hollow, absent of life and light. I literally was dying in my spirit, soul, and body, struggling to hold on in any way possible. I was lost, confused, in pain, and without hope. But God.

I began listening to all of Marci's audio teachings. I was blown away by her testimony, what she had endured, and how God was now using her to set others free. I was especially impacted by her talk entitled *The Wellspring of Life*, where she explains the breakdown of the heart being two chambers – soul and spirit – and how we so often feed the soul, while neglecting the spirit, regarding our health and life! Everything I had been doing was focused on my body and soul, while completely neglecting my spirit. I was using the wisdom of man, all the while completely ignoring THE answer laid out for us in God's Word.

I remember Marci saying in her 3rd post on muscle testing -- "It wasn't until I devoted the energies that once were directed at alternative medicine to seeking God's wisdom about health through the Bible that I found true and lasting healing." Those words penetrated my entire being. I knew I had to forsake everything I was doing in my attempt to get well and start pursuing the Lord with that same tenacity. I literally had spent ALL my energy seeking health and carrying out all the physical things to get well, while neglecting my walk with God, my marriage, and my children. All in vain.

I determined at that moment that all my energy was going to be spent in seeking His face. I stopped everything I was doing – yoga, naturopathic appointments, health protocols, detoxes, endless supplements, chiropractic, homeopathy, muscle testing, and every form of energy work. I threw it all out. I repented from these things, renounced them from my life, commanded Satan to leave, and closed all the open doors I had given to the enemy. I felt the demonic leave my home when I did this. I felt a tangible sense of fear as I renounced these things from my home and life. I remember decreeing 2 Timothy 1:7 until the enemy fled. He knew he was losing his grip on me.

I received God's gracious forgiveness and started over with the Lord. Scripture says, *Seek first the Kingdom of God and His righteousness, and all these things will be added unto you* (Matthew 6:33), and *Delight yourself in the Lord, and He will give you the desires of your heart* (Psalm 37:4). Broken and humbled, the Lord met me where I was and began to heal my shattered heart and body. For the first time in my life, I had come to the very end of myself. I couldn't do any of it on my own. I needed Jesus. I needed Him to set me free from me. I couldn't live this life without Him. On my own, look how deceived I had become. I grew up in a Christian home and always professed Christ, but I had never truly made Him Lord of my life. Oh, I thought I had, but I realized I had been running the show.

On April 17, 2018, I recommitted my life to the Lord. My entire life has radically changed! God gave me such a hunger for Him and His Word. I felt like a brand-new believer. I even got baptized again! The Lord gave me Romans 12:2, *Do not conform to the pattern of this world, but be transformed by the renewing of your mind. Then you will be able to test and approve what God's will is—his good, pleasing and perfect will.* I began devouring Scripture, and it came alive like never before! I started putting Scripture everywhere, meditating on His Word, and He began changing my mindset and my heart. God gave me a revelation of His deep love for me, and instead of feeling like I had disappointed Him or had to prove myself to Him, I came to know His love for me and my standing in Him because of Christ. As I pressed into Jesus, my body healed. As I learned my identity in Him and the hope that I have, I lost all the extra weight my body was carrying.

The Lord taught me about our spirit, soul, and body (1 Thessalonians 5:23), and how they all work together and function optimally when we put the health of our spirit first. Jesus MUST be first. It's how He made us. He comes in and fills us with hope, joy, peace, and purpose! I learned about spiritual warfare and how real our enemy is. I learned that the giftings and callings of God are irrevocable (Romans 11:29), and my life wasn't too far gone. He comes in, picks up the pieces and redeems us, no matter how far we've fallen (Psalm 103). Did it all happen overnight? No. It was a process. But the Holy Spirit – our Teacher, our Comforter – led me day by day and step by step.

It's now been almost 4 years since I read that article, and my life is truly transformed. I am not who I was. I am full of life and victory in Christ! He is truly my all in all. I have energy again, and He has renewed my youth like the eagles. Psalm 103:1-5 sums up what He has done for me! I pray my testimony encourages you to go after God with ALL your heart. He will not fail you. He loves you deeply and desires to meet you in your pain. He is not angry with you, nor does He condemn you. He longs to draw you close to His heart and heal you. Let Him. He will be everything your heart has ever desired. He will love you like no one else can. He will heal you – spirit, soul, and body – and help you get back on track with the good plans He has for you (Jeremiah 29:11-14).

Brooke from Kansas.

I was introduced to muscle-testing over 10 years ago. I got involved with this practice as I was searching for natural supplements to help my daughter with what her doctor believed to be allergies as well as for my son. I had been doing much praying to the Lord and reading about natural health, to also help myself with lifelong health challenges. When I attempted to purchase some supplements at a health store and was asking for some guidance regarding my daughter's symptoms, I was questioned about my daughter by the practitioner regarding details that only my husband and I could have known about her. I was then given recommendations to follow with a specific supplement. I was told that I would need to return in 3 months to receive guidance on how to, now, strengthen a system in her body. I followed the recommendations and was completely astonished by the results. I had an "awe" moment and thought this must be the answer to my prayers.

My health issues were normal to me, so I never really thought much about getting help until I got older. My early twenties are when I started on a path of wellness. I started becoming a little overwhelmed by the thought of marriage and children in light of the reality of my health issues. I was raised "medically-minded," and worked under that philosophy for 11 years. I personally became very disturbed under that philosophy and witnessing people close to me becoming pill-dependent and never really getting better added to my concerns. I was very determined not to be dependent on something.

Fast forward to 10-12 years ago, and that is when I got my initial consult with muscle-testing. I thought this route was good because of my daughter's results as well as the idea of taking the guesswork out of which supplements to buy as well as the dosage and duration. Like with my daughter, I was asked about things back from my childhood that could possibly be contributing to my health issues, which no one ever could have known. I wrote down the suggested recommendations to be followed, such as taking supplements or doing a type of homeopathic remedy. Some of the remedies seemed extremely odd but seemed justifiable when looking at the body through the lens of natural healing. This went on for several years because I felt that my health was improving.

I could not wrap my head around how I could get guidance over the phone vs being in person, but over time, I did start getting my follow-up consultations just over the phone. I was told that this method of muscle-testing was explained by quantum physics and told that God is the creator of energy. It seems that the common denominator of natural health and "energy" is to position your body so it can heal itself. Over time, I decided to take a class on this so that I could help myself and my children. I learned multiple types of muscle testing including sway testing and also how to use a pendulum. I eventually became pretty proficient. I was not only helping my immediate family but some extended family as well because the "treatments," overall, appeared to be having positive effects.

However, the longer I became involved, the more dependent I became on it because of the never-ending symptoms. It was explained to me that my symptoms were my body's way of healing itself by detoxing, cleansing, etc. Eventually, I felt as if I had a never-ending virus and weakness that often left me in bed. I started becoming very sensitive to people, things, and some environments. For example, I recall uncontrollably coughing at times when a person would come into contact with me.

In the meantime, it did occur to me very "quietly" in my soul that the Holy Spirit was no longer my "helper." During these years, I became consistently involved in our church's women's inductive Bible study. Over a course of several years God was getting my attention through our study of Hebrews, specifically, Chapter 4--"the believers' rest." I was becoming convicted of an unrestful heart through lifelong habits. In our study of Deuteronomy, I was being pressed by the Holy Spirit to question muscle-testing and that His Word was my answer to my health challenges. I brought my concerns to my husband, and he encouraged me to pray and to trust God's faithfulness. Half a year later, a dear sister in Christ asked me if I prayed whether I should be performing the treatment that I would conclude through muscle-testing. Sadly, my answer was, "no."

God started convicting me in the book of Deuteronomy, specifically, 18:10-11 as I was looking up definitions of the words. It reads as follows: *There shall not be found among you anyone who makes his son or his daughter pass through the fire, one who uses divination, a soothsayer, one who interprets omens, or a sorcerer, or one who casts a spell, or a medium, or a spiritist, or one who consults the dead.* Through an online search, Marci's lesson on YouTube, *11 Reasons Muscle Testing is*

Divination appeared. I listened right away and knew in my spirit that it was my confirmation from the Lord to stop muscle-testing.

This was the start of repentance. I was undone! I immediately threw away hundreds of dollars of supplements, resources, and paraphernalia that pertained to this practice. Within a few days, what seemed like a blockage in my stomach, left. I was so amazed, thankful, and encouraged! Another praise was that the depression I experienced on and off throughout my life was completely gone!

I read Marci's book, *Life to the Body-- Biblical Principles for Health & Healing*, only because the title contained the word, "biblical." Through prayer and a biblical principle that Marci talks about in her book, the Lord led me to deal with my deep, life-long, issue of control. God led me to more biblical teaching to better understand that I have had lifelong issues of fear and perfectionism as well; ultimately, uncovering the sin of pride, an unbelieving heart, and trusting in myself.

The last 14 months, God has also revealed to me through His Word, lifelong unrepented bitterness, worry, resentment, and discontentment. He has repeatedly brought to me through several people--*Be Still and Know That I Am God* Psalm 46:10. Currently, I am walking in and towards repentance by stopping my attempts to figure things out and allowing God, not Brooke, to lead me. My health has started to slowly improve. I am learning to be completely dependent on Him. Proverbs 3:5-6 describes the truth of what I am learning; *Trust in the Lord with all your heart and lean not on your own understanding; In all your ways acknowledge Him, And He shall direct your paths.* I encourage anyone who is currently involved in this practice or questioning it to pray and meditate over this verse and wait for His answer. He is faithful; I promise He will provide an answer.

Darlene from Texas

First and foremost, I am a believer and follower of Christ, a wife, and a mother. I was diagnosed with a platelet disorder in 2012. I was desperate for improvement in my health to avoid taking a chemo pill every day for the rest of my life as a form of treatment since the Lord hadn't removed my affliction. So, I took matters into my own hands and began to see a natural health practitioner who promised a more natural and healthier alternative with the use of Muscle Reflex Testing (MRT). After seeing her for about 9 months, my platelets went from 770,000 to 890,000. The practitioner I was seeing then referred me to her mentor whose office was 2 hours away from my home.

So, in February 2016 I went to the referral in desperation. The new practitioner wanted to see me every week. On some visits I'd be hooked up to a machine lying down and then have to stand up. Muscle Reflex Testing (MRT) was used every time to test supplements, and I was put on an autoimmune protocol. Within 2 months my platelets dropped to 680,000. Eventually, the Lord in His infinite mercy spoke to me in ways that I could understand that MRT was divination. The Lord first used a sermon on YouTube by Apologia Studios speaking about Modern Tools of the Occult (primarily Koren Specific Technique). I couldn't finish watching it from the conviction I was experiencing by the Holy Spirit, because what the video was describing was so similar to MRT.

I immediately messaged the first practitioner I had gone to about this sermon. She was agitated by my message and told me that she knew God was using her practice to help people. I reasoned that surely this practitioner, as a believer, wouldn't be seeking the help of demons. In my desperation and willful disobedience, I convinced myself yet again to keep going.

However, not long after that the Lord also brought to my attention the New Age's deceptive belief that energies in our bodies ultimately go back into the universe as a collective whole. The language that was used brought MRT to the forefront of my mind. I immediately googled "Is Muscle Reflex Testing apart of the occult?", which brought me to Marci Julin's testimony on her ministry website, called "Heart and Mind Ministries," where she detailed her experience with muscle testing. She shared how the Lord brought her out of using it and showed her that it is divination.

As I read Marci's testimony, I could see myself and my justifications for partaking in the practice, such as how it worked not making sense, and the internal conflict about it that I willingly ignored because I saw results. Though our stories are different to an extent, the Lord used it to convict me of my sin in using MRT, and in my brokenness I cried out to the LORD of hosts and repented for allowing my body to be used as a tool for divination, which is an abomination to Him.

Not only did I repent, but so did my husband. He prayed for protection from demonic influences over our family and home. The next day I threw out all supplements I had ever received via an appointment with a naturopath. I canceled my next appointment that was scheduled. I told them that the Lord made it clear that I could no longer partake in muscle testing. And we haven't looked back.

It was a lot to process. I had been dependent on MRT for over three years, and quite frankly enslaved and brought to poverty because of the costs. In spite of this, the Lord was so gracious to still provide for us and keep a roof over our head and expensive food in our bellies during our involvement with this sinful abomination. He is so faithful!

As I share this experience with others, they look at me like I am crazy, and some try to convince me that I would be dead if I hadn't gone to see the naturopaths. But we have stood firm because it is divination, and it's a sinful abomination against a HOLY God.

It's been over five years since the Lord brought me and my family out of MRT. I won't see practitioners if testing of any kind of "energies" is a part of their treatment. The biggest challenges for me the last few years has been having a good theology about what God says about healing, food, and supplements. He's been gracious to continually sanctify me in those areas. I still have my platelet disorder, but my numbers haven't gotten as high as they once were.

After repenting of MRT the Lord has truly blessed us in many ways. We were able to pay off debts early between numerous student loans and car notes. We were also blessed with two more daughters, one of which went to be with the Lord in 2019, and our youngest daughter who just recently celebrated her third birthday.

My heart is burdened to see friends and acquaintances using the same practitioners I once used, because there is only true freedom and healing in Christ alone and not in MRT. My encouragement to anyone reading this is, if you are currently involved with muscle testing, stop, and turn from it to the Lord. Don't try to justify using it. If you have been involved, and have already come to Him in repentance, pray and consider sharing your testimony publicly, out of love for your neighbor so that they may not be ensnared by this demonic practice.

Soli deo gloria

Johanna from Texas

We started seeing a chiropractic/wellness doctor here in TX after moving from Southern CA 5 years ago. We were away from our family doctor (in CA who we trusted) and wanted a more natural approach for help with our 12-year-old daughter who was diagnosed with Rheumatoid Arthritis. This was all new to us as she practiced muscle testing. Next thing you know, we were treating parasites, viruses, and allergies with a Wellness Pro machine in her office, which claims to use frequencies. She also used an acupuncture machine that she ran down my daughter's spine. The same doctor also started using hair and saliva samples to diagnose viruses and bacteria and telling us what codes need to be run off of that.

Later, I was diagnosed with type 1 diabetes, as well as hypothyroidism at age 42. I had much hesitation at the beginning, but then due to the results and the practitioner's reasoning, we justified that this must be OK. There are so many families in our church who see practitioners like her. We had bought a frequency machine and used it a lot at home and recently loaned it out to a family.

I continued to have a check in my spirit that this didn't seem right. Then at church, the woman who I loaned the frequency machine to told me that she had been asking her son's body what he had. I questioned her on how she was doing this. She said she was taking the spreadsheet that comes with the machine that lists the frequencies of bacteria and viruses and had her son put his finger on them one by one while asking and testing for it. She said she then asked how many times to run the frequency code, and it would tell her. At that moment I saw it for what it was. As we spoke inside our church building, I said to her, "That sounds like witchcraft."

That unnerving conversation then led my daughter, husband, and I on a search. We came across Marci's testimony. My daughter had also been considering natural health care, and I have had my reservations and concerns that she could be led astray. We have repented from muscle testing and have commanded anything unclean to leave our home in Jesus' name. It had been several years of bondage to running codes and worrying about it.

We continue to live in freedom from fear and worry after repenting for the use of these practices. It has been wonderful not to be under the bondage that came from the fear of feeling like we had to use the "wellness machine" or else... We are amazed at the path it would have continued to lead us down and realize the deception that is over so many in the church, (a strong delusion) not only with these alternative health practices but also with spiritual, biblical matters. It's like there is a veil that is covering eyes to see the truth of God's Word. This ultimately led us to another church which seems to be biblical (expository teaching) where God's Word is the authority not other's "revelation."

Gwendolyn from Tennessee

My story of deception in the New Age and the occult began, innocently enough, when trying to help my youngest son recover emotionally from a dog attack. In April 2016, I went for a weekend CARE (Center for Aromatherapy Research and Education) intensive course to learn about healing techniques that used essential oils. I was introduced to emotional (*Emotional Release*) and physical healing (*Raindrop Technique* and *Vitaflex*). While at the conference, I witnessed a woman receive an *Emotional Release* from a traumatic event during a class session. She had volunteered to be the recipient. She seemed to transform from a frightened, closed person to someone joyful and free in front of our eyes. All of us who witnessed it were amazed and moved by her response. We learned how to do this technique on ourselves and others. We practiced doing the *Raindrop Technique* on each other and saw demonstrations of *Vitaflex*. Every technique included essential oils and touch to supposedly restore the divine blueprint of perfection at a cellular level and release toxins that were physical, spiritual, and emotional. I put what I learned that weekend on the shelf for the next several months and didn't think too much about it.

The next winter I injured my hips trying to get back into shape during a Pilates class at the local gym. That whole next year of 2017 I was on and off crutches. Since I was supposed to be this health guru and expert in essential oils, I hid my pain from everyone but my immediate family. I just walked slowly. I never took the crutches or cane out in public and never asked for help or prayers.

Later in December of the same year, I won a trip to Utah from my essential oil business upline in the network marketing company I was in. A woman there was offering free sessions of *Raindrop Technique* - putting oils on the feet and back - that I had learned about at CARE. I had not had a *Raindrop* since the CARE classroom setting, so I immediately volunteered. I was barely managing to walk around. I had stubbornly refused to bring my cane.

I was excited to get a *Raindrop* because I had continued to suffer most of the year with this terrible hip pain. I had sat in a doctor's office that summer and was told I needed both hips replaced. At the age of fifty, I felt like my life was basically over. I could no longer do anything I enjoyed doing, like gardening, hiking, walking. I was careful to conceal my pain around others so I wouldn't in any way discredit the alternative health field I loved. I didn't want to be a bad example of what oils could or could not do.

While on the massage table getting this application of oils, I suddenly began to shake uncontrollably and sob as I lay on my stomach. I recognized it as a release of emotions like we had been taught about in the CARE class.

As the days passed, I had less and less pain, until I felt almost completely restored to health. I believed I really had experienced a miracle. I felt like I needed to know more about this and could help others if I became certified, but I didn't have much time. The extensive requirements had to be completed before the middle of April of 2018, because I only had two years from the initial CARE intensive I had gone to. It was cram time!

Sadly, as I look back on that, I realize it was all illusion and deception. There was no true release of trauma for the young woman at the CARE class, I was not healed of any emotional or physical pain when I received a *Raindrop* session. This relief of symptoms was temporary, as I would later learn.

To become certified and licensed I had to practice doing *Raindrop* (which included Emotional Release) and teach and train others to do the techniques of *Raindrop* and *Vitaflex*. I would need to pay for and pass an exam to demonstrate my knowledge at the end. Then I would pay for and go through the training to become a Licensed Spiritual Healer (LSH) to legally charge for the techniques. This fell under spiritual practices and not medical, although it is technically alternative medicine. It was during the LSH training that I learned muscle testing, although I recognized it as something I had learned about here and there from a few members of the essential oil network marketing group, although it was never called muscle testing.

Previously, in private or in essential oil classes taught by others, they had shown ways to find out if a person "needed" an essential oil. One way was using the whole body. It was explained that the body had an innate intelligence so that it "knew" truth at a cellular level. It could express a yes or no answer to a question by the whole body swaying forward or backward if the person held an oil bottle in both hands near the heart and asked themselves if the body needed it or not. This is as if one were using the body as a pendulum. In my ignorance, I did not recognize this as divination or an occult tool. I never asked myself, how in the world this was supposed to work.

In classes that I took for several weeks to become a LSH, we were taught several ways to use our fingers and hands to get yes or no answers to questions. It could be used more in depth than just whether an oil should be used, to also discover how many drops and when it should be used. It all went back to the body supposedly knowing the answer by innate intelligence and this was the way to tap into that knowledge.

The LSH classes were for anyone in the alternative medicine field, so the students could use muscle testing for all sorts of things. The instructor told us that we could test its veracity by having someone hide an object in the house and use the method to discover where it was hidden. I must say that this made me uncomfortable. I never did it but I do not doubt that it would work because I now believe that the information received was demonic.

God graciously saved me from these and many other occult practices that were part of the essential oil alternative medicine world. Not only had I done these things, but I had taught others to do them as well. The entire time I was involved in essential oils and the network marketing company, I thought I was doing the Lord's work and was part of a church. Most of my customers were Christians. The homeschool community was saturated with essential oil users, though not to the extent or in the ways I was using them. I thought that God had specially created the oils to be used for healing. I took verses out of context. I believed oils were there to remove the curse and restore the image of God in each cell. What a lie! I now know that essential oils can have aesthetic value in their pleasant aromas and some mild therapeutic qualities for skin care, but they are not the answer to every physical, mental, emotional, or spiritual health problem and must be used with utmost caution.

Raindrop uses a massive amount of essential oils undiluted on the spine and feet using shamanistic beliefs of energy fields. I have witnessed allergic reactions. We were taught that any negative response was healthy and simply "releasing toxins." I now attribute my so-called *Emotional Release* deliverance during *Raindrop* to demons pretending - playing a game to make me think the oils had some power of healing. Part of the deception is the illusion of control. Muscle testing makes one feel very powerful. There seemed to be no limit to what I could find out.

The hip pain also returned. I felt like I needed more and more sessions and oils to keep it at bay. It is today much improved on its own. The *Emotional Releases* of many I met who experienced the technique like the woman in class proved to be short-lived because continuing and even worse emotional bondage would appear after one trauma seemed vanquished. It was never enough. Finally, I shudder when I think of demonic activity using my body to give me "answers" to essential oil questions when doing muscle testing.

But God showed me my sin and now I know that He alone saves and, in His providence, heals now or later. His plan is always best. Repenting of muscle testing was part of God's forgiveness and restoration for me. I had spent years in deception and thousands of dollars, but I plan to use this story to help others be free from deception. God is putting my broken self back together in His time and sanctifying me into the image of His Son. To God be the glory!

Megan a Nurse Practitioner from Texas

My husband and I have recently taken a step of faith and started a functional medicine consulting business. Although I have always had a holistic approach in my work, God has been working on my heart for years, prompting me to change the way I practice medicine so that HE can be known as the Healer and receive all the glory while He changes the hearts of His people.

Over the past few years, I have met other providers, patients and friends who use energy healing modalities, especially muscle testing, *NAET*, and *ZYTO*'s *Evox* scans. I have never felt at peace about these methods and could sense that the Holy Spirit was helping me to discern the dangers of them. The confusing part is that many of those that are performing or receiving these services are Christians. I realized that I could not find a single person that also felt discomfort about this like I did.

One day I sat down and started searching the internet to try to get some answers. I typed in all sorts of combinations like "muscle and testing and Christian and energy..." and I ended up finding Marci's blog. Reading her posts about muscle testing addressed all my questions and concerns about these methods of healing. It was so refreshing to see all of the statements backed up by Scripture and to read her testimony of personal experience with muscle testing. I also read her book *Life to the Body* and have recommended it to many people.

As I continue to build out my practice, I have noticed that more and more of the AK methods are popping up, both in alternative practices but also in more traditional practices. They are getting harder to avoid. I have a friend who is a health coach, and very active in her faith, who uses *ZYTO* scans stating it is just a tool provided by the Holy Spirit. Just last week I met another Christian naturopath whose favorite method is *EVOX*. I am so thankful for all of Marci's work because it has helped me to stand firm and choose to call what is evil-evil, avoid allowing this stuff into my work, and teach others to stay far away from these methods.

Ruth Anne from Ontario, Canada

Muscle testing (body talk) was recommended to me by a family member to try for my chronic neck pain due to a pinched nerve. I had tried several other treatment types that were not working. I had suspicions that this was a New Age/Reiki practice, so I completed a quick online search to be sure it wasn't and didn't find anything suggesting it was demonic or anything else negative about it. Instead, I found information that supported the belief that it was a kinetic/movement form of therapy. Positive reviews were all that I could find on that initial search. I went ahead and booked an appointment. In hindsight, I should have spent more time digging in on my suspicions and researched more about the practice.

During the first appointment, I asked about Reiki and was assured it wasn't practiced in this type of healing. However, the practitioner spoke a lot about God, said a lot of logical prayers but also spoke about God being the divine in a way reminiscent of my Reiki involvement, which raised my suspicions. The session worked well, and I went a couple of weeks without pain, which was fabulous. I thought I had found a method of relief and so my worries were cast aside because of the results. The price of this treatment was high, so I waited another month before booking another appointment.

The 2nd appointment was very different. The practitioner wanted double the time and money and went into "sway tests," a full body muscle test and wanted to make sure I had crystal green, raw, Aventurine stones. I was told to carry them in my pocket and place them all over my house. My body and mind during this session went very weird. I felt a spiritual zapping. When I was in the presence of this lady, I felt magnetized to whatever she said or did. It was as though I was a zombie to her. When I got home, I wondered what the heck happened.

I didn't like what I experienced and started to do more research. I found out the stones were New Age, so I rid myself/house of them. I then found the blog that Marci Julin posted on the Heart and Mind Ministries website. I had the confirmation that the practice was New Age divination. Lastly, I did the sway test and point blank asked if the spirits being consulted were from Jesus Christ of Nazareth. The sway answer was no. My heart and mind sunk.

I am a born again Christian and felt so guilty of doing this practice. Prior to being born again, I had dabbled in Reiki and other New Age practices and my church led me through baptism and various renunciations, so I thought I had fully repented. Yet, I easily got sucked back in. I felt that I had betrayed God. I said a few prayers of forgiveness and got some close friends to pray over me. I wish that was all I needed to do, but that was not the case this time.

What followed was an unleashing of holy hell--spiritual war. Once I realized it was demonic, I stepped both feet back to my Jesus side of the spiritual war and the dark side fought back. I truly believe a portal was opened and unclean spirits began tormenting me and my family. I started with the absolute wrong thing to do. I called the Muscle test practitioner and demanded she "undo" what she did. The lady performed a "remote" session. (at a charge of course). The activity slowed a bit but then gained momentum. She admitted a portal door was opened and she didn't have the power to close. Scary.

I am writing this testimony over 2 ½ years past those body talk sessions, and I am now finally seeing the light at the end of the tunnel. The spirits have not entirely vacated yet. They are still trying to torment and bully, but it is much better than it was. These attacks convinced me to never ever visit these energy practices ever again! I discovered my view of hell and spiritual warfare was not serious prior to this. This situation has given me a new perspective. I have put on my spiritual armor and have not turned back.

I then did many things but what helped(s) the most is speaking to Jesus constantly--asking for everything needed and gaining guidance in the Bible. Also, I got the support of and help from church. There really aren't any formulas for the recovery. Jesus will meet you where you are and lead you through the paths of righteousness. Forgive yourself for doing this demonic practice. Don't let Satan deceive you that this is a guilty burden you must bear. And above everything else have no fear!!!

Fear is an invitation for the devil to torment you. You have authority, in Jesus' name, over the demons that torment you.

Get aligned with Jesus in prayer, find out who you are in Christ, trusting and having faith in Christ, loving Jesus. Encourage others and pray for others. Spread the word that new age is demonic. Love Jesus and love others.

Scripture that encourages me: Isaiah 62, Psalms 91, Psalms 107, Psalms 94, Psalms 18, Ephesians 6:10-18 Scripture is food – Jesus has prepared the table and it is time to eat!

Meg from Pennsylvania

I was hooked by essential oils right away. The most exciting part about them to me was that they were "pure" from God's creation. "Exactly as God made them." I made sure all my family had the oils they needed for anything that came up. I pulled many of my family members into helping me with my classes and helping me advertise. I believed everyone needed to know about these amazing products.

Meanwhile, the girl who had introduced essential oils to me was the daughter of a Christian Doctor of Natural Medicine (ND), and through her I learned incredible testimonies from her mother's clients – true miracles, such as healings from cancer. I became really excited, and even obsessed, with the concept of alternative medicine, or Natural Healthcare as a whole and decided to visit the ND to be screened by her electro-dermal screening machine. The day I did, I knew I wanted to become a Doctor of Natural Medicine myself and soon began a program to become a board-certified "Complementary and Alternative Healthcare Practitioner."

That's about the time things started to get weird. I learned the form of muscle testing called Sway Testing from my friends. Although there were hushed comments about the fact that this might be perceived as witchcraft, we proceeded with great seriousness. The swayed responses I received at first were dramatic. I was hooked! However, when I tried later to repeat the process for my parents, I felt nothing. My mom asked me if I'd prayed about it, which, in all honesty, I had not. After my husband went to sleep that night, I continued practicing sway testing, but then decided I should spend some time in prayer and reading the Word.

My passage for the day just happened to be Deuteronomy 18:10-11, where God forbids divination, witchcraft, and mediums. After finishing my devotions, I felt as though I should search online about muscle testing, and upon doing so, came across Marci Julin's blog post about muscle testing being divination. Through Bible study, the Holy Spirit and Marci's testimony, my eyes were opened. I immediately repented and at that late hour took my stand against Satan in the name of Jesus. To my surprise, the response was palpable, as though an evil force was staring me down in opposition and then suddenly it was gone.

Soon after this, I discovered that I was going to be learning about chakras, auras, and other occult practices that fell under the energy medicine umbrella in my Complementary and Alternative Healthcare program. I quickly walked away from the program and never looked back. For me, leaving muscle testing behind was simple. Quitting my school program and letting all the money and time I had spent be wasted was also okay.

But I was surprised to find out that even essential oils were not as safe as I had believed. It turns out, they were my "gateway drug." I realized the language I had been using all along for talking about oils, which I had learned by repeating the things I had heard, reflected traces of pantheistic, New Age doctrine. Previously, I did not even know what that was. But now I did.

In classes I would say things like: God made the oils in the plant to help the plants to heal by repairing their imbalances, and He also made the oils so that they could repair imbalances in our bodies as well. As Christians we can fall into a trap of believing that to trust in God's creation is the same thing as trusting in the God who made it. That is not the case, and the Bible tells us so. Romans 1:25 says, *They exchanged the truth about God for a lie and worshiped and served created things rather than the Creator – who is forever praised. Amen.*

At the same time, everything I said was also a subtle message to distrust medical professionals. Again, I was repeating what I had heard. I didn't necessarily distrust doctors myself, nor did I intend to cause others to do it. It was just implied by the general message of alternative medicine. So, at my very last essential oils class, I realized that before I ever talked about essential oils again, I would have to re-learn them. But no sooner did I think that than God revealed my essential oils business did not need re-vamped; it needed to end! And I needed to get rid of all my oils and everything having to do with them. And I DID have to tell all my team and all my customers that I had been deceived.

God revealed this to me using II Chronicles 33 – the story of King Manasseh of Judah. Manasseh led the people of Judah and Jerusalem astray into the occult and wouldn't listen to the Lord's warnings. After he was led away as a prisoner by the king of Assyria, Manasseh had a change of heart and repented. The Lord brought him back to Jerusalem, where he got rid of all the occult idols and told the people to serve the Lord, the God of Israel. He wrote a record of his sins, a confession, trying to warn others to not do as he had done.

From those parts of the story, God revealed to me that I was to get rid of the things that had been worship to other gods in my life, which included anything and everything from the essential oil company. Aromatherapy is one of those therapies of Alternative Medicine that arose within the Energy Medicine belief system. It is difficult to separate the physical aspects from the New Age philosophies that are an integral piece of the therapy.

God also revealed to me that I was to write a confession to warn others not to do as I had done, which I sent to my whole team and customers. If that wasn't humbling enough, there was more. I asked God if I could sell or give away my remaining essential oil products to any who could benefit from them. The Lord impressed upon my spirit that the answer was no.

For although King Manasseh had reformed his life, he had failed to utterly deface and destroy the images of the false gods he had made. The law for Israel was to destroy such with fire. Therefore, Manasseh's son Amon later found and resurrected the images. Because Manasseh had only removed the idols from the city, others still had access to them. His own son began to worship the idols. And since Amon did not repent, his guilt was even more severe than that of his father. He was killed. Perhaps if Manasseh had destroyed the idols, his son's life would have played out differently. When I understood God's directive to me, I determined to burn everything. It didn't feel foolish or dramatic. I felt free.

But there was still pain yet to come. There is always a cost for sin, and I had been disobedient to the Lord for years. Amon was not the only one who was influenced and corrupted by his father's original disobedience. Although Manasseh had done an about-face and used whatever power he had as king to try to reform the people, whom he himself had corrupted, he was only able to bring them from their false gods but not from their high places. The people worshipped the Lord God; only now, they sacrificed to Him in the high places. This was not living in obedience to God. This was using a demonic ritual to worship God. That is what Christians are doing who practice occult techniques but claim to have Christianized them. Praying while doing yoga, asking God for the answer when muscle testing, glorifying essential oils as miracles of God, attributing abilities to them that can only come from Him, like forgiveness. If it's only partial obedience, it's not really obedience.

So, no matter how hard he may have tried, King Manasseh could not carry out the reformation of the people as far as he had carried their corruption. Even when we do all we can to recover the people that have, by our example, been seduced and drawn away from God, we may never be able to recover them completely. Just like with Manasseh, when I tried to tell everybody that I had been wrong, it did not go as I hoped, and many continued in energy medicine. This still weighs heavily on me even years later. This is the cost of my disobedience. There are always consequences of sin.

It has now been several years since my involvement in energy medicine. It almost feels like it never even happened. Once I was set free, I spent some time trying to warn others, but then I lost interest in even talking about alternative medicine. I felt washed clean and new. I focused instead on what God really had for me. It felt so good to walk completely in His will again. Everything I do now with and for Jesus is more fulfilling in every way than worshipping Him in the high places could ever be. He calls us to be holy because He is holy. I am grateful beyond what I can express that He revealed the deception of energy medicine.

Karen from Illinois

Approximately 12 years ago, I noticed my health declining, but I was only in my early thirties. I would get blood tests, only to discover they were normal every single time. It was frustrating to not feel as healthy as my friends, as I suffered from a myriad of annoying symptoms. I had everything from gastric issues to body aches and pains on a daily basis. My quality of life was diminished and so I prayed for an answer daily.

My older sister told me that her chiropractor tried out this new thing called "muscle testing" on her. She knew of my suffering and said I should give it a shot. I went to my first appointment filled with hope.

My first impression of the practitioner was that she seemed a little "flighty." When she explained muscle testing to me, it sounded a little odd. That made me uneasy right at the start. Even though I always had an underlying feeling that something wasn't right, I was naïve and went along with whatever she said because I was desperate. I felt a bit better after a few metals detox treatments, and months of ingesting an array of whole food supplements. She had me use some homeopathy supplements as well. I was also eating healthier during this time, and I think that made the most difference. I never felt 100% better. My husband also visited her, and it helped him somewhat with his gastric issues. At some point, though, he decided it wasn't for him.

My uneasiness with her practices got me searching online for reviews from Christians who have tried muscle testing. I wanted other opinions besides my sister's, as she didn't think there was anything wrong with it. I found some interesting articles that were anti-muscle testing, calling it quack science, occultism, etc. I don't recall if there was a specific reason I stopped going, but I do remember feeling a strong sense that I was done there, and that I had been searching in the wrong place for healing.

I repented of these practices once I stopped going, but I still wasn't exactly sure how bad it really was for a Christian to be involved in. My family had been going through some major spiritual warfare during this exact same time because of the actions of a family member of mine, so my mind wasn't very clear. I was filled with anxiety and stress. Years later, when I found Marci's story, I was 100% positive I had made the right decision and that the Lord had led me away from muscle testing. I repented again, only because I was clearer of mind by this point and wanted the Lord to hear my sincerity.

I haven't noticed any struggles or difficulties following repentance. I have a number of health issues, and sometimes I wonder if I'd be feeling better if I had gone to the correct medical doctors instead of wasting 2.5 years of my life doing muscle testing and metal detox regimens with the chiropractor.

I feel that I am more aware of new age practices and now do my due diligence in researching something before getting involved in it. I was thankfully able to get my sister to stop doing the muscle testing as well.

I've learned to be more careful in choosing what alternative medicinal practices I take part in. I am more apt to push my medical doctor to take extensive blood tests and other tests to see if there is a medical reason for my ailments. If you seek the Lord earnestly about your ailments, he will provide the correct doctors in his timing.

I would encourage others to pray and seek the Lord when dealing with health problems, and He will provide the correct doctors and treatments. Leaning on alternative medicines and practices can be very harmful to your spiritual health, and even your physical health, by focusing so much on the wrong type of treatment and prolonging a health issue that very well could have been healed sooner if diagnosed correctly.

Dawn from North Dakota

I was sought out by someone who practices muscle testing. Last August I had several kidney stone attacks. I asked for prayer, as I ended up in the hospital twice. After my second hospital visit some friends of ours asked if they could visit us. We agreed and during the visit he began asking lots of questions about my health.

He explained that he had suffered severe illness several years ago and had been healed and had since begun treating others who suffer illness. He explained that what he did was similar to osteopathy. He said he manipulated organs and muscles to get everything back in sync. Since we've known this family for many years and they are Christians, I allowed him to work on me.

At first the sessions were short because I was in so much pain due to the stones. But as time went on sessions could last for hours. I would go home covered in bruises and would experience what he told me were detox symptoms for days. My head would be foggy, I would lose my balance, and I would have episodes of vomiting. He assured me that these were normal and told me that he had tested that I was detoxing heavy metals and chemicals. He then began testing me for allergies and recommended diet changes and supplements. I saw huge improvements. So I kept going back. There was always more that needed to be done. I eventually had him work on my husband and children.

Their family recently took in a young lady that had severe health issues. He and I had a conversation where I shared some concerns I had about how this situation might be affecting their family. He became very angry with me. Around the same time as our discussion, I started seeing things online about muscle testing and started to do some investigation. That's when I found Marci's talk on muscle testing being divination. I was immediately convicted. I knew that what I had been involved with was Satanic.

I had my husband listen and he agreed. He admitted that he had always been skeptical. Especially when I would call, and he would test me over the phone. We actually jokingly called it sorcery. Little did we know how right we actually were. Marci's YouTube video on energy medicine was also eye opening. It explained everything so well.

I had trusted him because he was a friend and a Christian. But the way he explained what he did really was energy medicine even though he didn't use occult words. I repented and my husband and I prayed. I then repented to my children for exposing them to something evil. I haven't spoken to my friend since our discussion. My husband said we need to cut ties because our friend has told us that he sees things about people, and my husband doesn't want to unknowingly partake in it.

I am thankful to my Lord and Savior for his Truth but especially for His forgiveness. His mercies are new every morning!

Vanessa from Colorado

Coming from a New Age background, I've always had the hardest time finding a health practitioner who did not integrate some spiritually questionable technique in their practice. Eventually I thought I found someone who seemed spiritually neutral. Nothing on her website indicated anything about NAET. She was very smart and knowledgeable about healing the gut, hormone balance, nutrition, etc. All the things I was seeking help on.

But, during my first (and only) visit, when she asked permission to introduce a method for treatment that some clients opt out of, my husband and I went on the alert! She gave a BIG disclaimer before showing us the muscle testing technique. When we questioned her on how muscle testing "works," she presented it in an almost convincing scientific way. But we knew this spiritually wasn't for us.

Even though she explained I did not have to do muscle testing to be treated by her, I was very uncomfortable about continuing, which led me to look further into the NAET world, where I'm so glad I found Marci Julin's testimony.

I would encourage even the strongest of discerning Christians to always be careful when you are in a place of need with your health. The enemy is subtle and wants to lure you into a place that seems spiritually neutral and safe. But we must test the spirit of all things, especially things that almost "scientifically" make sense. Always be on your guard and trust the Great Physician to lead you to His pastures of True healing for your body, soul, and spirit.

Melanie from New England

I was in my mid-thirties when I saw a new chiropractor for the first time. It was at this visit that I was muscle tested for a supplement. I had never heard of muscle testing and didn't understand the theory. Nonetheless, this began my ten-year journey into the muscle testing of my own body, through a proxy and by a machine as performed by a couple of chiropractors.

Soon I was being muscle tested for all sorts of potential allergies during nutrition sessions. I would bring assorted items to my appointments: containers of red wine, baggies of cat hair, tubes of facial cleanser, medication, etc. If I suspected that something was not agreeing with me, I was muscle tested for it. I asked my chiropractor who exactly she was speaking to, how did it work and so on. All the answers could be explained away, but, as a lifelong Christian, the whole practice gnawed at me. The practitioner explained that she was speaking to my body, my unconscious self, the Universe. Call it what you want, it seemed to be some sort of detached third party that she spoke to. I did an Internet search for: "what is muscle testing?", "should Christians' muscle test?", "validity of muscle testing," "applied kinesiology," etc. Muscle testing, or the practice of applied kinesiology, can be found on several quack-watch sites, but I didn't find anything that told me why I should stop, especially when I was seeing results.

I started to pray about it. "Lord, help me to read something if muscle testing isn't right for me." I also started to pray during my nutrition sessions. I would pray beforehand in the car and while on the table. I asked God that only the truth be told and that I wouldn't be given any supplements that my body didn't need. I prayed that the Holy Spirt would be present and would direct the chiropractor as she muscle tested me.

My husband and I had been attending a new church for about one year and really hit the ground running. My husband became a deacon, and I was asked to join the pastoral search committee. Life was busy and exciting until a particular night in July. I remember it vividly. I had just come home from a chiropractic adjustment and told my husband that I didn't feel quite right; I felt dizzy, as if my equilibrium was off in my head. It was very hard to explain the feeling. I suffered through the weekend. I felt horrible. I was off kilter, off balance, and felt just terrible. I researched everything I could regarding dizziness, yet I found no relief. I made an appointment with my primary care doctor. She was the first of eight doctors and specialists that I would see over the next ten months.

The search committee's work was extremely aggressive. It was physically, emotionally, and spiritually draining; yet I loved it. There was no time to feel sick. During this time, I learned how to deal with my daily dizziness, but I was desperate to find relief. It affected my vision, energy level, mood, desire to do things, and my entire vestibular system was out of whack. Shortly after all this happened, I called my chiropractor, and she told me to come back in; she would muscle test me to ensure nothing happened during my adjustment with her. She checked me out and sent me on my way. She advised me to schedule a nutrition session with her so that we could get to the bottom of the problem, and so I did.

During this session she asked my body many yes/no questions. This time it was different. I wasn't holding anything in my hand—we weren't testing anything. We were trying to understand the source of the dizziness. She decided on a supplement for me, confirmed that a new medicine my ENT prescribed was working, and home I went. During the next few weeks, I started to experience some relief. I was thrilled. Shortly after this I had another adjustment and felt woozy afterwards, but the worst was yet to come.

Incredible dizziness followed. It was different than before. It was extreme. I wasn't spinning; I never had that. This would come in waves and was frightening. My symptoms increased throughout the day. The stairs would move as I climbed them, I skipped a beat when I walked, and I felt airborne. I eventually developed strange neurological symptoms. I would get tingling in my extremities and feel odd all over. I was convinced I had MS. All my MRIs, cat scans, neurological and vestibular tests and dental scans came back normal. I was put on courses of antibiotics, tried eliminating foods, tried all kinds of allergy medicines and prayed so hard through it all. I thought I would never feel normal again.

I called my chiropractor's office. Her receptionist returned my call letting me know that she was fully booked but, that the chiropractor had muscle tested me through her, using her as a proxy from afar, and apparently, I was stressed and needed to relax. None of this made sense to me. Nonetheless, I made another appointment in the next couple of weeks. Again, the chiropractor asked my body a series of yes/no questions. She concluded through the questioning that the chiropractic adjustment caused my dizziness. The chiropractor said she should have read the warning signs leading up to this, headaches, and such. I was relieved that I didn't have MS or fibromyalgia or any other horrible disease that I feared, but I felt awful and sad and angry.

Shortly after this episode, I prayed a prayer I never had before. I asked the Lord to let me know if I had any areas of unconfessed sin in my life. Did He ever! Later that week I was sitting in my living room looking at my supplement basket. The word bondage came to my mind. I started thinking about my whole experience with muscle testing and realized I was in a losing cycle. I would be built up only to be torn down and left worse than before. I was in bondage to muscle testing and taking supplements. Why was I so symptomatic all the time? I decided enough was enough and that I would stop constantly running to the chiropractor. I cancelled my future appointments.

I once again conducted an Internet search and my eyes immediately fell to heartandmindministies.com and the subject line, Muscle Testing— Repackaged Divination. I couldn't read fast enough. Marci's words pierced my heart as she explained that my body had essentially been a conduit for the demonic, a human Ouija board. I threw away every supplement in my house and I confessed my sin of divination to the Lord.

The words, "there is freedom in Christ" kept running through my head. I was on the path to freedom and true healing. My husband and I met with our newly hired pastor and together we repented and renounced muscle testing. I wept through the whole thing. I can't say that muscle testing didn't weigh heavily on my mind in the days to come. It did. I yearned for it. I realized what was happening and what Marci said she had experienced—the desire to go back to it. I got out of bed and went downstairs and read my Bible. God gave me this verse that morning: I Peter: 2:24: "He himself bore our sins in his body on the tree, so that we might die to sins and live for righteousness; by his wounds you have been healed." God is enough.

Through much intercessory prayer from others, and my own confession, my strange symptoms left me. It didn't happen overnight, but they did leave. To this day, I don't know for sure what caused the severe symptoms. A couple of things indicate to me that they were, at the least, spiritually caused. For example, my longstanding anxieties left me once I stopped muscle testing. I also know that my physical symptoms began once I became very involved in a new church, joined the pastoral search team and started a Bible study in my home.

I believe that through muscle testing I gave the enemy a foothold into my life. Since I knew the Lord and prayed through it all, His protection was on me, but that didn't mean I wouldn't suffer physical or emotional or spiritual consequences. I am so thankful to the Lord for the physical symptoms that I experienced. Without them, I might still be a slave to this practice.

Lauri from Texas

So how did this born-again daughter of God, wife for 30 years, mother of 9 home-schooled children, Bible-teaching, discipleship ministry leader with a Type-A personality get involved with muscle testing? Well, I was first introduced to it by a Christian nutritionist in 2006 while seeking the best health options for our child with Lyme disease. He used muscle testing to determine her food allergies and what supplements to take. Several years later I learned about a muscle testing class taught by a Christian mother and eagerly took it in order to benefit our family's health and to save time and money by doing the testing myself instead of depending on other alternative health providers. Soon after, I was introduced to long-distance, proxy testing with *The Body Code & The Emotion Code* and began dabbling with that in order to help my daughter who by that time was in college and still struggling with her health.

I developed a short-cut method with *The Body Code*, which I believed was a blessing from God, and began using that on a bi-weekly basis to test all my family's health issues by "applying" nutrients or releasing emotions in order to bring their bodies back to a healthy balanced state. How often I tested depended on how busy I was with normal family duties. Once I became competent enough, occasionally I would offer free help to other non-family members struggling with health issues as a form of ministry. When Covid hit me in mid-December 2020, though, I began testing daily for myself and everyone in the home which really sharpened my abilities to the point that I was able to sense the answers even before conducting the test, something called clairvoyance.

Since I continued to struggle with Covid-related fatigue for weeks, I did little else besides sit in my bedroom and continue to test. If I became too fatigued while testing, I would simply place both of my hands on my salt lamp and get revitalized with enough "energy" to continue. During this time, I actually had the thought that I would be content to just sit there and test indefinitely and that could be my full-time ministry instead of continuing the discipleship ministry I was already involved in with my husband. But through a multitude of God-ordained events, the Lord nipped that thought in the bud using the prayer warriors in my life and His Word to show me the true path to take.

We started the discipleship ministry back up even before my strength was fully back because the Lord reminded me that when I am weak, He is strong. After this act of obedience, the Lord began to cause me to be unsettled about muscle testing. I was beginning to realize the similarities of fatigue that I would experience while testing to that which I felt during Covid and also to the fatigue caused by spiritual oppression. (I learned Corrie Ten Boom experienced great fatigue many times before she was to speak here in the U.S.)

The next event the Lord used to shake things up in my life was a 40-day intercessory prayer and fasting time intended for my daughter. I asked the Lord to give me a new Scripture each day to pray over her. I had never done anything like this before, and it was quite a time of spiritual stretching for me to be still and listen to the Spirit's leading in the Word. Near the end of this fast, a friend at my church approached me with desperation in her voice and asked if we could get together that week to find a biblical answer for muscle testing. She was extremely disturbed by what she had just encountered at a Young Living conference where they were teaching muscle testing. God used her request as a kick in my pants to quit playing around with my waffling thoughts about muscle testing and to truly come to a conclusion about it all.

My problem, however, was that I was so busy that week with planning for our ministry's spring festival and Gospel presentation. God knew that I lacked the time to dig and research, so in His graciousness He brought me just the right article I needed that matched my situation— Marci Julin's blog articles on muscle testing. After reading them, a heavy sense of conviction fell all over me. The realization hit me that I had been deceived! Me, the one who strongly advocates studying God's Word, obeying it, "when in doubt, don't!" Yes, even the one who prays daily with her husband! I was broken, humbled, and ashamed before the Lord, and I immediately sent a text to my husband and to two godly mentors saying this simple statement: "Pray for me. Long story short, I'm repenting of muscle testing. It's divination and an abomination to the Lord."

That simple text is what began the process of releasing the grip of spiritual oppression that the demonic realm had on me, and yet a huge battle ensued that I could sense. Confusion would cloud my thinking, and just as quickly after crying out to God, He would bring clarity. In time after much searching of my heart, I repented of 1) not listening to the still small voice of the Holy Spirit when doubts would rise (grieving the Spirit) 2) allowing the excuse to stand of being too busy to dig into the issue 3) taking matters into my own hands with our health instead of first going to the Lord 4) allowing myself to become a slave of muscle testing when it consumed much of my attention, energy and time—time that could have been used for the upbuilding of God's kingdom, not in attempting to control my own kingdom.

I was finally able to see how muscle testing fed so many of my sinful bents—my desire for control, my lack of patience and wanting answers to my health issues now, and my "I know-better-than-you" attitude, first towards my husband who wasn't as sensitive as I and then to others who were clueless about muscle testing. Also in hindsight, I realized that I had kept the information about my testing from most of my older mentors by believing the whispered lie; "They just would not understand." In reality, I was avoiding their discernment.

I also realized just how blessed I was to be in a time of prayer and fasting. It was this spiritual discipline that prepared my heart and made it more tender to the Spirit's conviction. This type of oppression with its strong deceptive qualities, I believe, requires strong measures. Of course, it was all part of God's sovereign plan, but I think I would still be testing right now if I had not spent an extended period of time in prayer and fasting, even though it was supposedly for my child.

I expected all of hell to wreak havoc on my family's health once I quit muscle testing, but God in His grace protected us. The first time my child asked me to test something for him, I refused and told him to pray instead and ask the Lord to help show us what the problem was. We, together with the Lord's help, discerned some bad food choices, the need for hydration, etc. Recently when the flu caused some concern with my mother's lungs, once again after prayer the Lord guided me to the right resources in order to help her heal by using the tried-and-true methods of nutritional healing—all God-given resources from His created nature for our use.

So, what have I learned through this journey thus far? I must depend on Jesus for everything—even my health! I need to know Him better every single day, listen to His voice, constantly keep my eyes on Him, and trust in His timing. My prayer is that He will take these ashes from my own life's story and make something beautiful in someone else's for His glory.

Appendix

Appendix A

Steps for Repentance & Standing Against the Enemy

Submit yourselves, then, to God. Resist the devil, and he will flee from you. Come near to God and he will come near to you. Wash your hands, you sinners, and purify your hearts, you double-minded. James 4:7-8

1. Submit yourself to God in confession & repentance

Before you do any rebuking of spirits, you must first confess your sin and tell God of your desire to repent. Ask for his protection and authority over demons. If your children are old enough to understand, and they have been a part of our transgression, then explain things to them in simple terms before including them when you follow James 4:7-8. Even though they are involved at your direction, they may personally need to repent as well. From my own son and the stories of others, it is apparent that children are vulnerable to Satan's influence. For instance, it is not uncommon for them to experience vivid, spiritually oppressive dreams as a result of their parents' imprudence. Make sure they are appropriately included in your family's repentance.

2. Stand against the devil, out loud, in the name of Jesus

Luke 4:35 / Luke 10:17 / Acts 19:13-16

It is clear from passages in the Gospels that the rebuking of evil spirits was done out loud. It is also clear from the NT that it is only the name of Jesus that has any authority over Satan. I strongly caution anyone who is not certain of their salvation (through the blood of Christ alone) about rebuking Satan. To be clear, we do not rebuke the devil, God does. Jude 1:9 says that even the archangel Michael did not dare to rebuke Satan but instead said, "The Lord rebuke you." According to Ephesians 6, we "stand" against the enemy in the power of Jesus. It is Christ's presence indwelling a believer that allows the individual to have authority over demons, and Acts 19:13-16 tells a story of caution for those who are not saved.

I have heard some teach that you must name the spirits to rebuke them, but this is not necessary according to almost all instances in the Bible, nor is it realistic to expect that the name(s) to use will be knowable in most cases. One other suggestion I have for women: If your husband has also been involved, I encourage you to discuss this with him and ask him, as the biblically mandated head of his family, to lead your family in taking this stand against Satan.

3. Eliminate ALL paraphernalia & literature from those practices regardless of the cost.

Acts 19:18-20 says, *Many of those who believed now came and openly confessed what they had done. A number who had practiced sorcery brought their scrolls together and burned them publicly. When they calculated the value of the scrolls, the total came to fifty thousand drachmas. In this way the word of the Lord spread widely and grew in power.*

As I have said, many people have contacted me through my website indicating that they have decided to repent of their involvement with muscle testing, and they have followed James 4:7-8 to do so. However, they stop short of completely eliminating every trace of related paraphernalia. It's very hard to give up things that cost a lot of money. However, that is exactly the model we see in Acts 19:18-20. To leave something behind gives the devil a continued foothold in your life and ground to stand on for ongoing temptation. Do not allow this to happen. With repentance comes healing, but repentance means completely turning from that sin. Don't think about it or dwell on it. Just do it!

For further Scriptural encouragement on the importance of completely eliminating (destroying) all things related to energy medicine, consider the example from II Chronicles 33 – the story of King Manasseh of Judah. (Meg from Pennsylvania discusses this example in her testimony.)

Appendix B

Muscle Testing (AK) Explained

Another name for muscle testing is Applied Kinesiology, and there are many variations in its methodology and application. It is used to test for allergies, diagnose conditions, determine emotional baggage, determine which supplements and how many to take, determine which materials to use in dental fillings, and even in veterinary care. It also seems to have become an integral part of the thriving market for essential oils. It is everywhere! All of these methods are based on the belief that the body knows what it needs. All we have to do is ask it.

Performing the muscle test is quite simple. The belief is that the body gives either a yes or no answer through muscle strength. Generally, the individual being tested holds a tiny amount of a suspected allergen (or other substance about which inquiry is to be made) in one hand while extending their other arm to their side at a right angle. The practitioner then places one hand on the individual's shoulder and uses the other hand to lightly press down on the extended arm.

In theory, if allergic to the substance being tested or if the substance would not be good for that individual, the individual's arm muscle will weaken, and the arm can easily be pressed down. If not allergic or the substance would be helpful to the body, the arm remains strong.

It is also possible to self-test using other techniques. Another variation of testing is surrogate testing, which is done through a parent of a young child and in cases where the individual is not capable of performing the strength test themselves. A further method of muscle testing that is practiced by especially "gifted" practitioners is done remotely via telephone. (In this method, there is absolutely no physical contact with the individual!)

Appendix C

NAET

NAET's developer, Devi S. Nambudripad, DC, LAc, RN, PhD, is described on her Web site as an acupuncturist, chiropractor, kinesiologist, and registered nurse who practices in Buena Park, California.[269] Nambudripad teaches her theories about disease in her book, Say Goodbye to Illness. Her website says the following: An allergy is defined in terms of what a substance does to the energy flow in the body. Allergies are the result of energy imbalances in the body, leading to a diminished state of health in one or more organ systems.[270]

NAET purports that allergies cause energy blockages, which are theoretically at the root of every health malady. AK is used to determine allergies. Her theory far surpasses any conventional view of allergies and includes everything imaginable, including the individual components of everything. It teaches that not only can you be allergic to milk, for example, but to the calcium in milk. The theory goes that if you are allergic to calcium, then your body cannot properly absorb that vital mineral, and calcium deficiency symptoms would ensue.

Each offending component, as well as milk itself must be treated. A simple treatment affecting the spine and key Chinese meridian pressure points can be performed in a matter of minutes that can supposedly "clear" the allergy. After the treatment, the individual is again muscle tested to determine if the allergy has been "cleared." If it has not, the treatment protocol is repeated until the muscle remains strong. If it does remain strong, then the individual is told to completely avoid the treated allergen for 25 hours. Afterwards, the individual is again muscle tested to confirm that the allergy is cleared.

The danger here is apparent—as in cases where the allergy may be life-threatening. One documented case of the worst-case scenario sadly came to pass and was reported in an Irish newspaper in 2009. Thomas Schatten, a 43-year-old man was treated by a chiropractor using NAET for his allergy to peanuts. Neither he nor the chiropractor recognized the beginning symptoms of anaphylactic shock that began during the treatment. Ninety minutes after returning home, the man died of anaphylactic shock.[271] It would appear muscle testing proved inaccurate in determining that this man's allergy was "cleared."

Unlike with Applied Kinesiology, the scientific studies on NAET are limited. The NAET company conducted one in-house study on people who were treated for milk allergies in 2006.[272] This study does appear to follow the typical protocol for a double-blind study, except that I could find no published scientific results for any aspect of the study. Instead, only a general conclusion is given that NAET effectively reversed the treated patients' allergies. Without supporting data, such a conclusion certainly seems questionable.

An in-house, single-blind pilot study was submitted to clinicaltrials.gov. and begun in 2005, whereby Nambudripad might *test the efficacy of* NAET *(Nambudripad's Allergy Elimination Technique) protocols for the treatment of Autism Spectrum Disorder in children between the ages of 3-10 years old, especially in the areas of improving language and communication skills.*[273] The study was a single blind study with approximately 60 children of various ages divided between two groups. One group received NAET treatments multiple times a week for one year, while the control group was monitored but received no treatments. The children continued to receive their medications deemed necessary prior to the trial.

Although the study concludes that *there were 23 NAET treated children who improved to the extent that they were able to function in regular school classes*, they also make an interesting observation: *In contrast, the severity of mood swings increased by a statistically significant 29% in the NAET treated children. Though the cause of this is not clear.*[274] Such a significant increase in mood swings in Autism certainly calls into question how effective such treatments really are. Further scrutiny and replication by an unbiased group would be helpful, as well as monitoring the ongoing condition of the children in years to follow.

Another study was conducted in 2011, which tested six children who were treated with the NAET protocol for peanut allergies.[275] Serum blood testing was done for IgE, IgG, and Tryptase (standard measurements for allergies). This single-blind study was completed without any control groups and with such a small number of participants that it is difficult to garner any meaningful conclusions. However, following 18 treatments per child, a progressive oral challenge was done. If any sign of reaction was noted, the treatment was repeated. Once no reaction was noted, the children's blood was retested. According to the data on the charts displayed in the study's abstract, four of the six children had the same or higher blood serum levels, indicating a worsening, not improvement. All of the children's serum levels indicated peanut allergy remained. The study concludes by expressing confusion over why the children did not demonstrate physical symptoms by the end of the oral challenge and yet blood levels remain unchanged. Two of the children did require treatment in the hours following the completion of the study.

This apparent improvement from severe to minor reactions is notable. Interestingly, the peanut study did trend in the same direction that I generally experienced while involved with NAET. Others and I who were treated with NAET most frequently seemed to benefit for a time, but it rarely lasted. As a result, the constant need for treatments keeps one bound to the practice and can potentially place participants in danger as they continue exposure to allergenic substances with misplaced confidence that they are cleared for exposure to them.

The final study I found was submitted to clinicaltrials.gov in August of 2014 and was sponsored by the National Taiwan University Hospital. This double-blind, controlled study proposed to test 80 individuals for crab and shrimp allergies. They state that traditional IgE and skin testing would be used to form a baseline for each of the participants and then proposed to retest after 6 months. It is unclear whether this study was ever completed. No results, data, or conclusions have been posted from the time of the study until April 2024.[276]

Appendix D

How to Know for Sure that You Will Go to Heaven

The Bible says in 1 John 5:13, *I write these things to you who believe in the name of the Son of God, that you may KNOW that you have eternal life* (emphasis mine). Salvation is not a process, nor should it be something that is questioned by the true believer. You are either saved from the eternal wrath of God or you are not. I would like to share with you from the Bible how you can know for sure. Your simple role in salvation is summarized by the word "believe," which John used 84 times in the Gospel of John and 7 times in 1 John. But what exactly are you to believe?

Let us start at the beginning with the truth that all have sinned and come short of God's perfect standard of holiness.[cxxxviii] If you have thought that simply being a good person will get you into heaven, then be aware that the Bible makes it clear your most righteous acts are filthy in God's sight.[cxxxix] You may be a "good person" compared to many others, but God's standard is perfection. Because we are born with a sin nature and continue to live by that nature, we are separated from God who is without sin (holy). What we earn by our sin is eternal death (separation from God in hell).[cxl]

God knew that we could never pay the debt owed for our sin, so He sent His sinless Son, Jesus, to take the wrath for sin by dying in our place.[cxli] Jesus, the very Son of God, took on human flesh but not human sinfulness and, therefore, became the spotless sacrifice (without moral flaw) for the sins of the world. His atoning blood satisfies God's wrath for

---

[cxxxviii] Romans 3:23 *For all have sinned and fall short of the glory of God.* (KJV)
[cxxxix] Isaiah 64:6a *All of us have become like one who is unclean, and all our righteous acts are like filthy rags.*
[cxl] Romans 6:23 *The wages of sin is death but the gift of God is eternal life in Christ Jesus our Lord.* (KJV)
[cxli] Romans 5:8 *But God demonstrates his own love towards us, in this, while we were yet sinners, Christ died for us.* (NIV)

all who believe in His name, thereby saving them from judgment.[cxlii] Jesus died, was buried, and raised on the third day. He was seen by many before ascending back up into heaven where He is preparing a place (heaven) for those who believe in Him for salvation.[cxliii] Acts 4:12 speaks of Christ being the ONLY means for salvation. *And there is salvation in no one else, for there is no other name under heaven given among men by which we must be saved."*

It is by the grace of God, not works (the things you do), that one is saved.[cxliv] Grace (unmerited favor) is not getting what you deserve (God's judgment or wrath) and, in its place, getting the free gift of eternal salvation. Such grace is only through God and separate from our works. That means if you have previously believed that Christ + something else would save you, you are not saved. Saving faith is in Christ's work at the cross only. Church attendance, good behavior, being raised in a Christian family, giving money to the church or those in need, praying a prayer, or going forward at an event and then living as though you are lord of your life will not save you. Salvation is in Christ alone through faith alone.

I ask people what they would say if they were to die and stand before God. Consider Jesus' words in Matthew 7:23-24 of what some will say at that time. *On that day many will say to me, 'Lord, Lord, did we not prophesy in your name, and cast out demons in your name, and do many mighty works in your name?' And then will I declare to them, 'I never knew you; depart from me, you workers of lawlessness.'* You see, many confuse grace with works. James 2:19 also says, *You believe that God is one; you do well. Even the demons believe—and shudder!* It is possible to have head knowledge without heart belief. Works follow true faith, not the other way around. Good works are done out of love and obedience to the Savior as Lord of your life.

If you have never placed your trust in Christ alone as your Lord and Savior, I urge you to stop right now and pray. It is not a prayer that saves you. It is faith, and God knows your heart. Prayer is simply a way to tell God that you are a sinner who is now believing in Jesus alone for salvation. Romans 10:9 says, *if you confess with your mouth that Jesus is Lord and*

[cxlii] 2 Corinthians 5:21 *God made him who had no sin to be sin for us, so that in him we might become the righteousness of God.* (NIV)

[cxliii] 1 Corinthians 15:3-6 and John 14:2-3

[cxliv] Ephesians 2:8-9 For by grace you have been saved through faith. And this is not your own doing; it is the gift of God, [9] not a result of works, so that no one may boast.

believe in your heart that God raised him from the dead, you will be saved.

The Bible promises in John 5:24 that when you do so, you immediately pass from death to life! *Truly, truly, I say to you, whoever hears my word and believes him who sent me has eternal life. He does not come into judgment, but has passed from death to life.* Have you heard this word and believed in Christ as your Lord and Savior? Then the one-time transaction between you and God has been made, and you will not go to hell. You are His treasured child and will be with Him for eternity.

God seals that transaction with the gift of the Holy Spirit to dwell in your heart and guide you in understanding God's Word.[cxlv] God promises that He will never leave you or forsake you.[cxlvi]

Now that you have become a believer, I encourage you to do a few things to help you grow in the faith. Keep an ongoing dialogue with God through prayer. Your prayers of confession of sin, thankfulness, praise, and requests are pleasing to God. We are instructed to pray to God the Father in the name of Jesus.[cxlvii] He wants to hear from His children! Prayer is your way to talk to God, and reading the Bible is His way to speak to you. I would encourage you to read it every day. To begin, I recommend reading Ephesians 2 and making a list of everything it says about who you are in Christ, the gifts God has given you, and what His plans are for you. After that read the book of Philippians (encouragement for believers) and then Luke (the life and work of Jesus) and then Genesis (how it all began). Along with prayer and reading the Bible, find a doctrinally sound church that will help you grow in your faith through fellowship with other believers and teaching from God's Word. The Bible commands believers to be a part of His body (the church), and trust me, you will need it! You have begun a new adventure! Go in peace.

[cxlv] John 16:13
[cxlvi] Hebrews 13:5
[cxlvii] John 14:13-18

Appendix E

11 Red Flags to Aid in the Discernment of Questionable Modalities

1. Is the information acquired by the practice the result of secret knowledge?
2. Do you have a sense of unease (lack of peace) with regard to the practice?
3. Have the results of alternative testing been verified through traditionally accepted methods (blood tests, x-rays, etc.) or do the alternative methods contradict traditional results?
4. Does the method used for testing or treatment ever occur through a surrogate, by telephone, or by a machine that has not been scientifically proven to consistently achieve valid results?
5. Is a mysterious gifting required to perform the alternative practice or does the presence of certain people interfere with the effectiveness of the diagnoses or treatment? (i.e. a spouse must leave the room)
6. Are the methods consistent with historically Satanic practices or chance? Are they considered New Age or tied to eastern religions?
7. Do the practices produce "bondage" in people?
8. Do the explanations for how it works use any of the following buzzwords: energy, quantum physics, chi, chakras, the subconscious, inner child, tapping, frequency, or talk of the body as though it is a separate entity-- "the body knows how to fix itself, the body doesn't lie," etc.?
9. Anything that uses muscle testing in any form is divination and, therefore, forbidden for the Christian.
10. Over time, does the general progression of symptoms worsen, even though there may be individual improvements? Are the symptoms that develop strange, include suicidal thoughts, or is there great fighting and strife in your home?
11. Have you developed symptoms characterized as Lyme Disease, EMF or mold sensitivity, heavy metal poisoning, parasites, dizziness, or brain fog but have not, through traditionally accepted testing, been shown to have these conditions?

Appendix F

Recommendations for Reaching a Friend Involved in Energy Medicine

Never forget that there is a battle by Satan for your friend's soul so pray for them accordingly. According to numerous passages like 1 Peter 2:9, believers are a kingdom of priests whose job is to intercede or stand in the gap for others. Let your love for your friend lead you to serious intercession for them. You cannot remove the veil of deception, but God can. Plead with Him!

2 Timothy 2:22-26 provides the perfect roadmap both in how to handle someone who is deceived and how to pray for them. It says,

Have nothing to do with foolish, ignorant controversies; you know that they breed quarrels. And the Lord's servant must not be quarrelsome but kind to everyone, able to teach, patiently enduring evil, correcting his opponents with gentleness. God may perhaps grant them repentance leading to a knowledge of the truth, and they may come to their senses and escape from the snare of the devil, after being captured by him to do his will.

In whatever method God directs you to make known your concerns, do not be drawn into quarrelling over the matter. Be gentle and kind. It would be easy to come across as harsh and uncaring in your zeal to free your friend from sin. Remember, most people involved in these practices stay involved because they are both deceived and suffering. Ripping off the Band-Aid may be the wrong approach for one who is already hurting.

Often those involved in energy medicine do not recognize that their health has actually gotten worse, even if there have been isolated instances of improvement. If you are aware of their worsening condition, it can be eye-opening to the individual to have it pointed out. In such a case, the individual will likely be defensive, so be prepared to drop the matter and allow the Holy Spirit to bring about further consideration at a later time. The same is true in pointing out that you notice they are in bondage to these practices. My friend did this for me over 10 years ago. She did not say much, but it was enough to get my attention. She also gave me a book to read. I WAS offended, and I did not read the book for a while, but God used both what she said and the book to powerfully set me free. I knew she loved me and was not acting all holier-than-thou, so eventually I listened and responded to what the Holy Spirit was trying to say to me.

I have had so many individuals reach out to me through the years. Quite a few have said that they were repenting of muscle testing because a friend dared to approach them about their sin and gave them my information. One woman said it took her a year to respond, but eventually God brought her back to what her friend pointed out.

Finally, after you have lovingly reached out to your friend in the manner in which God led you, pray according to 2 Timothy 2:26. "God, grant _____ (your friend's name) repentance leading to a knowledge of the truth, that he/she may come to his/her senses and escape the snare of the devil who has captured him/her to do his will." May God bless you as you stand unceasingly in the gap for your friend as an intercessor until God removes the veil.

Biblical Fasting for Discernment & Health

Reasons for fasting:

- **To end bondage:** Isaiah 58:6 *"Is not this the kind of fasting I have chosen: to loose the chains of injustice and untie the cords of the yoke, to set the oppressed free and break every yoke?*

  Daniel 9:2-3 *In the first year of his reign, I, Daniel, understood from the Scriptures, according to the word of the LORD given to Jeremiah the prophet, that the desolation of Jerusalem would last seventy years. So I turned to the Lord God and pleaded with him in prayer and petition, in fasting, and in sackcloth and ashes.*

- **For healing:** Isaiah 58:8-9 *Then your light will break forth like the dawn, and your healing will quickly appear; then your righteousness will go before you, and the glory of the LORD will be your rear guard. Then you will call, and the LORD will answer; you will cry for help, and he will say: Here am I.*

  Psalm 35:13 *Yet when they were ill, I put on sackcloth and humbled myself with fasting.*

- **To seek God's intervention:** Esther 4:16 *Go, gather together all the Jews who are in Susa, and fast for me. Do not eat or drink for three days, night or day. I and my attendants will fast as you do. When this is done, I will go to the king, even though it is against the law. And if I perish, I perish."*

  Ezra 9:21 *There, by the Ahava Canal, I proclaimed a fast, so that we might humble ourselves before our God and ask him for a safe journey for us and our children, with all our possessions.*

- **In humble repentance:** Nehemiah 9

- **To seek guidance:** <u>Acts 13:2</u> *While they were worshiping the Lord and fasting, the Holy Spirit said, "Set apart for me Barnabas and Saul for the work to which I have called them."*

Instructions for fasting:

- **No fighting or selfish pursuits:** <u>Isaiah 58:3-4</u> *'Why have we fasted,' they say, 'and you have not seen it? Why have we humbled ourselves, and you have not noticed?' Yet on the day of your fasting, you do as you please and exploit all your workers. Your fasting ends in quarreling and strife, and in striking each other with wicked fists. You cannot fast as you do today and expect your voice to be heard on high.*

- **Do it secretly:** <u>Matthew 6:16-18</u> *"When you fast, do not look somber as the hypocrites do, for they disfigure their faces to show others they are fasting. Truly I tell you, they have received their reward in full. But when you fast, put oil on your head and wash your face, so that it will not be obvious to others that you are fasting, but only to your Father, who is unseen; and your Father, who sees what is done in secret, will reward you.*

- **Or, with others:** <u>Acts 13:2</u> & <u>14:23</u>, <u>Esther 4:3</u> & <u>16</u>

The underlying purpose of biblical fasting is to humbly seek God's mercy, which is far more than merely not eating. By denying the demands of the body, we recognize our humble dependance on the LORD. Do you require special mercy in guidance, deliverance, healing, or a repentant heart? Throughout Scripture, we see fasting utilized as a special means for unique situations. It is not a time of punishing oneself for sin or so that God will forgive us (for this we already have upon confession), but so that we might request God's further mercy in light of the consequences of sin.

The time that would have been spent in feeding the flesh is spent instead on seeking God. When I have replaced meals with the bread of heaven (the Lord), I always discover that the struggle with hunger is minimal, unlike when I have fasted for purely physical reasons. Fasting is a spiritual discipline and should be treated as such.

Acknowledgments

During the two years of writing this book, a handful of people have come alongside to make its completion possible, and I am grateful for each one.

Seth, my amazing husband—You have made me into the writer I am by teaching me through your editing of all I have written through the years. You have the patience of Job! Your encouragement to me throughout the writing of this book has spurred me on to completion. I must not forget that it was you who came up with the name for this book, as well as numerous illustrations used in its pages, which provide clarity to otherwise murky topics. Thank you for generously sharing your time, skill, and keen mind in order to bring *Ouija Medicine* to completion. You will always be my hero.

Physics guru I am not, and yet God answered my prayers in providing one to come alongside me in editing the chapter on quantum mechanics. Thank you, Stephen Gollmer PhD, for your invaluable assistance and patience with me. May God bless you abundantly for how you willingly guided me in the writing of that chapter.

God blessed me with a prayer team of women who prayed throughout the writing of this book. Many times, when the task seemed impossible, your encouragement and prayers carried me through. Thank you, Mary, Michelle, Brittany, Melanie, and Angela.

Thank you to those who humbly and courageously share their stories in the pages of this book.

Finally, thank you to my son, Caleb, for using your graphic design skills to design a book cover once again. I am proud of you and the way you willingly share the gifts God has given you to further His kingdom.

About the Author

Born in southern California but primarily raised in the Atlanta area, Marci Julin is the second of four children. At a young age, she heard the Gospel in a Baptist Sunday school class and responded by placing her trust in Jesus Christ for salvation. When only 8 years old she felt the call of God to reach the lost with the Good News of Jesus Christ and had the unique privilege of spending her teenage summers on the mission field. That desire to see people come to saving faith in Jesus Christ never abated, but the realities of life prevented full-time service until she became an empty nester.

While attending Bryan College, a Christian liberal arts college in Dayton, Tennessee, she met Seth, and then married, him in 1991. Before the birth of their son, they moved to the Orlando, Florida area to be near family and continued to reside there for 25 years. Although she graduated from Bryan with a bachelor's degree in elementary education and a minor in Bible, Marci chose to be a homemaker and home-school their only child, Caleb, through the 7th grade. She then taught for two years at her son's classical Christian school.

In spite of always feeling God's hand on her life and desiring to please Him, Marci struggled with depression and trusting that God loved her personally due to many years of plaguing health problems. As a type A, driven person she continued pushing herself to her physical limits, always striving to be perfect in everything in order to win the approval of her Lord. It wasn't until God allowed her to become bedridden that she was forced to deal with her misconceptions about God and His deep, unfailing love for her. As the merciful Savior brought healing to her heart and mind through Scripture, He also brought complete physical healing. She wrote of this journey in her books, *When You Can't Trust His Heart* and *Life to the Body*. She now wholeheartedly agrees with the Psalmist when he says, *It was good for me to be afflicted so that I might learn your decrees. The law from your mouth is more precious to me than thousands of pieces of silver and gold* (Psalm 119:71-72).

Since her son, Caleb left home to attend Bryan College, Marci began Heart & Mind Ministries and has devoted her time to biblical teaching, writing, and speaking. Before the birth of Marci's first grandson, God orchestrated their move to beautiful north Georgia where they enjoy being near Caleb and his family. For over ten years Marci and Seth cared for his parents until both left behind the troubled minds of Alzheimer's for their eternal rewards in heaven.

Marci enjoys traveling and exploring the beautiful areas of God's amazing creation, running, gardening, beekeeping, and studying God's Word. More than anything, Marci longs to inspire others with a passion for God's Word and a love for her Savior.

- You can gain access to other teaching or contact her regarding scheduling her for speaking to a women's group on her website at
  https://www.heartandmindministries.com

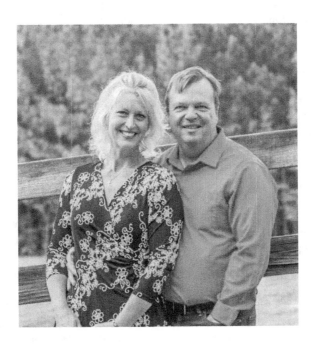

Index

End Notes

[1] Nambudripad, Devi S., *Say Goodbye to Illness*, Delta Publishing Co, Buena Park, CA, 2002.

[2] Ibid

[3] Fisher, Mary Insana and Shana Harrington , "Research Round-up: Manual Muscle Testing" (2015). Physical Therapy Faculty Publications. 47. https://ecommons.udayton.edu/dpt_fac_pub/47

[4] Kendall, Florence P, Modified from 1993, MACS FORM 04: MANUAL MUSCLE TESTING PROCEDURES, https://www.niehs.nih.gov/research/resources/assets/docs/muscle_grading_and_testing_procedures_508.pdf

[5] Fisher, Mary Insana and Harrington, Shana, "Research Round-up: Manual Muscle Testing" (2015). Physical Therapy Faculty Publications. 47. https://ecommons.udayton.edu/dpt_fac_pub/47

[6] International College of Applied Kinesiology (ICAP), 2018, *What Is Applied Kinesiology?*, https://www.icak.com/what-is-applied-kinesiology.html.

[7] Cuthbert SC, Goodheart GJ., Jr. On the reliability and validity of manual muscle testing: a literature review. *Chiropr Osteopat.* 2007;**15**:4. doi: 10.1186/1746-1340-15-4 On the reliability and validity of manual muscle testing: a literature review (nih.gov)

[8] Ibid

[9] Haas, Mitchell et al. "Disentangling manual muscle testing and Applied Kinesiology: critique and reinterpretation of a literature review." *Chiropractic & osteopathy* vol. 15 11. 23 Aug. 2007, doi:10.1186/1746-1340-15-11

[10] Thie, John F., Touch for Health, Healing the World One Balance at a Time, https://www.touchforhealth.us/about-us/

[11] Diamond, John, *Your Body Doesn't Lie*, Warner Books Edition, Harper and Row, Publishing, 10 East 53rd Street, New York, NY, 10022, 1980.

[12] John Diamond Healing from Within, *Three Papers in Honor of George Goodheart*, Presented at the International College of Applied Kinesiology

Conference, Detroit, MI, June 2007, Diamond, John MD, https://drjohndiamond.com/tributes/three-papers-in-honor-of-george-goodheart/.

[13] Energy Medicine Research Institute website, https://www.energymedicineri.com/dr-lisa-tully-phd-and-founder-energy-medicine-research-institute.html

[14] Website for Academy of Spiritual and Consciousness Studies, http://ascsi2.ning.com/page/ginette-nachman

[15] Ibid

[16] Schwartz, Stephan A, Jessica Utts, S James P Spottiswoode, Christopher W Shade, Lisa Tully, William F Morris, Ginette Nachman, *A double-blind, randomized study to assess the validity of applied kinesiology (AK) as a diagnostic tool and as a nonlocal proximity effect,* Mar-Apr 2014;10(2):99-108. doi: 10.1016/j.explore.2013.12.002. Epub 2013 Dec 18, https://pubmed.ncbi.nlm.nih.gov/24607076/

[17] Ibid.

[18] Ibid.

[19] Staehle, H.-J, M.J. Koch, T. Pioch, *Double-blind Study on Materials Testing with Applied Kinesiology, Journal of Dental Research,* Department of Conservative Dentistry, November 1, 2005, Volume: 84, issue: 11, page(s): 1066-1069, University of Heidelberg, Im Neuenheimer Feld 400, D-61920 Heidelberg, Germany;

[20] Wüthrich, B., *Unproven techniques in allergy diagnosis,* University of Zürich, Zürich. Switzerland, J Invest Allergol Clin Immunol 2005; Vol. 15(2): 86-90, http://www.jiaci.org/issues/vol15issue02/1.pdf.

[21] Ibid

[22] Ibid

[23] Pothmann, R, S von Frankenberg, C Hoicke, H Weingarten, R Lüdtke [Evaluation of applied kinesiology in nutritional intolerance of childhood], PMID: 11799301, DOI: 10.1159/000057250, Forsch Komplementarmed Klass Naturheilkd, 2001 Dec;8(6):336-44. [Evaluation of applied kinesiology in nutritional intolerance of childhood] - PubMed (nih.gov)

[24] Lüdtke, R, B Kunz, N Seeber, J Ring, *Test-retest-reliability and validity of the Kinesiology muscle test,* 2001 Sep;9(3):141-5. doi: 10.1054/ctim.2001.0455. PMID: 11926427, https://pubmed.ncbi.nlm.nih.gov/11926427/

[25] Kenney JJ, Clemens R, Forsythe KD. Applied kinesiology unreliable for assessing nutrient status. J Am Diet Assoc. 1988 Jun;88(6):698-704. PMID: 3372923.

[26] Hyman, Ray Ph.D., *How People Are Fooled by Ideomotor Action*, August 26, 2003, https://quackwatch.org/related/ideomotor/

[27] Haas, Mitchell et al. "Disentangling manual muscle testing and Applied Kinesiology: critique and reinterpretation of a literature review." *Chiropractic & osteopathy* vol. 15 11. 23 Aug. 2007, doi:10.1186/1746-1340-15-11

[28] Zuckerman, Arthur, *46 Placebo Effect Statistics: 2020/2021 Data, Examples & Implications*, Compare Camp website, May 27, 2020, https://comparecamp.com/placebo-effect-statistics/

[29] Ibid

[30] Jensen, Anne, The Oxford Studies: Part II — Results And Implications, June 16, 2017 http://gemskinesiology.com/2017/06/16/the-oxford-studies-part-ii-results-and-implications/

[31] *Pinocchio's Arm: A Lie Detector Test*, Scientific American, Science Buddies on March 10, 2016, https://www.scientificamerican.com/article/pinocchio-s-arm-a-lie-detector-test/

[32] Jensen AM, Stevens RJ, Burls AJ. *Estimating the accuracy of muscle response testing: two randomised-order blinded studies*. BMC Complement Altern Med. 2016 Nov 30;16(1):492. doi: 10.1186/s12906-016-1416-2. PMID: 27903263; PMCID: PMC5131520.

[33] Diamond, John, *The Thymus and the Heart Chakra,* YouTube video, February 25, 2020, *https://www.youtube.com/watch?v=e5cR_flLit8*

[34] Pollack, Robert, Edward Kravitz, Nutrition in Oral Health and Disease, Philadelphia, PA: Lea & Febiger, 1985 (p 310).

[35] Diamond, John, *Dr. George Goodheart: The Nature of A Genius Dr. George Goodheart: The Nature of A Genius,* taken from the website, John Diamond,

Healing from Within, https://drjohndiamond.com/tributes/dr-george-goodheart-nature-of-a-genius/

[36] Diamond, John, *Three Papers in Honor of George Goodheart*, Presented at the International College of Applied Kinesiology International Conference, Detroit, Michigan—June 9, 2007, https://drjohndiamond.com/tributes/three-papers-in-honor-of-george-goodheart/

[37] "Divination." Merriam-Webster.com Dictionary, Merriam-Webster, https://www.merriam-webster.com/dictionary/divination. Accessed 8 Aug. 2021.

[38] Gruss, Edmond C., The Ouija Board: Doorway to the Occult, Moody Press, Chicago, 1975.

[39] https://www.williamfuld.com/biography.html

[40] D.R. Linson, "Washington's Haunted Boy," Fate, April 1951, reprinted in Exorcism: Fact Not Fiction (New York: New Amer. Lib., 1974), p.13.

[41] Gruss, Edmond C., The Ouija Board: Doorway to the Occult, Moody Press, Chicago, 1975.

[42] *Baltimore Sun*, May 17, 1959.

[43] Ibid.

[44] Koch, Kurt E., *Demonology Past and Present*, Kregel Publications, Grand Rapids MI, 1973, (p 88-90).

[45] Parker Brothers, *The Weird and Wonderful Ouija Talking Board Set*, instruction leaflet, p.2.

[46] Gage, Greg. *How to Control Someone Else's Arm*, Ted Talk, March 2015, https://www.ted.com/talks/greg_gage_how_to_control_someone_else_s_arm_with_your_brain/transcript#t-200416

[47] Ibid.

[48] http://www.energymedicineuniversity.org/emfield.html

[49] Srinivasan, TM, IJOY, *Energy Medicine*, International Journal of Yoga, 2010 Jan-Jun; 3(1).

[50] Baron, Marci, Namavar, Roxanna, *What Everyone Should Know About Energy Healing,* https://www.mindbodygreen.com/0-23890/what-everyone-should-know-about-energy-healing.html.

[51] Shakespeare, William, *Romeo and Juliet,* Act 2 Scene 2.

[52] Feinstein, David Ph.D, Eden, Donna, *Six Pillars of Energy Medicine, Clinical Strengths of a Complementary Paradigm,* https://edenenergymedicine.com/six-pillars-of-energy-medicine/

[53] Ibid

[54] Hunt, V. Electronic evidence of auras, chakras in UCLA study. *Brain/Mind Bulletin*, 1978;3(9):1-2.

[55] Feinstein, David Ph.D., Eden, Donna, *Six Pillars of Energy Medicine, Clinical Strengths of a Complementary Paradigm,* https://edenenergymedicine.com/six-pillars-of-energy-medicine/

[56] Ibid

[57] Ibid

[58] Ibid

[59] Hall, Harriet, MD, *A review of Energy Medicine: The Scientific Basis, by James L. Oschman,* reprinted from Skeptic Magazine 2005, January 14, 2006, http://quackfiles.blogspot.com/2006/01/review-of-energy-medicine-scientific.html

[60] Caridad, Carlos, June 25, 2019, https://www.youtube.com/watch?v=oLfP5Z8BguE

[61] http://quantumreflexanalysis.com/

[62] Davis, Tim, *Explainer: What Is Wave-Particle Duality,* July 27, 2012, https://theconversation.com/explainer-what-is-wave-particle-duality-7414

[63] *What Is Quantum Physics?*, Caltech, Science Exchange, https://scienceexchange.caltech.edu/topics/quantum-science-explained/quantum-physics

[64] Lincoln, Don Ph.D., "What is Quantum Mechanics Really All About?" https://www.youtube.com/watch?v=K0VY9_hB_WU

[65] *What Is Quantum Physics?*, Caltech Science Exchange, https://scienceexchange.caltech.edu/topics/quantum-science-explained/quantum-physics

[66] Jade, What is the Schrodinger Equation, Exactly?, Up and Atom, https://www.youtube.com/watch?v=QeUMFo8sODk

[67] Sanders, Laura, *Everyday Entanglement, Physicists Take Quantum Weirdness Out Of The Lab,* Science News, November 5, 2010 At 5:01 Pm, https://www.sciencenews.org/article/everyday-entanglement

[68] Lincoln, Don Ph.D., "Quantum Entanglement: Spooky Action at a Distance," https://www.youtube.com/watch?v=JFozGfxmi8A

[69] Siegfried, Tom, *Quantum Spookiness Survives Its Toughest Tests-- Entanglement's Weirdness Leads To New View On Emergence Of Spacetime,* January 27, 2016 At 8:00 Am, Science News, https://www.sciencenews.org/blog/context/quantum-spookiness-survives-its-toughest-tests

[70] Ibid

[71] Carroll, Robert Todd, PHd., *Vibrational Medicine*, http://www.skepdic.com/vibrationalmedicine.html

[72] Plante, Amber, *How the human body uses electricity*, University of Maryland Graduate School, Gazette, February 2016, https://graduate.umaryland.edu/gsa/gazette/February-2016/How-the-human-body-uses-electricity/

[73] Pereda, A. Electrical synapses and their functional interactions with chemical synapses. *Nat Rev Neurosci* **15,** 250–263 (2014). https://doi.org/10.1038/nrn3708

[74] CA: A Cancer Journal for Clinicians, Questionable methods of cancer management: Electronic devices, March/April 1994 https://doi.org/10.3322/canjclin.44.2.115

[75] Zimmerman, Jacquelyn W et al. "Targeted treatment of cancer with radiofrequency electromagnetic fields amplitude-modulated at tumor-specific frequencies." *Chinese journal of cancer* vol. 32,11 (2013): 573-81. doi:10.5732/cjc.013.10177

[76] Pasche B, Erman M, Hayduk R, et al. Effects of low energy emission therapy in chronic psychophysiological insomnia. *Sleep.* 1996;19:327–336.

[77] Aaron RK, Ciombor DM, Simon BJ. Treatment of nonunions with electric and electromagnetic fields. *Clin Orthop Relat Res.* 2004;419:21–29

Hall, Harriet MD, *A review of Energy Medicine: The Scientific Basis by James L. Oschman*, London: Churchill Livingstone, an imprint of Harcourt Publishers Limited, 2000. 274 pp. ISBN 0-443-06261-7, MDhttp://quackfiles.blogspot.com/2006/01/review-of-energy-medicine-scientific.html

[78] Costa FP, de Oliveira AC, Meirelles R, Machado MC, Zanesco T, Surjan R, Chammas MC, de Souza Rocha M, Morgan D, Cantor A, Zimmerman J, Brezovich I, Kuster N, Barbault A, Pasche B. Treatment of advanced hepatocellular carcinoma with very low levels of amplitude-modulated electromagnetic fields. Br J Cancer. 2011 Aug 23;105(5):640-8. doi: 10.1038/bjc.2011.292. Epub 2011 Aug 9. PMID: 21829195; PMCID: PMC3188936.

[79] Stupp R, Wong ET, Kanner AA, Steinberg D, Engelhard H, Heidecke V, Kirson ED, Taillibert S, Liebermann F, Dbalý V, Ram Z, Villano JL, Rainov N, Weinberg U, Schiff D, Kunschner L, Raizer J, Honnorat J, Sloan A, Malkin M, Landolfi JC, Payer F, Mehdorn M, Weil RJ, Pannullo SC, Westphal M, Smrcka M, Chin L, Kostron H, Hofer S, Bruce J, Cosgrove R, Paleologous N, Palti Y, Gutin PH. NovoTTF-100A versus physician's choice chemotherapy in recurrent glioblastoma: a randomised phase III trial of a novel treatment modality. Eur J Cancer. 2012 Sep;48(14):2192-202. doi: 10.1016/j.ejca.2012.04.011. Epub 2012 May 18. PMID: 22608262.

[80] *UK - Soundwaves effectively and precisely treat prostate cancer*, 2/7/2022 12:33:30 PM, https://menafn.com/1103651362/UK-Soundwaves-effectively-and-precisely-treat-prostate-cancer

[81] *Ultrasound Can Selectively Kill Cancer Cells*, February 4, 2020, https://www.caltech.edu/about/news/ultrasound-can-selectively-kill-cancer-cells

[82] Perkins, Robert, *Ultrasound Can Selectively Kill Cancer Cells*, February 4, 2020, https://www.caltech.edu/about/news/ultrasound-can-selectively-kill-cancer-cells

[83] https://en.wikipedia.org/wiki/Pseudoscience

[84] https://www.spinepluschiropractic.com/bioresonance-therapy-history-science-behind-treatment/

[85] https://www.nasa.gov/mission_pages/sunearth/news/gallery/schumann-resonance.html

[86] QRA Testing | Heise Health Clinic (drheise.com)

[87] https://www.toppr.com/guides/physics-formulas/resonant-frequency-formula/

[88] Hall, Harriett, MD, BioCharger's Claims Are Too Silly to Take Seriously, Science Based Medicine, January 21, 2020, https://sciencebasedmedicine.org/biochargers-claims-are-too-silly-to-take-seriously/

[89] Randall JM, Matthews RT, Stiles MA. Resonant frequencies of standing humans. Ergonomics. 1997 Sep;40(9):879-86. doi: 10.1080/001401397187711. PMID: 9306739.

[90] Carroll, Robert Todd, PHd., *Vibrational Medicine*, http://www.skepdic.com/vibrationalmedicine.html

[91] https://www.physicsforums.com/threads/how-can-you-measure-frequencies-in-the-human-body.901612/

[92] https://en.wikipedia.org/wiki/Pseudoscience

[93] https://www.biologicalmedicineinstitute.com/albert-abrams /

[94] Ibid

[95] Bailey, David M., "The Rise and Fall of Albert Abrams", *Oklahoma State Medical Association.* Retrieved from the Digital Public Library of America <http://www.archive.org/details/journalofoklahom7111okla> .

[96] Ibid

[97] Ibid

[98] Ibid

[99] Jarvis, William T. Ph.D., *Radionics and Albert Abrams, M.D. Quackwatch*, February 1, 2002, https://quackwatch.org/ncahf/articles/o-r/radionics/

[100] Ibid (The original source cited is no longer accessible. Flaxman, N.: A Cardiology Anomaly: Albert Abrams (1863-1924), Bull. Hist. Med. 27: 252-268, 1953.)

[101] [101]Jarvis, William T. Ph.D., *Radionics and Albert Abrams, M.D. Quackwatch*, February 1, 2002, https://quackwatch.org/ncahf/articles/o-r/radionics/

[102] Ibid

[103] Our Abrams Investigation—I, Author(s): the Staff, *Scientific American* , Vol. 129, No. 4 (OCTOBER 1923), p. 230, https://www.jstor.org/stable/10.2307/24974666

[104] Lescarboura, Austin C. "Our Abrams In▯estigation-II." *Scientific American*, vol. 129, no. 5, Scientific American, a division of Nature America, Inc., 1923, pp. 306–70, http://www.jstor.org/stable/24974707.

[105] Ibid

[106] Lescarboura, Austin C. "Our Abrams Investigation—X." *Scientific American*, vol. 131, no. 1, Scientific American, a division of Nature America, Inc., 1924, pp. 16–70, http://www.jstor.org/stable/24975119.

[107] Brown, Edward, *New choices for healing ourselves, Interview with Richard Gerber*, https://www.share-international.org/archives/health-healing/hh_ebnewch.html

[108] Carroll, Robert Todd, PHd., *Radionics*, http://www.skepdic.com/radionics.html

[109] Barrett, Stephen, M.D., *Be Wary of Radionics Devices*, December 27, 2011, https://quackwatch.org/device/reports/radionics/

[110] *The Kabbalah And Controversy Of Ruth B Drown*, Wired Alchemy, Aetheric Technologies & Consciousness, July 6, 2021, http://wiredalchemy.com/the-kabbalah-and-controversy-of-ruth-b-drown/

[111] CA: A Cancer Journal for Clinicians, Questionable methods of cancer management: Electronic devices, March/April 1994 https://acsjournals.onlinelibrary.wiley.com/doi/epdf/10.3322/canjclin.44.2.115

[112] Ibid

[113] Smith, Ralph Lee, *The Incredible Drown Case (1968),* Chirobase--Your Skeptical Guide to Chiropractic History, Theories, and Practices, https://quackwatch.org/chiropractic/hx/drown/

[114] Ibid

[115] Drown, Ruth, *Drown Radio Therapy*, Journal of Borderland Research, Vol 17, Number 7, https://borderlandsciences.org/journal/vol/17/n07/Drown_Radio_Therapy.html

[116] *The Kabbalah And Controversy Of Ruth B Drown*, Wired Alchemy, Aetheric Technologies & Consciousness, July 6, 2021, http://wiredalchemy.com/the-kabbalah-and-controversy-of-ruth-b-drown/

[117] Smith, Ralph Lee, *The Incredible Drown Case (1968),* Chirobase--Your Skeptical Guide to Chiropractic History, Theories, and Practices, https://quackwatch.org/chiropractic/hx/drown/

[118] Ibid

[119] Ibid

[120] Jarvis, William T. Ph.D., *Rife Devices, National Council Against Health Fraud Archive--Enhancing Freedom of Choice through Reliable Health Information,* December 29, 2000,

[121] *History—Dr. Royal Raymond Rife,* https://www.biologicalmedicineinstitute.com/royal-raymond-rife

[122] Brown, C N, *The Rife Microscope in the Science Museum Collection*, April 7, 1993, https://www.rife.de/science-museum-report.html

[123] http://barry-lynes.com/

[124] Marsh, John, personal letter from John Marsh to Christopher Bird, August 23, 1982, http://www.rifevideos.com/royal_rife_documents.html

[125] Question #2 in Royal Raymond Rife's 1961 trial deposition, https://rifevideos.com/dr_royal_rife_deposition_1961.html

[126] Marsh, John, personal letter from John Marsh to Christopher Bird, August 23, 1982, http://www.rifevideos.com/royal_rife_documents.html

[127] CA: A Cancer Journal for Clinicians, Questionable methods of cancer management: Electronic devices, March/April 1994 https://acsjournals.onlinelibrary.wiley.com/doi/epdf/10.3322/canjclin.44.2.115

[128] Brown, C N, *The Rife Microscope in the Science Museum Collection*, April 7, 1993, https://www.rife.de/science-museum-report.html

[129] Rife, Royal R., *Royal Rife in His Own Words*, https://www.rifevideos.com/Video/mp4/Royal_rife_in_his_own_words.mp4

[130] Brown, C N, *The Rife Microscope in the Science Museum Collection*, April 7, 1993, https://www.rife.de/science-museum-report.html

[131] Alberts B, Johnson A, Lewis J, et al. Molecular Biology of the Cell. 4th edition. New York: Garland Science; 2002. Looking at the Structure of Cells in the Microscope. Available from: https://www.ncbi.nlm.nih.gov/books/NBK26880/

[132] Rife, Royal R., *Royal Rife in His Own Words*, https://www.rifevideos.com/Video/mp4/Royal_rife_in_his_own_words.mp4

[133] Ibid

[134] Marsh collection, Rife audio CD's, https://www.rifevideos.com/pdf/a_history/the_rife_machine_report_a_history_of_rifes_instruments_and_frequencies.pdf

[135] Smith, Jeff, *Royal Raymond Rife: Into the Micro Beyond,* Long-Ago In San Diego, Feb. 15, 2012, https://www.sandiegoreader.com/news/2012/feb/15/unforgettable/

[136] *Filterable Bodies Seen With the Rife Microscope, Science News,* Vol.4 #1978, December 11, 1931, https://static1.squarespace.com/static/6120fd6cda3b62095f7499c9/t/615c945af41afa655c8a7a9d/1633457243076/Science+Review+of+California+microscope+demonstration+Dec+1931.pdf

[137] Question #72 in Royal Raymond Rife's1961 trial deposition, https://rifevideos.com/dr_royal_rife_deposition_1961.html

[138] Brown, C N, *The Rife Microscope in the Science Museum Collection*, April 7, 1993, https://www.rife.de/science-museum-report.html

[139] Ibid

[140] Ibid

[141] Ibid

[142] *The Rife Machine Report- A History of Rife's Instruments & Frequencies*, January 2022 edition, https://www.rifevideos.com/pdf/a_history/the_rife_machine_report_a_histor y_of_rifes_instruments_and_frequencies.pdf

[143] Ibid

[144] Lynes, Barry, *The Cancer Cure That Worked—Fifty Years of Suppression*, Marcus Books, Ontario, Canada, 1987.

[145] Hood, Del, *Scientific Genius Dies; Saw Work Discredited*, The Daily Californian, August 1971, https://rifevideos.com/scientific_genius_dies_saw_work_discredited.html

[146] *The Rife Machine Report- A History of Rife's Instruments & Frequencies*, January 2022 edition, https://www.rifevideos.com/pdf/a_history/the_rife_machine_report_a_histor y_of_rifes_instruments_and_frequencies.pdf

[147] Ibid, p.308.

[148] Dr. Stafford letter to Dr. Jeppson, April 1, 1958, *The Rife Machine Report- A History of Rife's Instruments & Frequencies*, January 2022 edition, https://www.rifevideos.com/pdf/a_history/the_rife_machine_report_a_histor y_of_rifes_instruments_and_frequencies.pdf

[149] John Marsh collection, Dr Stafford's report on using the AZ-58, page 4, www.rife.org

[150] Crane, John, *The Crane Report*, https://www.rife.de/the-crane-report.html

[151] Burbank, Theodora, *The BackBlog: Elisha Perkins and the Metallic Tractors*, Warren Anatomical Museum, Harvard Countway Library, February 2, 2020, https://countway.harvard.edu/news/backblog-elisha-perkins-metallic-tractors

[152] CA: A Cancer Journal for Clinicians, Questionable methods of cancer management: Electronic devices, March/April 1994 https://acsjournals.onlinelibrary.wiley.com/doi/epdf/10.3322/canjclin.44.2.115

[153] Haygarth J: Of the Imagination, As Cause and As Cure, of Disorders of the Body, Exemplified by Fictitious Tractors and Epidemical Convulsions. London, Cruttwell, 1800.

[154] CFR - Code of Federal Regulations Title 21, December 22, 2023, https://www.accessdata.fda.gov/scripts/cdrh/cfdocs/cfcfr/CFRSearch.cfm?fr=1 01.93

[155] Barrett, Stephen, M.D., *Quack "Electrodiagnostic" Devices*, February 14, 2018, https://quackwatch.org/related/electro/

[156] Hall, Harriet, M.D., *Frequencies and Their Kindred Delusions*, Science-Based Medicine, April 5, 2011, https://sciencebasedmedicine.org/frequencies-and-their-kindred-delusions/

[157] Hall, Harriet, M.D., *BioCharger's Claims Are Too Silly to Take Seriously*, January 21, 2020, https://sciencebasedmedicine.org/biochargers-claims-are-too-silly-to-take-seriously/

[158] https://biocharger.com/science-behind-the-biocharger/

[159] *Wikipedia*, Alexander Gurwitsch, https://en.wikipedia.org/wiki/Alexander_Gurwitsch

[160] https://somavedic.com/pages/science#shopify-section-template--14254231846975__science-pdf-section

[161] Brice, August, https://techwellness.com/blogs/expertise/does-somavedic-work-emf-protection-crystals

[162] Ibid

[163] Johansson, Olle, PhD., https://techwellness.com/blogs/expertise/does-somavedic-work-emf-protection-crystals

[164] Somavedic—An interview with Ivan Rybjansky the inventor of the Somavedic device, https://youtu.be/X8iW_WnBUJI?si=lpkp5BQD2SECD9J1

[165] Ibid (18-19 minute marker)

[166] Hall, Harriet, MD, *Amino Neuro Frequency: Just More "Embedded Frequencies" Silliness,* October 3, 2017,

https://sciencebasedmedicine.org/amino-neuro-frequency-just-more-embedded-frequencies-silliness/

[166] https://luminas.com/

[167] Hall, Harriet, MD, *Amino Neuro Frequency: Just More "Embedded Frequencies" Silliness,* October 3, 2017, https://sciencebasedmedicine.org/amino-neuro-frequency-just-more-embedded-frequencies-silliness/

[168] https://luminas.com/

[169] https://luminas.com/clinical-study/

[170] Gorsky, David, MD & PhD, *Luminas Pain Relief Patches: Where the words "quantum" and "energy" really mean "magic",* Respectful Insolence, https://www.respectfulinsolence.com/2018/08/17/luminas-pain-relief-patches/

[171] https://www.respectfulinsolence.com/2018/08/17/luminas-pain-relief-patches/

[172] https://www.energytouchschool.com/what-is-energytouch-healing

[173] https://taopatch.co/

[174] https://taopatch.co/pages/research

[175] Pinches, Samuel, PhD, *TaoPatch – Is it a scam?,* July 13, 2020, https://painreliefpatchreviews.com/taopatch/taopatch-is-it-a-scam/

[176] Ibid

[177] Ibid

[178] Oliveira, Arnaldo. (2016). Electroacupuncture According to Voll: Historical Background and Literature Review. Meridians: The Journal of Acupuncture and Oriental Medicine. 3. 5-10, 40.

[179] Barrett, Stephen, M.D., *Quack "Electrodiagnostic" Devices*, Quackwatch, February 14, 2018, https://quackwatch.org/related/electro/ Quack "Electrodiagnostic" Devices

[180] Wikipedia, original source, Boucsein, Wolfram (2012). Electrodermal Activity. Springer Science & Business Media. p. 4. ISBN 9781461411260. Retrieved 16 April 2015.

[181] Ibid

[182] Wikipedia, original source, Pflanzer, Richard. "Galvanic Skin Response and the Polygraph" (PDF). BIOPAC Systems, Inc. Archived from the original (PDF) on 18 December 2014. Retrieved 18 August 2017.

[183] Wikipedia, original source, Brown, Barbara (November 9, 1977). "Skin Talks - - And It May Not Be Saying What You Want To". Pocatello, Idaho: Field Enterprises, Inc. Idaho State Journal. p. 32. Retrieved 8 April 2015.

[184] Wikipedia, original source, Boucsein, Wolfram (2012). Electrodermal Activity. Springer Science & Business Media. p. 7. ISBN 9781461411260. Retrieved 10 April 2015.

[185] Wikipedia, original source, Matté, James Allan (2000-01-01). Examination and Cross-examination of Experts in Forensic Psychophysiology Using the Polygraph. J.A.M. Publications. ISBN 9780965579421.

[186] Barrett, Stephen, MD, The Fakery of Electrodermal Screening, Skeptical Inquirer, Volume 41, No. 5, September / October 2017, https://skepticalinquirer.org/2017/09/the-fakery-of-electrodermal-screening/

[187] https://itovi.com/ (March 2024)

[188] Barrett, Stephen, M.D., *iTOVi scanning: Another Test to Avoid*, March 7, 2017, https://quackwatch.org/device/reports/itovi/

[189] Barrett, Stephen, M.D., Close Examination of a ZYTO Electrodermal Screening System, August 26, 2017, https://quackwatch.org/device/reports/zyto/momed/

[190] https://zyto.com/what-is-a-biosurvey

[191] https://zyto.com/virtual-items (March 2024)

[192] Warning Letter CMS 652316, Zyto Technologies, June 21, 2023, https://cdn.centerforinquiry.org/wp-content/uploads/sites/33/2023/07/13201012/zyto_warning_letter_2023.pdf

[193] https://www.zyto.com/wp-content/uploads/2020/11/Advanced-Scan-Full-Report-Sample.pdf

[194] https://zyto.com/what-is-a-biosurvey (March 2024)

[195] Barrett, Stephen, M.D., Close Examination of a ZYTO Electrodermal Screening System, August 26, 2017, https://quackwatch.org/device/reports/zyto/momed/

[196] Ibid

[197] Barrett S. Close Examination of a ZYTO Electrodermal Screening System. Mo Med. 2017 Jul-Aug;114(4):238-244. PMID: 30228598; PMCID: PMC6140073.

[198] Thomas, William E., M.D., *Hahnemann's Allergy to Quinine,* *https://www.angelfire.com/mb2/quinine/allergy.html* and Pheifer, Samuel, M.D., *Healing at Any Price?,* Milton Keynes, England: Word Limited, 1988.

[199] Ullman, Dana MPH, "A Condensed History of Homeopathy," Excerpted from Discovering Homeopathy: Medicine for the 21st Century, North Atlantic Books, A Condensed History of Homeopathy – Homeopathic.com

[200] Ankerberg, John and John Weldon, *Can You Trust Your Doctor? The Complete Guide to New Age Medicine and Its threat to Your Family*, Wolgemuth & Hyatt, Publishers, Inc. Brentwood, TN, 1991.

[201] Browning, William W., A.B., LL.B., M.D., *Modern Homeopathy: Its Absurdities and Inconsistencies (1894),* July 30, 2019, Hahnemann, Samuel, M.D., Organon, French translation, p. 323. https://quackwatch.org/homeopathy/history/browning/

[202] Hahnemann, Samuel, M.D., *Materia Medica*, Vol 2., trans., Charles J. Hempel, 1879, New York, William Radde, 1886.

[203] F. Dantas, P. Fisher, H. Walach, F. Wieland, D.P. Rastogi, H. Teixeira, D. Koster, J.P. Jansen, J. Eizayaga, M.E.P. Alvarez, M. Marim, P. Belon, L.L.M. Weckx, "A systematic review of the quality of homeopathic pathogenetic trials published from 1945 to 1995", Homeopathy, Volume 96, Issue 1, 2007, ISSN 1475-4916, https://doi.org/10.1016/j.homp.2006.11.005.

[204] Ibid

[205] Ankerberg, John and John Weldon, *Can You Trust Your Doctor? The Complete Guide to New Age Medicine and Its threat to Your Family*, Wolgemuth & Hyatt, Publishers, Inc. Brentwood, TN, 1991, excerpt from Oliver Wendall Holmes, *Homeopathy*, ref. 3. Pp.221-243.

[206] Ulman, Dana and Stephen Cummings, "The Science of Homeopathy," New Realities, Summer, 1985.

[207] NCAHF Position Paper on Homeopathy, November 10, 2020, https://quackwatch.org/ncahf/pp/homeop/

[208] Barrett, Stephen M.D., "Homeopathy: The Ultimate Fake," August 25, 2016, https://quackwatch.org/related/homeo/

[209] Ibid

[210] Browning, William W., A.B., LL.B., M.D., *Modern Homeopathy: Its Absurdities and Inconsistencies (1894)*, July 30, 2019, https://quackwatch.org/homeopathy/history/browning/

[211] Ibid

[212] Laslof, Leslie J., *Wholistic Dimensions of Healing: A Resource Guide*, Garden City, NY: Dolphin/Doubleday, 1978.

[213] Grossinger, Richard, *Planet Medicine: From Stone Age Shamanism to Post-Industrial Healing*, Garden City, NY: Anchor Press/Doubleday, 1980.

[214] Ankerberg, John and John Weldon, *Can You Trust Your Doctor? The Complete Guide to New Age Medicine and Its threat to Your Family*, Wolgemuth & Hyatt, Publishers, Inc. Brentwood, TN, 1991.

[215] DeSmedt, Evelyn, et.al., *Life Arts: A Practical Guide to Total Being—New Medicine and Ancient Wisdom*, New York, NY: St. Martin's Press, 1973.

[216] Pheifer, Samuel, M.D., *Healing at Any Price?*, Milton Keynes, England: Word Limited, 1988.

[217] Ibid

[218] Ibid

[219] Bopp, H.J., M.D., *Homeopathy*, Down, North Ireland: Word of Life Publications, 1984.

[220] Pheifer, Samuel, M.D., *Healing at Any Price?*, Milton Keynes, England: Word Limited, 1988.

[221] Hahnemann, Samuel, M.D., *Organon of Medicine*, 6th Edition, reprint, New Dehli, India: B. Jain Publishers, 1978.

[222] Ibid

[223] Ibid

[224] Grossinger, Richard, *Planet Medicine: From Stone Age Shamanism to Post-Industrial Healing*, Garden City, NY: Anchor Press/Doubleday, 1980.

[225] Field, Robert, "The Spiritual Medicine of Homeopathy," April 21, 2020, https://www.resonanceschoolofhomeopathy.com/blog/the-spiritual-medicine-of-homeopathy

[226] Hahnemann, Samuel, M.D., *The Organon of the Healing Art* (5th edition),

[227] Ulman, Dana, *A Modern Understanding of Homeopathic Medicine, excerpt from Discovering Homeopathy: Medicine for the 21st Century,* North Atlantic Books, 1990. https://homeopathic.com/a-modern-understanding-of-homeopathic-medicine/

[228] Browning, William W., A.B., LL.B., M.D., *Modern Homeopathy: Its Absurdities and Inconsistencies (1894),* July 30, 2019, https://quackwatch.org/homeopathy/history/browning/

[229] Ibid

[230] Ibid

[231] NCAHF Position Paper on Homeopathy, November 10, 2020, https://quackwatch.org/ncahf/pp/homeop/

[232] Browning, William W., A.B., LL.B., M.D., *Modern Homeopathy: Its Absurdities and Inconsistencies (1894),* July 30, 2019, https://quackwatch.org/homeopathy/history/browning/

[233] NCAHF Position Paper on Homeopathy, November 10, 2020, https://quackwatch.org/ncahf/pp/homeop/

[234] Ankerberg, John and John Weldon, *Can You Trust Your Doctor? The Complete Guide to New Age Medicine and Its threat to Your Family*, Wolgemuth & Hyatt, Publishers, Inc. Brentwood, TN, 1991.

[235] Hahnemman, Samuel, M.D., *The Chronic Diseases, Their Peculiar Nature and Their Homeopathic Cure—Theoretical Part*, trans., Louis H. Tafel, New Dehli, India: Jain Publishers, 1978.

[236] Park, Robert, Ph.D., "Alternative Medicine and the Laws of Physics," Volume 21, #5, September/October 1997, https://skepticalinquirer.org/1997/09/alternative-medicine-and-the-laws-of-physics/

[237] NCAHF Position Paper on Homeopathy, November 10, 2020, https://quackwatch.org/ncahf/pp/homeop/

[238] Ibid

[239] Hall, Harriet M.D., A review of Energy Medicine: The Scientific Basis by James L. Oschman. London: Churchill Livingstone, an imprint of Harcourt Publishers Limited, 2000.

[240] Ibid

[241] Ibid

[242] Ulman, Dana, *A Condensed History of Homeopathy, excerpt from Discovering Homeopathy: Medicine for the 21st Century,* North Atlantic Books, 1990. A Condensed History of Homeopathy – Homeopathic.com

[243] Carpenter, Mary, "Homeopathic Chic," *Health*, March, 1989.

[244] Field, Robert, *The spiritual Medicine of Homeopathy* April 21, 2020, https://www.resonanceschoolofhomeopathy.com/blog/the-spiritual-medicine-of-homeopathy

[245] Ankerberg, John and John Weldon, *Can You Trust Your Doctor? The Complete Guide to New Age Medicine and Its threat to Your Family*, Wolgemuth & Hyatt, Publishers, Inc. Brentwood, TN, 1991.

[246] Hahnemann, Samuel, M.D., *Organon of Medicine*, 6th Edition, reprint, New Dehli, India: B. Jain Publishers, 1978.

[247] Robert, Herbert, M.D., *Art of Cure by Homeopathy: A Modern Testbook*, reprint, New Dehli, India: B. Jain Publishers, 1976.

[248] Field, Robert, *The spiritual Medicine of Homeopathy* April 21, 2020, https://www.resonanceschoolofhomeopathy.com/blog/the-spiritual-medicine-of-homeopathy

[249] "Permeable to bad science:" Journal retracts paper hailed by proponents of homeopathy, https://retractionwatch.com/2019/06/11/permeable-to-bad-science-journal-retracts-paper-hailed-by-proponents-of-homeopathy/

[250] Gaertner, Katharina, Michael Teut, and Herald Walach, "Is Homeopathy Effective for Attention Deficit Disorder? A meta-analysis," June 2022, https://static-content.springer.com/esm/art%3A10.1038%2Fs41390-022-02127-3/MediaObjects/41390_2022_2127_MOESM1_ESM.pdf

[251] "Paper on homeopathy for ADHD retracted for 'deficiencies,'" https://retractionwatch.com/2023/11/01/paper-on-homeopathy-for-adhd-retracted-for-deficiencies/

[252] Morice, Alyn, *Adulterated "Homoeopathic" Cure For Asthma*, April 12, 1986DOI: https://doi.org/10.1016/S0140-6736(86)90976-1)

[253] Frass M, Lechleitner P, Gründling C, Pirker C, Grasmuk-Siegl E, Domayer J, Hochmair M, Gaertner K, Duscheck C, Muchitsch I, Marosi C, Schumacher M, Zöchbauer-Müller S, Manchanda RK, Schrott A, Burghuber O. Homeopathic Treatment as an Add-On Therapy May Improve Quality of Life and Prolong Survival in Patients with Non-Small Cell Lung Cancer: A Prospective, Randomized, Placebo-Controlled, Double-Blind, Three-Arm, Multicenter Study. Oncologist. 2020 Dec;25(12):e1930-e1955. doi: 10.1002/onco.13548. Epub 2020 Nov 7. Erratum in: Oncologist. 2021 Mar;26(3):e523. PMID: 33010094; PMCID: PMC8108047.

[254] Oncologist. 2022 Dec; 27(12): e985. Published online 2022 Oct 31. doi: 10.1093/oncolo/oyac221, PMCID: PMC9732219PMID: 36314553, https://www.ncbi.nlm.nih.gov/pmc/articles/PMC9732219/

[255] Ernst, Edzard, Guest post by Norbert Aust and Viktor, "Michael Frass' research into homeopathy for cancer: 'numerous breaches of scientific integrity,'" October 27, 2022, Weisshäuplhttps://edzardernst.com/2022/10/michael-frass-research-into-homeopathy-for-cancer-numerous-breaches-of-scientific-integrity/

[256] NHMRC Information Paper: Evidence on the effectiveness of homeopathy for treating health conditions. National Health and Medical Research Council. 2015. Canberra: National Health and Medical Research Council, March 2015.

[257] Wagenknecht A, Dörfler J, Freuding M, Josfeld L, Huebner J. Homeopathy effects in patients during oncological treatment: a systematic review. J Cancer Res Clin Oncol. 2023 May;149(5):1785-1810. doi: 10.1007/s00432-022-04054-6. Epub 2022 Jun 22. PMID: 35731274; PMCID: PMC10097733. https://pubmed.ncbi.nlm.nih.gov/35731274/

[258] Ernst E. A systematic review of systematic reviews of homeopathy. Br J Clin Pharmacol. 2002 Dec;54(6):577-82. doi: 10.1046/j.1365-2125.2002.01699.x. PMID: 12492603; PMCID: PMC1874503, https://www.ncbi.nlm.nih.gov/pmc/articles/PMC1874503/

[259] Gorsky, David, Ph.D., M.D., "Clinical trials of homeopathy versus 'respect for science,'" *Science-Based Medicine,* March 9, 2015, https://sciencebasedmedicine.org/prior-plausibility-versus-homeopathy-and-an-unethical-trial-at-the-university-of-toronto/

[260] Paine, Thomas, *The Age of Reason*, January 27, 1794.

[261] Ernst, Edzard, M.D., Ph.D., "Why I changed my mind about homeopathy" Tue 3 Apr 2012 10.28 EDT https://www.theguardian.com/science/blog/2012/apr/03/homeopathy-why-i-changed-my-mind

[262] Ankerberg, John and John Weldon, *Can You Trust Your Doctor? The Complete Guide to New Age Medicine and Its threat to Your Family*, Wolgemuth & Hyatt, Publishers, Inc. Brentwood, TN, 1991.

[263] Field, Robert, *The spiritual Medicine of Homeopathy* April 21, 2020, https://www.resonanceschoolofhomeopathy.com/blog/the-spiritual-medicine-of-homeopathy

[264] Bopp, H.J., M.D., *Homeopathy*, Down, North Ireland: Word of Life Publications, 1984.

[265] Ankerberg, John and John Weldon, *Can You Trust Your Doctor? The Complete Guide to New Age Medicine and Its threat to Your Family*, Wolgemuth & Hyatt, Publishers, Inc. Brentwood, TN, 1991.

[266] Bopp, H.J., M.D., *Homeopathy*, Down, North Ireland: Word of Life Publications, 1984.

[267] Dhakal A, Sbar E. Jarisch Herxheimer Reaction. [Updated 2022 Apr 28]. In: StatPearls [Internet]. Treasure Island (FL): StatPearls Publishing; 2022 Jan-. Available from: https://www.ncbi.nlm.nih.gov/books/NBK557820/

Butler T. The Jarisch-Herxheimer Reaction After Antibiotic Treatment of Spirochetal Infections: A Review of Recent Cases and Our Understanding of Pathogenesis. Am J Trop Med Hyg. 2017 Jan 11;96(1):46-52. doi: 10.4269/ajtmh.16-0434. Epub 2016 Oct 24. PMID: 28077740; PMCID: PMC5239707.

[268] "20 words that once meant something very different," Jun 18, 2014 / TED Guest Author, https://ideas.ted.com/20-words-that-once-meant-something-very-different/

[269] Barrett, Stephen MD, Nambudripad's Allergy Elimination Technique (NAET) and Its Variants," *Chirobase*, May 13, 2017, https://quackwatch.org/chiropractic/dd/naet/

[270] Nambudripad, Devi, "What is NAET?" NAET Web site, accessed Oct 11, 1999, reprinted by Stephen Barrett, MD, Nambudripad's Allergy Elimination Technique (NAET) and Its Variants," *Chirobase*, May 13, 2017, https://quackwatch.org/chiropractic/dd/naet/

[271] "O'Halloran, Georgina. Man died an hour after being treated for peanut allergy," *Irish Independent*., April 25, 2009, https://www.independent.ie/irish-news/courts/man-died-an-hour-after-being-treated-for-peanut-allergy/26531233.html

[272] Milk ALLERGY ELIMINATION THROUGH NAET (Nambudripad's Allergy Elimination Techniques). ClinicalTrials.gov Identifier: NCT00328731, May 19, 2006.

[273] *An Autism Study Using Nambudripad's Food Allergy Elimination Treatments,* ClinicalTrials.gov ID NCT00247156, Sponsor Nambudripad's Allergy Research Foundation, Information provided by Nambudripad's Allergy Research Foundation, Last Update Posted 2008-06-26 https://clinicaltrials.gov/study/NCT00247156?cond=autism&intr=NAET&rank=2 #study-overview

[274] Jacob Teitelbaum, MD; Devi S. Nambudripad, MD, PhD, DC, LAc; Yvonne Tyson, MD; Ming Chen, MD; Robert Prince, MD; Mala M. Moosad, RN, LAc, PhD; Laurie Teitelbaum, MS, *Improving Communication Skills in Children With Allergy-related Autism Using Nambudripad's Allergy Elimination Techniques: A Pilot Study*, https://www.naet.com/media/776/autism-naet-full-study-imcj_10_5_teitelbaum-published.pdf

[275] Abstract: "Biomedical Analyses of a Holistic Peanut Allergy Treatment: NAET." Proceedings of The National Conference On Undergraduate Research (NCUR) 2011 Ithaca College, New York , March 31 - April 2, 2011, Brady Vincent and Dayne Bonzo, Medical Laboratory Sciences, Weber State University, Ogden, Utah, Faculty Mentor: Dr. Yasmen Simonian PhD, MLS (ASCP)CM, https://www.naet.com/pdfs/peanutAllergy.pdf

[276] Randomized Double-Blind Placebo-Controlled Crab or Shrimp Allergy Reduction Study Using Nambudripad Allergy Elimination Techniques, ClinicalTrials.gov Identifier: NCT02208414, Verified August 2014 by National Taiwan University Hospital, First Posted : August 5, 2014, Last Update Posted : August 5, 2014, https://classic.clinicaltrials.gov/ct2/show/NCT02208414.

Made in the USA
Las Vegas, NV
13 November 2024

11767302R00201